FIBROID UTERUS
Surgical Challenges in
Minimal Access Surgery

FIBROID UTERUS
Surgical Challenges in Minimal Access Surgery

Edited by

Rooma Sinha, MD
Honorary Professor, Gynecology
Associate Professor Macquarie University, Sydney Australia
Senior Consultant Gynecologist
Minimal Access & Robotic Surgeon
Apollo Health City, Hyderabad, India

Arnold P. Advincula, MD
Levine Family Professor of Women's Health
Vice-Chair, Department of Obstetrics & Gynecology
Chief of Gynecologic Specialty Surgery, Sloane Hospital for Women
Medical Director, Mary & Michael Jaharis Simulation Center
Columbia University Medical Center
New York-Presbyterian Hospital
New York, New York

Kurian Joseph, MD, DGO
Senior Gynecologist & Endoscopic Surgeon
Director, Joseph Hospitals
Chennai, India

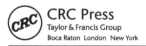

CRC Press
Taylor & Francis Group
Boca Raton London New York

CRC Press is an imprint of the
Taylor & Francis Group, an **informa** business

First edition published 2021
by CRC Press
6000 Broken Sound Parkway NW, Suite 300, Boca Raton, FL 33487-2742

and by CRC Press
2 Park Square, Milton Park, Abingdon, Oxon, OX14 4RN

© 2021 Taylor & Francis Group, LLC

CRC Press is an imprint of Taylor & Francis Group, LLC

Library of Congress Cataloging-in-Publication Data

ISBN: 978-0-367-24732-4 (hbk)
ISBN: 978-0-429-28411-3 (ebk)

Typeset in Palatino
by SPi Global, India

We dedicate this book to all women who place their implicit faith in us and to all the gynecological surgeons who are constantly updating their skills to provide the best care to these women.

Contents

Foreword

It is with great pleasure that I write a foreword for this book edited by Rooma Sinha, Arnold P. Advincula, and Kurian Joseph, my dear friends and colleagues in endoscopic surgery on the global floor over the last 30 years.

The three editors have lived on the cutting edge of advanced laparoscopic conventional and robotically assisted surgery from the beginning of video laparoscopy onward. In the years following 1990, we often met at international meetings of our various endoscopic societies. We were all learning from each other, teaching beginner and advanced courses at the AAGL, ESGE, ISGE, APAGE, IACE, and so on, and have continuously worked as leaders to advance the surgical care of women.

In this book, the editors focus on fibroids as challenges in minimal access surgery (MIS) and the authors discuss in detail diagnostic and therapeutic possibilities of today with modern technically, highly developed instruments, rich experience, and surgical skills. Besides these purely surgical aspects, the importance of indications and presurgical diagnostics including good imaging techniques are detailed along with limits as well as problems, which are openly eluded to. Tissue morcellation and possible nonrecognition of sarcomas are carefully discussed.

The editors have been able to recruit a large number of top clinicians/scientists in the field of gynecology and surgical procedures to contribute chapters to this book. The impressive list of authors guarantees readers not only up-to-date information on each aspect of fibroid treatment but also shows that the opinions and surgical tips have passed the critical eyes of world-renowned doctors in academic medicine.

The 22 chapters focus on surgical challenges of fibroid diagnosis and treatment, reflecting the early approaches of Victor Bonney (1872–1953), via Kurt Semm's first laparoscopic myomectomies in the early 1970s to today's conventional laparoscopic and robotically assisted myomectomies. They also leave space for the recognition of effective medical and imaging-guided fibroid-destroying drugs and techniques to further develop into practical therapeutical tools for additional treatment possibilities of uterine fibroids.

The book is really a landmark of 2021 for all possibilities of myomectomies in hysteroscopic and laparoscopic surgery gathered by a global forum of authors under the editorship of three international experts in the field.

Liselotte Mettler
Prof. Dr. med. Dr. h.c. mult
University Clinics of Schleswig Holstein, Kiel
Kiel, Germany

Preface

Fibroid "myomas" are among the most common tumors in women and impacts their lives from puberty to menopause. Minimal Access surgery is the most effective surgical treatment today. This book aims to discuss the surgical challenges we face as surgeons while treating them. The editors have attempted to provide a panoramic yet focused body of learning in the evaluation of fibroids and the surgical nuances in their treatment across various presentations of fibroid uterus. In the present day, the well-informed patient requires extensive counseling before surgery. For surgeons, the learning curve is steep for the minimal access surgical techniques for fibroid uterus; hence, this book will be a virtual ready reckoner for them.

The book comprises 22 of chapters and addresses issues like the challenges in obtaining proper consent before surgery; using different imaging modalities to locate fibroids and choosing the correct technique using hysteroscopy, laparoscopy, and robotic surgery in various presentations. A practical discussion on when to convert into a laparotomy is also included. Unusual presentations of fibroids are also reviewed, and the newer problem of parasitic fibroids is considered. The dreaded complications of secondary hemorrhage and rupture uterus have been included. The techniques of handling myomas during cesarean section has been discussed. Use of newer technology, the robotic surgical techinques in doing myomectomy and hysterectomy is discussed by experienced surgeons.

Contributions from experts in this field from India and abroad provide readers practical tips for surgery in various scenarios of fibroid uterus. We hope this book will provide insights to all gynecological surgeons and be a learning experience for budding surgeons.

We wholeheartedly thank all authors for their wonderful contributions, excellent illustrations, and practical tips. Thank you for sparing your time to do so.

It is said **"If the book is true, it will find an audience that is meant to read it."** And we hope this book will serve its purpose to make you a better surgeon.

Editors

Rooma Sinha, MD, is one of the leading Minimal Access & Robotic Gynecological surgeon in India. She is currently affiliated with Apollo Hospitals, Hyderabad. She has a flair for gynecological surgeries and has a reputation amongst her patients and colleagues alike for performing difficult and complex surgeries. She has been in clinical practice for the last 25 years. Observerships at Strong Memorial Hospital, University of Rochester, NY, USA, for minimal access surgery and at Mercy Hospital for Urogynecology in Melbourne, Australia, added international perspectives to her skills. Since 2012, she has updated her surgical skills to offer robotic-assisted surgery to her patients and has become one of the leading and most experienced robotic surgeons in India.

She has been awarded as Honorary Professor, Apollo Health Education & Research Foundation and Conjoint Associate Professor at Macquarie University in Sydney, Australia, and is the Clinical Lead Specialist in Gynecology for the Macquarie MD program. She is the lead faculty in the Fellowship program in Minimal Access & Robotic Surgery at Apollo Hospitals, Hyderabad. She believes she constantly learns while mentoring young surgeons in the field of Minimally Invasive & Robotic Surgery. Actively involved in teaching and publications, she has over 30 papers and chapters in books and national and international journals.

Her career began at St. Xavier's School in Bokaro Steel City, India, where she not only topped Indian School Certificate exams but received awards as DUX of the school and the "Best Influence Award" for her ability to inspire and influence her schoolmates. She was elected Vice Captain of school and Vice President of the Social Service League, which groomed her for social responsibility. She completed her graduation and postgraduation in medicine with seven distinctions and gold medals at the Institute of Medical Sciences, Benaras Hindu University, Varanasi, India. Pursuing a special interest, she did a postgraduate diploma in medico-legal systems from Symbiosis, Pune. She is board certified from the National Board (DNB), a Member of the National Academy of Medical Sciences (MNAMS), India, and a Fellow of Indian College of Obstetrics & Gynecology (FICOG).

Some awards to her credit are a FIGO Fellowship, the Asia Oceania Federation of Obstetrics & Gynecology (AOFOG) Shan Ratnam-Young Gynecologist Award, a Kamini Rao Yuva Oration award, and a Vasant Shahben Scholarship for overseas studies. She was awarded for excellence in the field of medicine by FICCI, Legend in the field of gynecology by Times Healthcare Achievers, and Best Gynecologist Laparoscopic & Robotic Surgeon by Hi9.

Being a team leader, Dr. Rooma brings with her an incredible work ethic to the operating room. She is punctual, efficient, skilled, and quick. Actively involved in spreading public awareness about gynecological conditions, especially about endometriosis.

What makes Dr. Rooma go on? The smiles on the faces of the women whom she treats are a treat to her. This gives her the energy and enthusiasm to carry on.

Arnold P. Advincula, MD, is a leader in minimally invasive surgical techniques and one of the world's most experienced gynecologic robotic surgeons. He has published and taught extensively in the area of minimally invasive surgery as well as developed surgical instruments in use worldwide. Dr. Advincula is a board-certified obstetrician-gynecologist and a fellow of both the American College of Obstetricians and Gynecologists and the American College of Surgeons.

After graduating with honors from the Temple University School of Medicine, Dr. Advincula completed an ob-gyn residency and a minimally invasive surgery fellowship at the University of North Carolina - Chapel Hill. He went on to spend 10 years at the University of Michigan, where he rose to the rank of Professor. During his tenure there, he served as Director of the Minimally Invasive Surgery Division and Fellowship program. He also founded the Endometriosis Center at Michigan. In 2009, Dr. Advincula joined Florida Hospital Celebration Health as Director of the Center for Specialized Gynecology. While in Florida, he served as the Director of the Celebration Health Endometriosis Center and established an AAGL-accredited Fellowship in Minimally Invasive Surgery. He was also Medical Director of Gynecologic Robotics at Florida Hospital as well as Professor of Obstetrics & Gynecology at the University of Central Florida College of Medicine. Additionally, Dr. Advincula was the Education Institute Director of the Nicholson Center, an advanced medical and surgical simulation training facility in Celebration, Florida. Prior to leaving Florida Hospital, Dr. Advincula helped launch central Florida's first Women's Institute.

In 2014, Dr. Advincula accepted the position of Levine Family Professor, Vice Chair of Women's Health & Chief of Gynecology at the Sloane Hospital for Women, Columbia University Irving Medical Center/New York Presbyterian Hospital. Dr. Advincula brings 20 years of clinical expertise, innovation, and leadership to the position. In addition to his departmental responsibilities, he also serves as Co-director of the AAGL-accredited Fellowship in Minimally Invasive Surgery. Shortly after his arrival to New York City, Dr. Advincula accepted the role of Medical Director of the Mary & Michael Jaharis Simulation Center for the Columbia University Vagelos College of Physicians & Surgeons. Despite his busy clinical and administrative schedule, Dr. Advincula not only has helped guide the growth of the simulation center across all health-care disciplines but also continues to leverage his expertise in simulation-based medical education to help elevate the training of medical students, residents, fellows, and physicians worldwide in advanced surgical techniques and optimized clinical care. Dr. Advincula serves on numerous editorial boards, including OBG Management, where he manages a widely viewed video education channel. Dr. Advincula has served on the board of the Society of Gynecologic Surgeons in addition to 18 months as President of the AAGL, where he helped rebrand the strategic direction of a global minimally invasive gynecologic surgery society of nearly 8000 members.

Kurian Joseph, MD, DGO, was a student from Stanley Medical College in Chennai, where he did his postgraduate work at the Madras Medical College. After receiving his MD, he was trained at various centers of excellence on endoscopy and fertility management. He worked with his father, Prof. A.K. Joseph, and developed a good obstetric and gynecology practice. He is trained in Laser Endoscopy surgery and was one of the first in India to do so. Dr. Joseph was in the forefront of the National Laparoscopic Tubal ligation program and set up and trained many doctors in laparoscopic tubal ligation. He started the first public–private partnership program in endoscopy with the German GTZ and Karl Storz under the UN University (Bonn) to train endoscopists in smaller towns to effectively use the instruments.

He started the Joseph Nursing Home, which later became the Joseph Hospitals as a tertiary care center for women with advanced obstetric care and one of South India's best endoscopy centers. Most advanced gynecological surgeries from difficult endometriosis to radical hysterectomies are performed at his center. His hospital was recognized as the training center at different times by Federation of Obstetrics & Gynecology Societies of India (FOGSI), AOFOG, and the International Society of Gynecological Endoscopy (ISGE).

Dr. Kurian was elected Vice President of the FOGSI and President of the AOFOG and today is a board member of the ISGE. He has also served as a member of the scientific committee of the FIGO conference at Vancouver.

He has delivered numerous guest lectures in India and around the world and has published multiple articles in endoscopy and obstetrics.

Contributors

Arnold P. Advincula
Department of Obstetrics and Gynecology
Sloane Hospital for Women
Mary and Michael Jaharis Simulation Center
Columbia University Medical Center/New York
    Presbyterian Hospital
New York, New York

Ibrahim Alkatout
Kiel School of Gynaecological Endoscopy
University Hospitals Schleswig-Holstein,
    Campus Kiel
Kiel, German

Chetna Arora
Division of Gynecologic Specialty Surgery
Columbia University Medical Center/New York
    Presbyterian Hospital
New York, New York

Anupama Bahadur
Additional Professor, Obstetrics and Gynecology
AIIMS
Rishikesh, India

Abhishek Chandavarkar
Apeksha Maternity and Nursing Home
Thane, India

Latika Chawla
Assistant Professor, Obstetrics and Gynecology
All India Institute of Medical Sciences
Rishikesh, India

Anupama Deenadayal
Mamata Fertility Hospital
Secunderabad, India

Mamata Deenadayal
Mamata Fertility Hospital
Secunderabad, India

Aarti Deenadayal Tolani
Mamata Fertility Hospital
Secunderabad, India

Hema Desai
Mamata Fertility Hospital
Secunderabad, India

Suhasini Donthi
Mamata Fertility Hospital
Secunderabad, India

Malacarne Elisa
Department of Maternal Fetal Medicine
Infertility and IVF Center
University of Pisa
Pisa, Italy

Braganti Francesca
Department of Maternal Fetal Medicine
Infertility and IVF Center
University of Pisa
Pisa, Italy

Sergio Haimovich
Unit Del Mar University Hospital
Barcelona, Spain

and

Department of Gynecology Ambulatory Surgery
Hillel Yaffe Medical Center
Hadera, Israel
and
Technion - Israeli Technology Institute
Haifa, Israel

Fouzia Hayat
Kokilaben Dhirubhai Ambani Hospital
Mumbai, India

Nutan Jain
Department of Obstetrics and Gynecology
Vardhman Super Speciality Hospital
Muzaffarnagar, India

Kadambari
Mamata Fertility Hospital
Secunderabad, India

Manish Y. Machave
Ruby Hall Clinic
Pune, India

Antonio Malvasi
Department of Obstetrics and Gynecology, GVM
    Care & Research Santa Maria Hospital, Bari,
    Italy. Laboratory of Human Physiology, Phystech
    BioMed School, Faculty of Biological & Medical
    Physics, Moscow Institute of Physics and
    Technology (State University), Dolgoprudny,
    Moscow Region, Russia.

Manou Manpreet Kaur
The Royal Marsden Hospital
London, United Kingdom

Liselotte Mettler
Prof Emeritus UKSH, Kiel, Germany
Honorary Patron Kiel School of Gynecological
    Endoscopy

Olarik Musigavong
Chaophya Abhaibhubejhr Hospital
Prachin Buri, Thailand

Aditi Parikh
Total Health Care Centre
Mumbai, India

Ravikant Prasad
Department of Radio Diagnosis
Apollo Hospital
Hyderabad, India

Alphy S. Puthiyidom
Mediclinic Welcare Hospital
Dubai

Bana Rupa
Department of Gynecology and Minimal Access
    Surgery
Apollo Hospital
Hyderabad, India

Anshumala Shukla Kulkarni
Consultant Laparoscopic & Robotic Surgeon
Kokilaben Dhirubhai Ambani Hospital
Mumbai

Neha Singh
Department of Gynecology and Minimal Access
    Surgery
Apollo Hospital
Hyderabad, India

Shalini Singh
Department of Obstetrics and Gynecology
Vardhman Super Speciality Hospital
Muzaffarnagar, India

Rooma Sinha
Honorary Professor, Gynecology
Associate Professor Macquarie University
Sydney, Australia

and

Senior Consultant Gynecologist
Minimal Access & Robotic Surgeon
Apollo Health City
Hyderabad, India

Anjali Sonawane
Total Health Care Centre
Mumbai, India

Michael Stark
The New European Surgical Academy (NESA)
Berlin, Germany
and
The Charite University Hospital
Berlin, Germany

and

Re-Source Medical Institute
Zurich, Switzerland

Sunita R. Tandulwadkar
Department of Obstetrics and Gynaecology
and IVF and Endoscopy Department
Ruby Hall Clinic
and
IVF and Endoscopy Department
Dr. D. Y. Patil Medical College
and
Solo Clinic and Solo Stem Cells
Pune, India

Andrea Tinelli
Department of Obstetrics and Gynecology
"Veris delli Ponti" Hospital
Scorrano, Lecce, Italy
and
Division of Experimental Endoscopic Surgery,
    Imaging, Technology and Minimally Invasive
    Therapy
Vito Fazzi Hospital
Lecce, Italy

and

Laboratory of Human Physiology
Phystech BioMed School
Faculty of Biological and Medical Physics
Moscow Institute of Physics and Technology
    (State University)
Dolgoprudny, Moscow Region, Russia

Prakash Trivedi
Total Health Care Centre and Aakar IVF Centre
Mumbai, India
and
Fortis Hospital Mulund
Mumbai, India

Soumil Trivedi
Total Health Care Centre and Aakar IVF Centre
Mumbai, India

Marina Vinciguerra
Department of Obstetrics and Gynecology
Azienda Ospedaliera Universitaria Policlinico di Bari
School of Medicine
University of Bari Aldo Moro
Bari, Italy

Cela Vito
Department of Maternal Fetal Medicine
Infertility and IVF Center
University of Pisa
Pisa, Italy

1 Counseling and Consent Challenges in a Woman with Fibroid Uterus

Rooma Sinha and Bana Rupa

CONTENTS

INTRODUCTION

Fibroids are a common occurrence in women of all ages. Many are asymptomatic and are incidentally diagnosed on ultrasound examinations. Counseling these women regarding the need for intervention or observation depends on various factors. The physician's knowledge and availability of resources play important roles in counseling. Furthermore, the patient's concerns and expectations influence the treatment modality. When either a non-invasive or invasive procedure is being discussed, the consent of the procedure by the patient will depend on her rapport with the doctor and the non-verbal clues that she receives from him or her.

Informed consent is the concept when a well-informed patient takes a decision after being explained all the facts along with the pros and cons of all reasonable alternatives to treat the same disease. Justice Cardozo stated in 1914, "every human being of adult years and sound mind has a right to determine what shall be done with his own body" [1]. An article by Entwistle et al. discusses various aspects of how informed consent about procedures should be discussed with patients as they have a right to be involved in decisions about their care [2]. Once provided all the information about the procedures and the alternatives available, they can exercise their choice in the final decision making. Many surgical procedures today can be carried out by a variety of methods, each having their advantages and disadvantages [2]. One needs to tailor the advice to each woman, depending her unique circumstances and desires. With the sufficient information provided to her, she can participate in the decision making regarding her care.

ASYMPTOMATIC FIBROIDS AND NOT PLANNING PREGNANCY
Observation or Intervention?

The question is when to suggest observation and when to suggest treatment for these women. There are no definite guidelines about the management of asymptomatic fibroids. Most of these patients with smaller fibroids can be counseled to observe with watchful expectancy. Any intervention should be clinically justified, and regression near menopause is expected. The decision to offer treatment in asymptomatic patients will depend on fibroid volume and the patients' concern about malignancy. Often, high-volume fibroids, even though asymptomatic, are counseled for surgical management, either myomectomy or hysterectomy, depending on a patient's choice.

Discussing all of these aspects while planning the treatment is imperative. Reasons for intervention in an asymptomatic fibroid could be to exclude malignancy or enhance fertility and reduce adverse pregnancy outcomes. However, in general, small asymptomatic fibroids are best left alone and should be kept in observation.

ASYMPTOMATIC FIBROIDS AND PLANNING PREGNANCY

These women may not be infertile at present or may have been trying to conceive but

1

are not able to get pregnant. Observations that myomectomy may improve fertility have been reported in the literature, but there is no clear-cut demonstration that removing fibroids results in pregnancy. Sometimes, a diagnosis of asymptomatic fibroids can cause anxiety in these women. They may begin to correlate some non specific complaints with the presence of these fibroids. They get concerned about the impact of these on future ability to conceive or impact on pregnancy. They are worried that these fibroids will continue to grow and that they will eventually need a hysterectomy and wonder whether they should be taking any therapy to stop the growth.

Young women with fibroids but a uterine size of less than 14 weeks should be encouraged to try to conceive spontaneously. Those who have not been able to conceive can benefit from removal of fibroids and should be counseled for myomectomy, especially if the fibroids are rapidly growing, they are submucosal in location, or she fails to conceive within 6 months. However, one must make it clear to the patient that removing fibroids does not guarantee a pregnancy. It could also justify counseling for intervention in asymptomatic fibroids to anticipate and avoid problems related to increase in size or development of complications during subsequent pregnancy.

PREGNANCY WITH FIBROIDS

Most women remain asymptomatic when they conceive with fibroids if their pregnancies remain uncomplicated with other problems as well. In general, about 10–40% of patients with myomas and pregnancy will present with a myoma-related complication [3]. The woman should be counseled that there is an increased chance of miscarriages as the miscarriage rates are significantly reduced after myomectomy [4]. Owing to the presence of fibroids, malpresentations, preterm labor, and intrauterine growth restriction are not uncommon. Patients can also present with persistent pain during the course of pregnancy.

WOMEN WITH SUBMUCOSAL FIBROIDS

It should be made clear in counseling that hysteroscopic removal of fibroids will result in improvement in heavy menstrual bleeding (HMB) but does not guarantee pregnancy. Large submucous fibroids can require two-stage surgical resection and this should be explained and consent should be taken before surgery. Operative hysteroscopic surgeries have some inherent complications like fluid overload, venous gas embolism, and hemorrhage and these can happen during surgery and this

should be explained and appropriate consent taken. Asymptomatic submucosal fibroids, when removed, can increase the chance of conception and the patient should be counseled accordingly.

FIBROIDS IN PERIMENOPAUSAL AGE AND BEYOND

The natural course of fibroids in this age group is unpredictable. Asymptomatic women can be counseled to observe and regularly monitor for either development of new symptoms or signs of rapid increase in the size of fibroids. Regular ultrasound exams are needed for follow-up in such situations. To women in this age group, treatment for symptomatic fibroids should be advised. Women who want a myomectomy during the perimenopausal and postmenopausal age group must be informed that there is a possible risk of lurking sarcoma in the fibroid. Although the possibility is low, it is there nevertheless. Hence, the patient should be counseled for hysterectomy rather than myomectomy in this age group.

CONSENT BEFORE MYOMECTOMY

The number and locations of the fibroids and the possibilities of their removal should be clearly explained to the patient. The smaller fibroids may not be accessible for removal and may grow in size in subsequent years. The risk of hemorrhage and the need for blood transfusion should be explained and consent should be taken. Owing to bleeding, a hysterectomy may need to be carried in life-saving situations but the possibility of this is rare. The symptom of HMB and dysmenorrhea may persist after surgery as many times there can be an associated adenomyosis that will cause such symptoms, and the proposed surgery addresses only the removal of fibroids. The myoma may recur or a new one may develop, requiring future surgical intervention. Yoo et al. reported myoma recurrence rates of 11.7%, 36.1%, 52.9%, and 84.4% at 1, 3, 5, and 8 years, respectively, after laparoscopic myomectomy [5], and Nezhat et al. reported recurrence rates of 31.7% and 51.4% at 3 and 5 years, respectively [6]. The recurrence rate increases with increasing postoperative years, and women planning pregnancy after myomectomy must be counseled regarding this fact. Reed et al., in their analysis of 628 women, reported that 21.8% had a second surgery, 74.8% of which were hysterectomies [7]. The cumulative rates of incidence of a second surgery were 23.5% at 5 years and 30% at 7 years [7]. The above mentions recurrence rates and the cumulative chance of a subsequent surgery for myoma should be explained and noted in the informed consent.

The uterine scar on myomectomy takes at least 3 months to heal; hence, the patient should be counseled not to attempt pregnancy before 3 months and preferably after 6 months. She should be informed of the risk of uterine rupture or the increased need for cesarean section in future pregnancy, especially after minimally invasive myomectomy. Additionally, uterine scars after myomectomy can have abnormal placentation (acreta, increta, percreta, and previa) and associated complications.

CONSENT BEFORE HYSTERECTOMY FOR FIBROID UTERUS

Hysterectomy is the most common recommendation a woman receives when her fibroids are diagnosed. It has permanent consequences and this may be the reason doctors suggest or the reason for patients to prefer it. It permanently eliminates uterine fibroids and there is no worry of recurrence or need for subsequent surgery. Some may even choose hysterectomy over newer, conservative techniques, such as uterine artery embolization or high-intensity focused ultrasound, as the long-term effects of such treatments are not fully known. Counseling for women who choose hysterectomy should be focused on intraoperative hemorrhage requiring blood transfusion, which can be needed in 23 out of every 1000 hysterectomies. Potential damage to the bladder or ureter (7 in 1000) or long-term disturbance to the bladder function, though very uncommon, should be discussed. There is also potential risk of bowel injury in about 4 in 10,000 hysterectomies. Development of pelvic abscess/infection and deep vein thrombosis or pulmonary embolism can also present as complications in the postoperative period. There is an additional risk of blood vessel injury during trocar entry if laparoscopic hysterectomy is being planned. Conversion to laparotomy during a laparoscopic procedure should be explained during counselling. To complete the procedure safely, conversion may become necessary in case of an intraoperative surgical difficulty or complication. The benefits and risks of conserving ovaries should be explained and consent taken before surgery regarding conservation of both ovaries/single ovary (right/left) or removal of both ovaries.

LAPAROSCOPY/LAPAROTOMY

Individualized care should be kept in mind when planning the route of surgery, be it myomectomy or hysterectomy. The counseling and decision should be based on the clinical situation and the expertise of the surgeon on a case-by-case basis. A safe and efficient surgery is of paramount importance for a good outcome

whether by open or minimal access surgery and this should be kept in mind for counseling. The intraoperative or postoperative gynecological outcome is similar regardless of whether it is achieved by laparoscopy or laparotomy, according to a meta-analysis published in *Human Reproduction* by Chapron in 2002 [8]. There is no difference in the risks of readmission, second procedure, and blood transfusion, according to this meta-analysis [8]. The route can also be determined on the basis of medical and surgical history regarding the presence of scars or mesh. All women considering hysterectomy or myomectomy should receive details regarding the risks and benefits of laparoscopic versus open hysterectomy or myomectomy. An open conversation with the patient will help her to decide the route of surgery she would like to have and then to give informed consent. However, there is no denying the fact that the laparoscopic approach has several advantages over laparotomy and this should be kept in mind when counseling women for hysterectomy or myomectomy. In a systematic review, the data show that laparoscopic myomectomy was associated with less hemoglobin drop, reduced operative blood loss, and diminished postoperative pain [9]. Most patients fully recovered by 2 weeks with fewer overall complications. However, they reported longer operating time with laparoscopic myomectomy [9]. These data and one's own surgical skill should be kept in mind while counseling women with fibroids needing surgery.

RISK OF SARCOMA OR MALIGNANCY DURING MYOMECTOMY/ HYSTERECTOMY

There is no reliable investigation in the preoperative period to distinguish uterine fibroids from sarcoma. The diagnosis is often retrospective when the final pathology report is available [10]. With a low incidence of sarcoma in patients with fibroids, it may seem a waste of time to many surgeons to discuss this at the time of surgery. However, many patients are very concerned regarding a cancer risk and this concern might nudge them to decide for hysterectomy rather than myomectomy in the presence of fibroids. Eighty percent of 1142 women who were due to undergo hysterectomy reported fear of developing cancer of the uterus if they did not undergo this surgery [11]. It is important for the surgeon to discuss these risks with the patient even if the surgery planned is for presumed benign fibroids. The challenge remains as to how to convey this information without scaring the patient. The trick lies in the way the surgeon presents and frames the information and reassures the patient while communicating with her. The patients may change their decision and consent depending on subtle differences in the way the information is presented to them. In a randomized study, when patients were informed that a cardiac procedure was "99% safe" instead of that 1 in 100 in patients will have complications, more patients consented for the procedure [12]. This should be followed with an honest discussion regarding the strategy the surgeon would use if morcellation were needed at the time of the surgery. The pros and cons of cold knife morcellation with small incisions versus the pros and cons using an electromechanical morcellator should be conveyed to the patient and her consent taken before surgery.

REFERENCES

1. Schloendorff v. New York Hospital 149 App. Div. 915. Mary E. Schloendorff, *Appellant v. the Society of the New York Hospital*, Respondent. 211 N.Y. 125; 105 N.E. 92; (1914 N.Y.) LEXIS 1028. 1914.

2. Entwistle V, Williams B, Skea Z, MacLennan G, Bhattacharya S. Which surgical decisions should patients participate in and how? Reflections on women's recollections of discussions about variants of hysterectomy. *Soc Sci Med.* 2006;62(2):499–509.

3. Ouyang DW, Economy KE, Norwitz ER. Obstetric complications of fibroids. *Obstet Gynecol Clin North Am.* 2006;33(1):153–169.

4. Maddalena S, De Giorgi O, Pesole A, Crosignani PG. Determinants of reproductive outcome after abdominal myomectomy for infertility. *Fertil Steril.* 1999;72(1):109–114.

5. Yoo E-H, Lee PI, Huh C-Y, Kim D-H, Lee B-S, Lee J-K, et al. Predictors of leiomyoma recurrence after laparoscopic myomectomy. *J Minim Invasive Gynecol.* 2007;14(6):690–697.

6. Nezhat FR, Roemisch M, Nezhat CH, Seidman DS, Nezhat CR. Recurrence rate after laparoscopic myomectomy. *J Am Assoc Gynecol Laparosc.* 1998;5(3):237–240.

7. Reed SD, Newton KM, Thompson LB, McCrummen BA, Warolin AK. The incidence of repeat uterine surgery following myomectomy. *J Women's Heal.* 2006;15(9):1046–1052.

8. Chapron C. Laparoscopic surgery is not inherently dangerous for patients presenting with benign gynaecologic pathology: results of a meta-analysis. *Hum Reprod.* 2002;17(5):1334–1342.

9. Jin C, Hu Y, Chen X-C, Zheng F-Y, Lin F, Zhou K, et al. Laparoscopic versus open myomectomy—a meta-analysis of randomized controlled trials. *Eur J Obstet Gynecol Reprod Biol.* 2009;145(1):14–21.

10. Gaetke-Udager K, McLean K, Sciallis AP, Alves T, Maturen KE, Mervak BM, et al. Diagnostic accuracy of ultrasound, contrast-enhanced CT, and conventional MRI for differentiating leiomyoma from leiomyosarcoma. *Acad Radiol.* 2016;23(10):1290–1297.

11. Gallicchio L, Harvey LA, Kjerulff KH. Fear of cancer among women undergoing hysterectomy for benign conditions. *Psychosom Med.* 2005;67(3):420–424.

12. Gurm HS, Litaker DG. Framing procedural risks to patients: is 99% safe the same as a risk of 1 in 100? *Acad Med.* 2000;75(8):840–842.

2 Preoperative Ultrasound Imaging in Fibroid Uterus

Mamata Deenadayal, Anupama Deenadayal, Hema Desai, and Aarti Deenadayal Tolani

CONTENTS

INTRODUCTION

"The uterus is such a reproductive organ that it should bear something, if not a child then a fibroid" is an age-old saying. Fibroids, also known as leiomyomas, are the most common tumors of the uterus. They consist of smooth muscle and varying degrees of fibrous connective tissue and appear in 70% of women by age 50. The 20–50% who are symptomatic have considerable social and economic impact with severe menorrhagia, pelvic pain, infertility, dysmenorrhea, and pressure symptoms on the surrounding organs. Submucous fibroids lower the pregnancy rates by 70%, and surgical removal appears to improve pregnancy rates. The surgical removal of symptomatic intramural fibroids should be a well-calculated decision, weighing the consequences of medical versus surgical management. Women with no fibroids or with subserous fibroids appear to have similar pregnancy outcomes.

Ultrasonography (USG) is a cost-effective and easily accessible modality to identify, locate, and completely evaluate all fibroids of varying sizes. Accurate fibroid mapping enables appropriate management (medical, surgical, or conservative management). For women of reproductive age who wish to preserve fertility, the standard treatment for symptomatic myomas is myomectomy. Pelvic USG is a valuable tool in preoperative evaluation (within 2 weeks prior to myomectomy) and should be systematically performed. Patient selection is crucial before performing laparoscopic myomectomy as a relationship between surgical complications and number, size, and location of myomas has been demonstrated. Therefore, precise preoperative evaluation is required to determine the optimal surgical approach and complexity. Owing to its safety, wide availability, and low cost, pelvic USG, both transvaginal and transabdominal, is typically the primary tool in assessment of uterine pathology and is considered valuable for diagnosis and characterization of myomas.

SETTINGS ON THE MACHINE

Listed below are salient points related to technique and knobs of the ultrasound machine:

1. *Probe*: A convex transabdominal probe (3.5–5 MHz) is used to give a panoramic view of the uterus on an adequately filled bladder. Since fibroids grow over time, most of the symptomatic fibroids that we see in our routine practice are large and mostly diagnosed transabdominally (transabdominal sonography, or TAS). A high-frequency transvaginal probe (5–9 MHz) gives a better resolution to identify and map fibroids, especially the smaller ones.

2. *Pre-set*: Today, on every machine, the optimum settings for a transvaginal sonography (TVS) and abdominal ultrasound can be pre-set (before performing the scan) to improve the quality of the scan and reduce the time to optimize the image.

3. *Depth*: The examination begins at a deeper plane for better orientation and then the depth is slowly decreased as needed to individually characterize each fibroid.

4. *Gain*: It should be adjusted so that fluid is black, tissues are mild gray, and some bits of the image are white. The brightness of the near, middle, and parts of the image can be changed for a clear image by using the gain knobs.

TYPICAL FEATURES OF FIBROIDS ON ULTRASOUND

- Fibroids can be hypoechoic, isoechoic, hyperechoic, or mixed echoic (Zaloudek and Hendrickson 2002) (cystic degeneration, hyalinization, and myxoid change) (Figure 2.1)

- Edema within these tumors is also another type of degenerative process, which, when less severe, is often referred to as hydropic change (Hendrickson and Kemson et al. 1980) or hydropic degeneration (Clement et al. 1992). Cyst formation can be an exaggeration of this process and is associated with increasing amounts of edematous fluid in them. Cystic change is recognized as a degenerative phenomenon (Coard and Plummer 2007)

- Linear stripy fan-shaped internal shadowing ("rain in the forest" appearance)

- Edge shadows: Significant shadowing from the edge of the lesion beyond the serosa of the uterus (Figure 2.2)

- Calcification: Posterior acoustic shadowing

- Peripheral calcification: Eggshell appearance and cavitation

CLASSIFICATION OF FIBROIDS

There are two main classifications in use:

1. These are the European Society for Gynecological Endoscopy fibroid classification and FIGO (International Federation of Gynecology and Obstetrics) classification. FIGO classification of myomas is the most routinely used classification in fibroid mapping on USG (Figure 2.3).

2. The STEPW (size, topography, extension, penetration, wall) classification system is used to decide partial or complete fibroid removal on hysteroscopic myomectomy of submucous myomas.

The submucous myomas are scored on the basis of their size, topography, proportion of

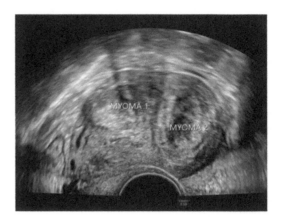

Figure 2.2 2D sagittal section of the uterus on transvaginal sonography (TVS) shows two well-defined myomas, isoechoic with the surrounding myometrium and casting typical edge shadow on gray scale.

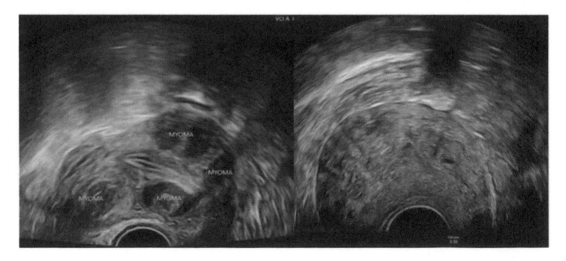

Figure 2.1 Fibroid and adenomyosis on ultrasound: the ultrasound image on the *left* shows sagittal section of the uterus with multiple fibroids. The ultrasound image on the *right* shows a sagittal section of the uterus with adenomyosis.

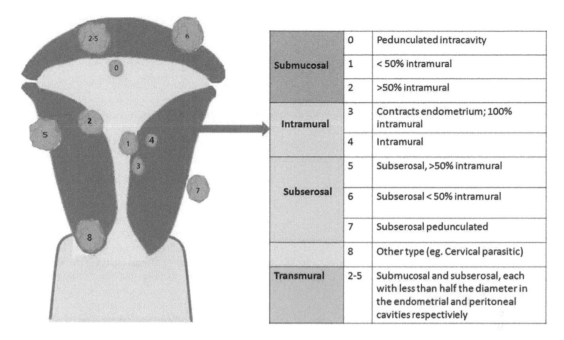

Submucosal	0	Pedunculated intracavity
	1	< 50% intramural
	2	>50% intramural
Intramural	3	Contracts endometrium; 100% intramural
	4	Intramural
Subserosal	5	Subserosal, >50% intramural
	6	Subserosal < 50% intramural
	7	Subserosal pedunculated
	8	Other type (eg. Cervical parasitic)
Transmural	2-5	Submucosal and subserosal, each with less than half the diameter in the endometrial and peritoneal cavities respectively

Figure 2.3   International Federation of Gynecology and Obstetrics (FIGO) classification of fibroids.

extension of the base, percentage of penetration into the myometrium, and location of the myoma in the lateral wall. Based on the total score, the complexity of the surgery can be defined and therapeutic options suggested (Figures 2.4, 2.5, and 2.6). As per the FIGO classification, it is a grade 1 submucous myoma, and as per STEPW classification, the score is 8, meaning it is a complicated mass to operate on hysteroscopy (Figure 2.7).

ULTRASOUND MODALITIES TO MAP THE FIBROIDS

2D Transvaginal and Transabdominal Ultrasound

Both TAS and TVS should be carried out as they complement each other. Although TVS is more sensitive in the diagnosis of small leiomyomas, TAS is essential in a large uterus since TVS is suboptimal in such situations. In TVS of a patient with a large cervical fibroid, the

STEPW Classification of Submucous Myomas

Number	Size in centimeters	Topography	Extension of the base	Penetration	Lateral wall
0	<2	Low	<1/3	0	+1
1	>2–5	Middle	>1/3–2/3	<50%	
2	>5	Upper	>2/3	>50%	
Score	+	+	+	+	+

Score	Group	Complexity and therapeutic option
0–4	I	Low-complexity hysteroscopic myomectomy
5–6	II	High-complexity hysteroscopic myomectomy Consider gonadotropin-releasing hormone use? Consider two-step hysteroscopic myomectomy.
7–9	III	Consider alternative to the hysteroscopic technique.

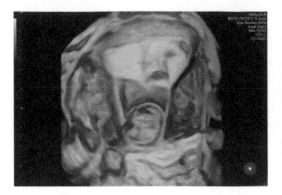

Figure 2.4 3D reconstruction of a uterine cavity—a virtual hysteroscopy. A 3D reconstructed image of a submucous myoma in the lower pole of the uterus.

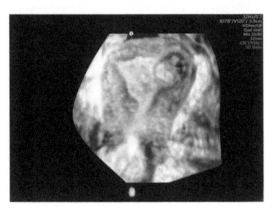

Figure 2.5 A 3D transvaginal sonography (TVS) coronal section of a rendered image of the uterus: showing an International Federation of Gynecology and Obstetrics (FIGO) stage 1 submucous fibroid with a less than 50% extension in to the myometrium and a STEPW (size, topography, extension, penetration, wall) score-4 indicating low complexity and possible hysteroscopic myomectomy.

assessment of structures above as it is prevented by the shadows. Hence, an additional TAS is necessary to properly visualize the structures around it to preoperatively assess additional pathologies and evaluate the best mode of treatment. TAS is difficult in obese patients, and an additional TVS or (in certain cases) a transrectal scan might be indicated (Sabrina et al. 2015). Large leiomyomas can occasionally obstruct the ureters and cause secondary hydronephrosis. Therefore, an ultrasound examination should include the assessment of the urinary tract whenever a large pelvic mass is identified (Figure 2.7) (Sabrina 2015). The kidneys need to be evaluated for hydronephrosis.

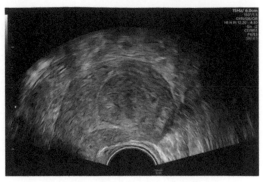

Figure 2.6 2D transvaginal sonography (TVS) sagittal section of the uterus showing a well-defined myometrial mass in the upper part of the uterus distorting the endometrial cavity and the endomyometrial junction. The 3D coronal image can further clarify the location and allow precise grading of the submucous myoma as per STEPW (size, topography, extension, penetration, wall) classification.

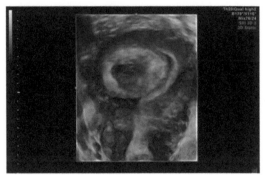

Figure 2.7 This shows a transvaginal sonography (TVS) 3D coronal-rendered image of the uterus, showing a large submucous fibroid more than 5 cm in size in the lateral wall and extending across the upper, middle, and lower corpus of the uterus with less than 50% myometrial extension.

3D Ultrasonography

- A 3D ultrasound is very useful for volume measurement of uterine leiomyomas and vascularity assessment by using vascularity index or vascularity volume display (Makris et al. 2007).

- A 3D reconstruction gives a clear picture regarding the outer contour of the uterus, shape of the uterine cavity, junctional zone, and relation of myometrial pathology to the endometrium and serosa.

- In patients with a distorted endometrium on 2D ultrasound, 3D hysterosonography may demonstrate submucosal leiomyomas, help distinguish between a pseudopolyp and endometrial polyp, and allow for accurate assessment of intrauterine abnormalities (Makris et al. 2007; Muniz et al. 2002).

- In a 3D-rendered coronal image, a walk through the image will show how anterior or posterior the fibroid is located.

Role of MRI in Fibroid Mapping

MRI is the preferred method for accurately characterizing pelvic masses (Weinreb et al. 1990). Submucosal, intramural, and subserosal fibroids, including the small fibroids and cervical location, are well demonstrated. MRI should be considered when there are more than five fibroids or the uterus is larger than 375 cc. The diagnosis of uterine leiomyomas on USG is usually reasonably straightforward, although focal adenomyosis can mimic a leiomyoma and a pedunculated uterine leiomyoma sometimes can be mistaken for an adnexal mass (Weinreb et al. 1990). When there is doubt about the origin of a pelvic mass at USG, further evaluation with MRI should be carried out. MRI sequences should include axial and sagittal T1W and T2W images (Rha et al. 2003).

Other Methods of Mapping Fibroids
Elastography

Elastography is an ultrasound-based imaging modality that assesses tissue stiffness. Given that endometrial polyps derive from soft endometrial tissue and submucosal fibroids from the hard muscle and fibrous tissue, elastography seems to be a perfect tool in differentiating such intramural masses.

Sonohysterography

Another modality that can add value and complement the traditional sonographic evaluation is 2D and 3D sonohysterography. In patients with a distorted endometrium on 2D USG, 3D hysterosonography will demonstrate submucosal leiomyomas, help distinguish between pseudopolyp and endometrial polyp, and allow for accurate assessment of intrauterine abnormalities (Yang et al. 2003). A 3D TVS can be combined with saline infusion into the uterine cavity to complement diagnostic hysteroscopy for the assessment of a submucosal leiomyoma. Three-dimensional saline contrast sonohysterography can provide even more information than conventional 3D TVS in such cases (Makris et al. 2007; Muniz et al. 2002).

STEPS FOR FIBROID MAPPING
Vaginal Entry

- Evaluate the vaginal wall at the entry as you begin the TVS. The appearance of bladder mucosa and its mobility and adherence to the uterus are noted.

- The cervix is examined for any abnormalities. Nabothian cysts, single or multiple, are common findings in the cervix on USG.

Evaluating the Uterus

a. The uterus is observed in the axial, coronal, and sagittal planes. With the depth setting, at least three fourths of the screen must be occupied by the uterus to avoid missing any pathologies (Figure 2.8).

b. While the uterus is being observed in various planes, if any pathology (e.g., fibroids) is identified, the following points are noted.

c. Is the location of the fibroid fundal, below the fundus, or cervical in the axial (transverse) plane while moving the probe to assess the uterus from the fundus of the uterus through both the cornuae, down to the cervix until the external os? Observe the relation of the fibroids to the endometrial echo in the coronal plane while moving the probe from the front of uterus to the back.

d. Record if the fibroid is in the anterior or posterior wall in the sagittal plane? Measure the distance from the serosa and the endometrium for each fibroid.

e. A 3D coronal view further enhances the visualization of the position of the fibroid.

f. In asymmetry of the anterior and posterior walls, the thickness of each wall is noted (including junctional zone) for follow-up to assess the progress of the pathology.

g. The total number of fibroids observed is documented.

Location of Each Fibroid in the Uterus

To identify the location of a fibroid in the uterus, it is important to delineate the endometrial cavity and identify the reference plane. Tracing from the cervical canal upward to the endometrial cavity in challenging cases is very helpful. Once the endometrial stripe is marked out, it is easy to locate the fibroids (Figure 2.9).

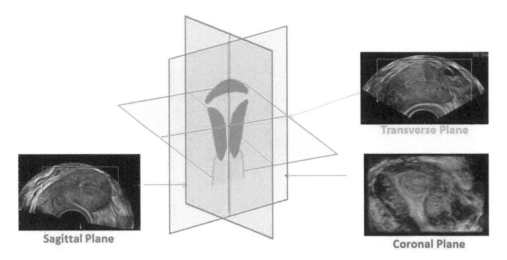

Transverse Plane

Sagittal Plane

Coronal Plane

Figure 2.8 A pictorial explanation of the different planes in which the uterus is observed during ultrasound.

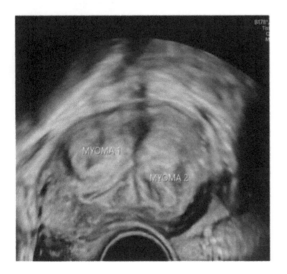

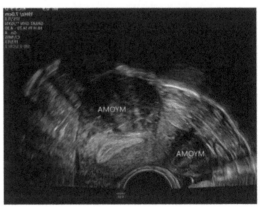

Figure 2.10 Ultrasound image showing a subserosal fibroid.

Figure 2.9 This sagittal section of the uterus on transvaginal sonography (TVS) shows a well-defined mass in the myometrium distorting the endometrial cavity and endomyometrial junction. A 3D assessment will help in further mapping the location of the fibroid in the uterus.

Position of the Fibroid

1. Anterior, posterior, or lateral wall.
   In anterior wall fibroids, the relationship to the bladder and any infiltration of the bladder wall must be documented.
2. Fundal, upper corpus, mid-corpus, lower corpus, cervix, cornual
   - Fundal – Any cornual distortion is looked for
   - Cornual – On the right or the left cornu
3. Cervical – Anterior or posterior aspect of the cervix

HOW TO MEASURE FIBROIDS ON ULTRASOUND SCAN

- Fibroids should be measured in three orthogonal planes.

- Ill-defined lesions are difficult to measure. In such cases, the probe should be rotated in different planes until a clear border can be observed. If required, try measuring the fibroid on power Doppler considering the circumferential flow at the border (and mention this in the report).

- The volume of each fibroid is calculated and mentioned.

Echogenicity

- The myometrium is used as standard for comparison of echogenicity of a lesion. Isoechoic lesions are difficult to define.

- Fibroids can be hyperechoic (white on the screen), hypoechoic (gray on the screen), anechoic (black on the screen), or a mixture.

- The reason for heterogenicity of a fibroid could be myometrial cysts or shadowing.

- A localized lesion may be a fibroid or an adenomyoma and, when diffuse, may be an adenomyosis.

- A fibroid usually shows edge shadows because of its well-defined margins.

Relationship of the Fibroid to the Endometrium

- Fibroid mapping is the term used to understand the relationship of the fibroid to the serosa and the endometrium, noting the exact distance between them. This information is useful for surgical management of fibroids and assessing possible complications. Fibroids are best seen in the secretory phase of the cycle on USG.

- The FIGO classification of fibroids helps the surgeon decide between a hysteroscopic or a laparoscopic approach for myomectomy.

Endomyometrial Junction

- Junctional zone: It is the innermost layer of the myometrium. It is the hypoechoic, dark.

- Halo just beyond endometrial margin. It is best viewed by 3D-rendered images using volume contrast imaging.

- Distortion of the endomyometrial junction may occur because of a submucous myoma or an intramural myoma close to the endometrial cavity.

Vascularity of the Fibroids

- Power Doppler is more sensitive in detecting flow in small vessels and low velocity flows. Color Doppler ultrasound typically shows circumferential vascularity. However, leiomyomas that are necrotic or have undergone torsion lack blood flow. Adenomyosis has intralesional flow.

- Vascular morphology is best seen on power Doppler (pulse repetition frequency of 0.3–0.6) and a 3D high-definition glass body display.

- Subjective color scoring from 1 (absent flow) to 4 (abundant flow) is used. Spectral flow analysis to assess the flow resistance which is estimated by the flow indices—resistance index (RI) or pulsatility index (PI)—is assessed. Flow velocity that is estimated by the peak systolic velocity (PSV) is also necessary.

- Doppler helps in identifying the site of origin of the fibroid by looking for the pedicle sign.

- Combined gray scale and color Doppler ultrasound helps in distinguishing a uterine leiomyosarcoma from a leiomyoma.

- When the diameter of the myoma is at least 8 cm with marked central vascularity with RI of less than 0.42 and PSV of more than 42 with presence of cystic degeneration, the diagnosis of a leiomyosarcoma should be considered. The prevalence of leiomyosarcoma is estimated to be 0.12 per 1000 surgeries. The sensitivity of ultrasound to diagnose a uterine sarcoma preoperatively was 85.7% (95% confidence interval [CI] 57.2–98.2), and the specificity was 99.5% (95% CI 98.7–99.8).

REPORTING IN A CASE OF FIBROID UTERUS

A systematic and detailed reporting method helps the clinician in making crucial decisions.

1. Location and number:

   - Wall (anterior/posterior/lateral)

   - Position (fundal/upper corpus/lower corpus/cervix)

   - Type (subserous/intramural/submucous/transmural) fibroid

2. Distance of fibroid from the endometrium and serosa:

   - X cm from the endo or serosa. Relevant 2D and 3D images should be provided

3. Diagrammatic representation of the fibroids in one or more planes

4. Measurement of the fibroids in three orthogonal planes

5. If the uterus is riddled with fibroids or mapping is suboptimal, it should be mentioned and the relevant fibroids (if possible) should be numbered (as F1, F2, and so on), measured, and mapped

6. Vascularity of the fibroid should be mentioned

CONCLUSION

Ultrasound has been shown to be an adequate and cost-effective means of evaluating size, number, and location of fibroids. Ideally, both TAS and TVS should be performed for precise location, and 3D ultrasound is very good for volume measurement, vascularity assessment, and spatial orientation of the fibroids. Ultrasound-assisted calculation of the volume of the uterus and fibroid can be useful in the estimation of surgical time.

MRI can be an add-on when there are five or more fibroids and when the origin of large pelvic masses needs to confirmed. A 3D saline contrast sonohysterography provides more information and is complementary in the assessment of intrauterine abnormalities. Knowledge of the variety of the fibroids enables an accurate diagnosis and appropriate treatment. Fibroids need to be differentiated from adenomyosis and endometrial polyps. Although most myomas are benign, 0.23–0.7% of apparently benign uterine leiomyomas are confirmed as leiomyosarcomas on the basis of the pathological examination. So it is always important to look at a myoma with suspicion and be more careful when a patient presents with a pelvic mass that has had a recent or rapid increase in size and use Doppler (2D and 3D) to further assess such suspicious masses clinically.

Variants of leiomyomas occur when they undergo cystic degeneration, hyalinization, or calcification. In such situations, coming to a diagnosis is sometimes difficult. Magnetic resonance imaging can be used in this situation for an accurate diagnosis.

Understanding various methods available to assess simple, straightforward, and atypical fibroids is essential. Mapping these fibroids in detail in the above-mentioned systematic manner gives the treating surgeon the necessary information to decide on the modality of treatment and prepare him or her to counsel the patient about the pathology and prognosticate treatment plans.

REFERENCES

Clement PB, Young RH, Scully RE. Diffuse perinodular, and other patterns of hydropic degeneration within and adjacent to uterine leiomyomas. Problems in differential diagnosis. *Am J Surg Pathol.* 1992;16:26–32.

Coard K, Plummer J. Massive multilocular cystic leiomyoma of the uterus: an extreme example of hydropic degeneration. *South Med J.* 2007;100:309–312.

Hendrickson MR, Kemson RL. Surgical pathology of the uterine corpus. In: Bennington J, editor. *Major problems in pathology.* Philadelphia (PA): WB Saunders;1980:473–484.

Makris N, Kalmantis K, Skartados N, Papadimitriou A, Mantzaris G, Antsaklis A. Three-dimensional hysterosonography versus hysteroscopy for the detection of intracavitary uterine abnormalities. *Int J Gynaecol Obstet.* 2007;97:6–9.

Muniz CJ, Fleischer AC, Donnelly EF, Mazer MJ. Three-dimensional color Doppler sonography and uterine artery arteriography of fibroids. *J Ultrasound Med.* 2002;21:129–133.

Rashid SQ, Chou Y-H, Tiu C-M. Ultrasonography of uterine leiomyomas. *J Med Ultrasound.* 2016;24(1):3–12.

Rha SE, Byun JY, Jung SE, Lee SL, Cho SM, Hwang SS, et al. CT and MRI of uterine sarcomas and their mimickers. *Am J Roentgenol.* 2003;181:1369–1374.

Weinreb JC, Barkoff ND, Megibow A, Demopoulos R. The value of MR imaging in distinguishing leiomyomas from other solid pelvic masses when sonography is indeterminate. *Am J Roentgenol.* 1990;154:295–9.

Yang T, Pandya A, Marcal L, Bude RO, Platt JF, Bedi DG, et al. Sonohysterography: principles, technique and role in diagnosis of endometrial pathology. *World J Radiol.* 2013;5:81–7.

Zaloudek C, Hendrickson MR. Mesenchymaltumors of the uterus. In: Kurman RJ, editor. *Blaustein's pathology of the female genital tract.* 5th ed. New York (NY): Springer; 2002:561–615.

3 MRI before Myomectomy

How Can It Help You?

Ravikant Prasad

CONTENTS

MAGNETIC RESONANCE IMAGING (MRI) SCANNERS AND HARDWARE

The magnetic resonance imaging (MRI) scanner is basically identified by its magnetic strength, which is denoted by Tesla (or simply "T"). A wide range of scanners with various magnetic strengths are available, starting as low as 0.2 T up to 6 T. Very low and very high magnetic strengths are of no clinical use. A low-strength magnetic field MRI scanner will produce images of low resolution and take a very long time for each sequence of scan. Scanners of very high magnetic strength (more than 3 T) are not very safe in the present clinical scenario, just because of their very high magnetic strength. Hence, present-day radiology units are using 1.5- or 3-T MRI scanners. A 3-T MRI scanner is advantageous in terms of image resolution and speed of scan and can perform some special sequences. In the present context of gynecological imaging, 1.5- and 3-T scanners are comparable.

The next important factor is availability of radiofrequency (RF) coils that are suitable for a given human anatomy. A suitable abdominal coil (torso coil) is essential to perform proper abdomen and pelvic scan.

MRI PULSE SEQUENCES

The fundamental requirement to obtain an image from any tissue in the body is the presence of hydrogen atoms in the tissue. MRI uses the magnetic property of hydrogen to generate images. So the tissues that contain abundant hydrogen produce high signals and hence a good image. The tissues that contain less hydrogen appear dark and hence will not produce good signals. The above statement is just a simplified rule of thumb.

As we use magnetic properties of the hydrogen atom in the tissues in MRI, we are able to manipulate magnetic field properties by the use of RF coils that are placed in close proximity to the part to be scanned. By doing so, we can generate images of different shades of gray, black, and white. To this manipulation of magnetic field property, we have given different terms, which we call sequences.

SEQUENCES IN MRI

A good number of sequences are available in MRI scanning. The basic and fundamental sequences that are used are T1, T2, PDW (proton-density weighted), and IR (inversion recovery).

MRI sequences that are commonly used in female pelvis scans are the following:

- T1-weighted (T1W) sequence
- T2-weighted (T2W) sequence
- Fat suppression

- Post-contrast

- Diffusion-weighted image

There are various other sequences that are named differently by different vendors.

Planes of Imaging

The unique ability of MRI is to acquire images in orthogonal and non-orthogonal planes. Computed tomography (CT) can acquire only in the axial plane. Later, those images are reconstructed in coronal and sagittal planes.

Descriptive Terminology

There are multiple shades of gray, black, and white in generated MR images, and we use terms like hyper-, hypo-, intermediate, iso-, and mixed intensity to describe these shades. These terms are relative to the surroundings.

For the sake of understanding, hyperintense means appearing bright, hypointense means appearing dark, intermediate intensity refers to shades of gray, isointense means appearing similar to the surrounding tissue, and mixed intensity means multiple shades within the lesion.

APPEARANCE OF VARIOUS TISSUES IN DIFFERENT SEQUENCES

Unlike the CT scan, the MRI scan has different shades of gray, black, and white. This causes significant confusion in the interpretation of MRI images by an untrained eye.

T1W images depict excellent anatomy. These images more or less resemble CT scan images. Only a few structures are hyperintense (bright) on a T1W image: fat, blood, gadolinium (MR contrast), melanin, protein-containing structures, or lesions. Hyperintensity on T1W images can also be seen in specific

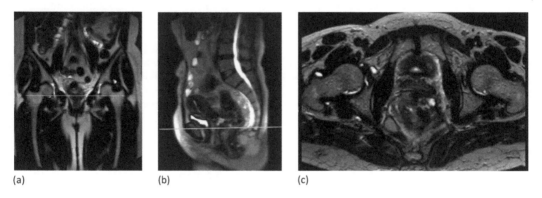

(a)   (b)   (c)

Figure 3.1   (a) Coronal plane. (b) Sagittal plane. (c) Axial/transverse plane.

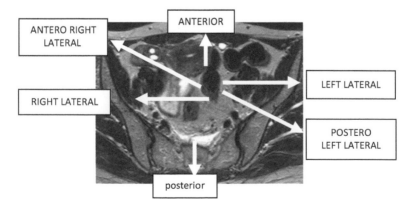

Figure 3.2   Descriptive terms in the axial plane.

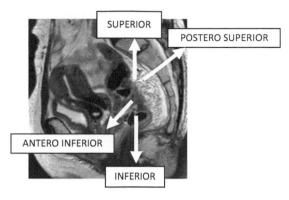

Figure 3.3 Descriptive terms in the sagittal plane.

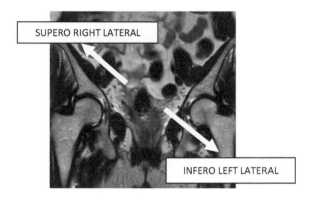

Figure 3.4 Descriptive terms in the coronal plane.

MRI artifacts and accumulation diseases. Most of the fluids (except blood) appear hypointense on T1W images.

T2W images are useful in identifying abnormal areas easily. In this sequence, fluid appears hyperintense and hence any lesions that contain fluid can be easily picked up on this sequence. Fat also appears hyperintense but less hyperintense than on T1W images. Hemorrhage has variable appearance in its different stages of evolution in both T1W and T2W images. In the context of this chapter, one should look for endometriosis where blood of different ages may be visualized. Most of the time, an endometrioma contains subacute hemorrhage, which is hyperintense on T1W images. This can be differentiated from fat, which is also hyperintense on T1W images, by using a fat-suppressed sequence in which fat gets suppressed and hence appears dark but subacute hemorrhage remains hyperintense.

As we noticed in the above paragraphs, fat and hemorrhage appear hyperintense in both T1W and T2W sequences. So we can use a fat-suppressed sequence in which fat will appear dark, thereby confirming the presence of fat in the given image. There are different types of fat-suppressed sequences but the most commonly used are short inversion time inversion recovery (STIR) and spectral attenuated inversion recovery (SPAIR). These fat-suppressed sequences can be T1W or T2W sequences.

Collagenous tissues (ligaments, tendons, and scars) are hypointense (dark) on all sequences.

The easiest way to identify T1W and T2W sequences is to look for fluid-filled structures (cerebrospinal fluid, gallbladder, and urinary bladder). If the fluid is hyperintense, it is a T2W image; if it is hypointense, it is a T1W image.

TABLE 3.1: The appearance of various tissues in different magnetic resonance imaging (MRI) sequences, in reference to pelvic structures

	No signal (dark)	Low signal	Intermediate signal	High signal (bright)
T1-weighted image	Air, calcium, cortical bone, flowing blood in a vessel, chronic hematoma	*FLUIDS* ligaments, tendons	Altered blood, proteneceous collections	Fat, subacute hematoma, MRI contrast and melanin
T2-weighted image	Air, calcium, cortical bone, flowing blood in a vessel, chronic hematoma	Ligaments, tendons	Fat, liver, pancreas, muscle	Fluids like cerebrospinal fluid (CSF), urine, bile, pus, etc.
Fat-suppressed image	Air, calcium, cortical bone, flowing blood in a vessel, chronic hematoma	*FAT*, ligaments, tendons	liver, pancreas, muscle	Fluids like CSF, urine, bile, pus, etc.

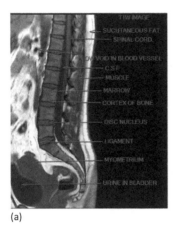
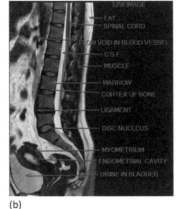
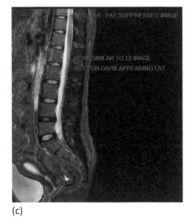

(a)   (b)   (c)

Figure 3.5 Routine magnetic resonance imaging (MRI) sequences in the sagittal plane to identify the appearance of different structures in different sequences. (a) T1-weighted (T1W) image. (b) T2-weighted (T2W) image. (c) T2W fat-suppressed image.

To identify a fat-suppressed sequence, we have to look at the subcutaneous fat. If it is hypointense, it is a fat-suppressed sequence.

If the fluid is hyperintense and the subcutaneous fat is hypointense, it is a T2 fat-suppressed sequence. When the fluid and subcutaneous fat are hypointense, we are dealing with a T1 fat-suppressed sequence. The appearance of various tissues in different sequences, particularly in reference to a pelvic scan, is illustrated in Table 3.1.

DIFFUSION-WEIGHTED IMAGING

Diffusion-weighted imaging (DWI) is currently indispensable in radiology. Diffusion refers to the random movement of molecules in a substance: the Brownian motion. DWI is a very fast technique where the diffusion behavior of hydrogen molecules is determined under different field strengths. DWI is an ultrafast T2W sequence. Because it is a fast sequence, the images that are acquired are of poor resolution but they are very sensitive to the molecular (hydrogen) motion.

The interpretive terms in this sequence are "restricted" and "facilitated."

The degree of hydrogen motion depends mainly on the following:

1. Cellularity of the tissue; more cellularity, less (restricted) diffusion.

2. Cytotoxic edema: This is edema (within the cell) due to ion pump failure (mostly secondary to anoxia). This causes restricted diffusion.

MRI TECHNIQUE

Patient Preparation

The patient should fast for at least 4 hours and empty the bladder and bowels just before examination to reduce blurring from motion artifacts due to bowel peristalsis and bladder motion. Other measures may include antispasmodics, such as hyoscine butylbromide 20–40 mg intramuscular/intravenous (IM/IV). Use of intravaginal (60 mL) and intrarectal (200 mL) ultrasound gel may be of benefit in defining the anatomy in the low pelvis where bladder neck, urethra, vaginal walls, labia, anorectal walls, perineal body, and sphincters can pose a challenge.

MRI Protocol

A phase-array surface coil is used to increase the signal-to-noise ratio. A basic imaging protocol must include a high-resolution, free-breathing T2W sequence in the axial, sagittal, and coronal planes and an axial T1W imaging sequence with and without fat suppression. For benign disease, fast breath-hold sequences are often enough despite slightly decreased resolution. However, evaluating pelvic malignancies requires long-duration, high-resolution, T2W fast spin-echo sequences. Three-dimensional gradient recalled echo T1W imaging sequences and fat-saturated T1W imaging sequences are specifically necessary to characterize fat or hemorrhage within the adnexa when there is clinical suspicion of dermoid or endometriosis. Other optional sequences depending on indication include diffusion imaging, dynamic contrast-enhanced MRI.

DWI improves the detection and potentially the characterization of small uterine tumors. Protocols should be optimized and tailored to address a specific indication for pelvic imaging.

Planning for Axial and Coronal Sections for the Body and Cervix of the Uterus

MRI images of two different patients showing proper planning technique for axial and coronal planes for the uterus.

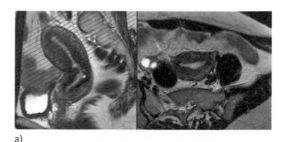

a)

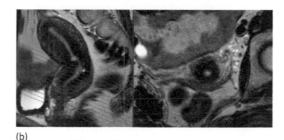

(b)

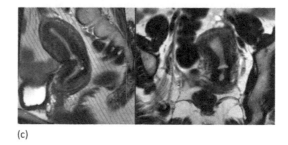

(c)

Figure 3.7 (a) Planning axial scan for uterine body. Scan plane should be perpendicular to the endometrial cavity on sagittal planner. (b) Planning axial scan for uterine cervix. Scan plane should be perpendicular to the endocervical canal on sagittal planner. (c) Planning coronal scan should be parallel to the endometrial cavity and endocervical canal.

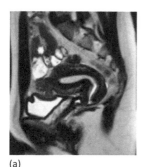

(a)

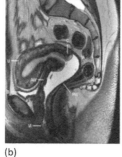

(b)

Figure 3.6 Magnetic resonance imaging (MRI) T2-weighted image of uterus in the sagittal plane (a) without and (b) with intravaginal ultrasound gel.

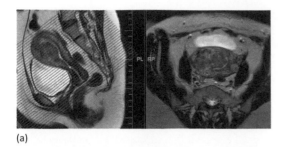

(a)

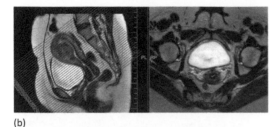

(b)

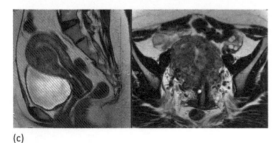

(c)

Figure 3.8 (a) Planning axial scan for uterine body. Scan plane should be perpendicular to the endometrial cavity on sagittal planner. (b) Planning axial scan for uterine cervix. Scan plane should be perpendicular to the endocervical canal on sagittal planner. (c) Planning coronal scan should be parallel to the endometrial cavity and endocervical canal.

NORMAL UTERINE ANATOMY ON MRI

The uterus can be divided into the uterine corpus and cervix. On T1W imaging, the entire uterus is isointense to muscle and different anatomic zones cannot be identified. The premenopausal uterine corpus on T2W images shows three distinct zones:

- The central high-signal intensity endometrium and secretions measure 3–6 mm in the proliferative phase and 5–13 mm in the secretory phase.
- The middle low-signal intensity junctional zone (JZ) measures 2–8 mm and is the innermost layer of the myometrium (less water and more smooth muscle).
- The outer intermediate-signal intensity of the myometrium.

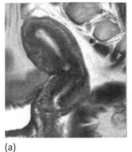 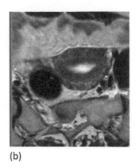

(a) (b)

Figure 3.9 Premenopausal uterine corpus on T2-weighted images (T2WI) show three distinct zones in sagittal (a) and axial (b) planes.

CBA

The postmenopausal uterus has an indistinct zonal anatomy, and the JZ is not consistently visualized.

The cervix on T2W image shows the following distinct zones:

- Central hyperintense mucosa: High-signal intensity endocervical mucosa and glands. Combined thickness of zones 1 and 2 is 2–3 mm.
- Hypointense fibrous stroma is 3–8 mm thick.
- Outer intermediate-signal intensity loose stroma.

MRI FOR FIBROIDS

Leiomyomas are the most common benign uterine tumors and are usually asymptomatic, but symptoms may range from abnormal bleeding to mass effect, infertility, second-trimester abortions, torsion, infection, acute degeneration, or sarcomatous degeneration. They can be classified by their location as submucosal, intramural, subserosal, or cervical.

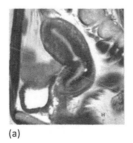 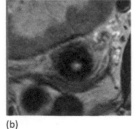

(a) (b)

Figure 3.10 Cervix on T2-weighted image (T2WI) shows three distinct zones in sagittal (a) and axial (b) planes.

International Federation of Gynecology and Obstetrics Classification of Myomas

The International Federation of Gynecology and Obstetrics (FIGO) classification system of myomas introduced by Munro et al. in 2011 is based on the relationship of the fibroid with the uterine wall. According to this classification, type 0 to type 8, the last one representing fibroids, which cannot otherwise be classified, have been proposed; whereas for a subset of fibroids, two numbers may be applicable, the first one referring to the relationship with the endometrium and the second one with the perimetrium. This possibility can indirectly imply the size of a myoma, which, for instance, extends throughout the uterine wall protruding into the uterine cavity and concurrently distorts the outline of the uterus (type 2–5).

- Type 0: Pedunculated intracavitary
- Type 1: Submucosal < 50% intramural
- Type 2: Submucosal ≥ 50% intramural
- Type 3: Entirely intramural, contacting the endometrium
- Type 5: Subserosal ≥ 50% intramural
- Type 6: Subserosal < 50% intramural
- Type 7: Subserosal pedunculated
- Type 8: Any other type like cervical, originating from the round ligament or parasitic

MRI provides a more accurate determination of location, number, size, degree of degeneration, malignant transformation, and other associated findings that are important in decision making for treatment options. Table 3.2 shows the relevant finding on MRI for each characteristic of fibroids.

TABLE 3.2: Characteristics of fibroids and their relevant findings on magnetic resonance imaging (MRI) sequences

Features of leiomyomas on MRI

Characteristic	Finding
Shape	Well-defined, round or oval
Appearance on T1-weighted images	Isointense to abdominal wall muscle
Appearance on T2-weighted images	Homogeneously hypointense. Degenerating fibroids are of mixed intensity
Enhancement on gadolinium contrast-enhanced images	Yes (can be variable), enhancement indicates viability
Diffusion-weighted images (high b value) and comparison with apparent diffusion coefficient (ADC) map	Hypointense compared with normal smooth muscle with similar appearance on ADC maps suggesting no restricted diffusion

Advantages of Using MRI

- Number, size, and location of fibroids:

  MRI is very accurate in identifying the number, size, and location of fibroids, which helps in planning treatment.

- Type of degeneration:

  Degenerating fibroid may show heterogeneous high-signal intensity on T2W images with lack of contrast enhancement.

  Hemorrhagic (red) degeneration of pregnancy or after uterine artery embolization demonstrates high-signal areas on T1W images. Table 3.3 describes the appearance of the various types of degeneration of fibroids on different MRI sequences.

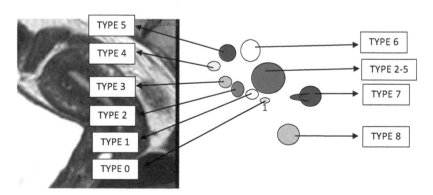

Figure 3.11 International Federation of Gynecology and Obstetrics (FIGO) classification system of myomas introduced by Munro et al. in 2011 on the basis of the relationship of the fibroid with the uterine wall.

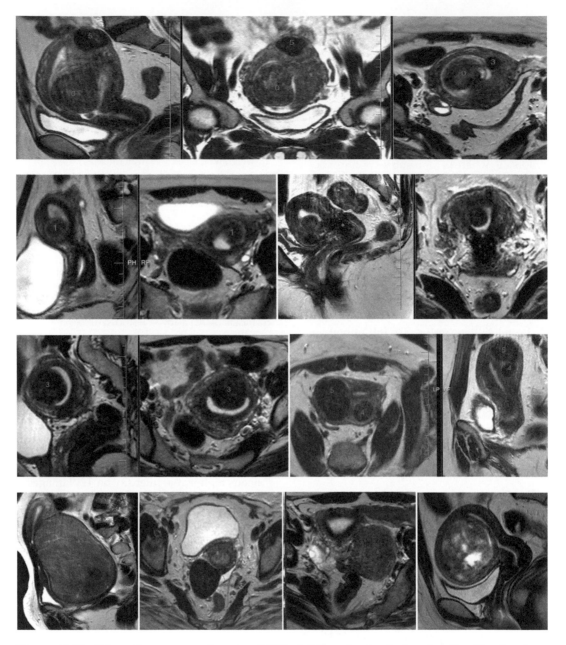

Figure 3.12 Magnetic resonance imaging (MRI) of different patients showing fibroids of various sizes and location. The numbering of the lesions is done in accordance with the International Federation of Gynecology and Obstetrics (FIGO) classification.

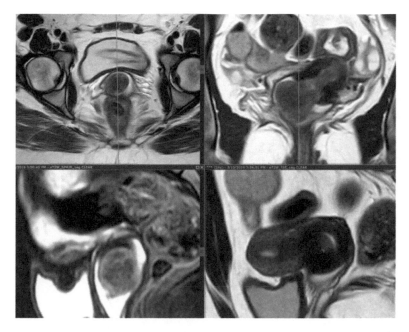

Figure 3.13 Magnetic resonance imaging (MRI) of uterus in different planes with ultrasound gel in vagina showing a cervical fibroid projecting into the upper vagina.

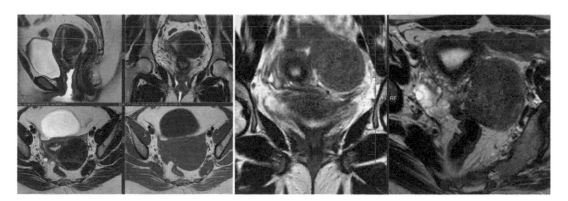

Figure 3.14 Magnetic resonance imaging (MRI) of two different patients clearly depicting the location of the fibroid (a) type 5 fibroid and (b) type 8 broad ligament fibroid.

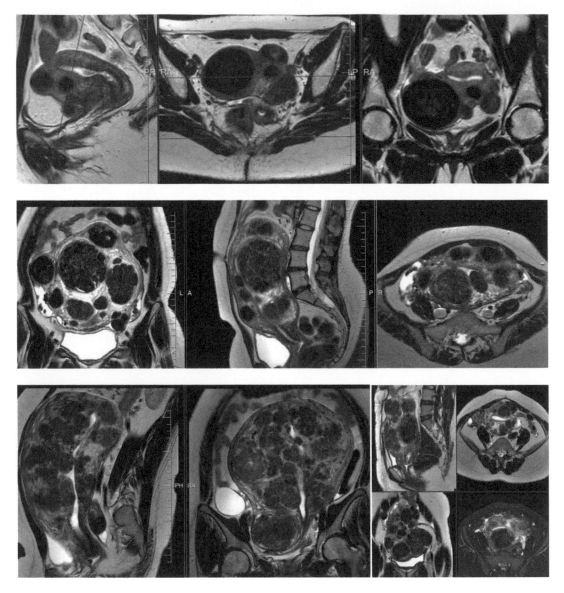

Figure 3.15 Magnetic resonance imaging (MRI) of uterus in different planes clearly depicting the number, size, and location of multiple fibroids. The relationship between the fibroids and endometrium is also well delineated.

TABLE 3.3: Appearance of the various types of degeneration of fibroids on different magnetic resonance imaging (MRI) sequences

Features of degenerating leiomyomas MRI

Degeneration type	Overall shape	T2-weighted images	T2-weighted images	Early enhancement	Restriction on diffusion-weighted imaging
Hyaline	Round or oval	Hypointense or isointense	Hypointense	Minimal or none	No
Cystic	Round or oval	Hypointense	Hyperintense	None	No
Myxoid	Round or oval		Markedly hyperintense	Progressive	No
Carneous, red, or uterine artery embolization–associated	Round or oval	Peripheral or diffuse hyperintensity	Peripheral or diffuse hypointensity	None	No
Calcific	Amorphous, central, or peripheral	Hypointense	Hypointense	None	No

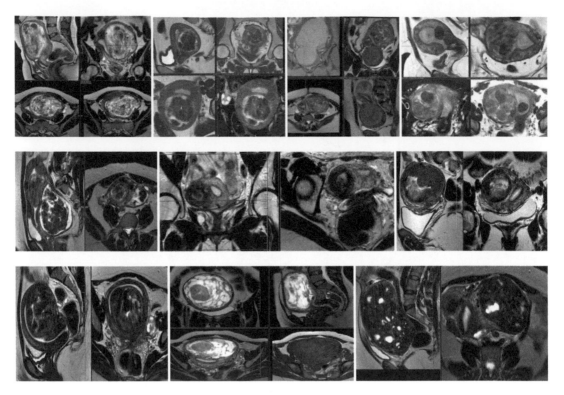

Figure 3.16 Magnetic resonance imaging (MRI) of different patients showing different types of degeneration of fibroids.

DIFFERENTIATING FIBROID FROM ADENOMYOSIS

Adenomyosis constitutes endometrial stroma and glands within the myometrium in women of reproductive age and may be microscopic, focal (adenomyoma), or diffuse. Adenomyosis is usually asymptomatic but may cause pain and dysfunctional uterine bleeding. MRI is a highly accurate non-invasive technique for the diagnosis with a high sensitivity (78–88%) and specificity (67–93%).

Direct Signs of Adenomyosis on MRI

1. *Microcysts*: Round cystic foci varying from 2 to 7 mm in diameter that are embedded in the myometrium are pathognomonic of adenomyosis in half of the cases.

   These small cystic spaces represent islets of ectopic endometrium accompanied by cystic glandular dilatation. They are usually located within the JZ; however,
they can be seen in the myometrium as well. They are hyperintense on T2 sequence and hypointense on T1 sequence the majority of times. But whenever they turn hemorrhagic because of hormonal influence, they can be hyperintense on T1W images.

2. *Adenomyoma*: An adenomyoma represents a group of endometriotic glands within the myometrium. This group of glands appears like a myometrial mass. The differentiation between fibroids and adenomyoma can be well appreciated on MRI evaluation, as illustrated in Table 3.4.

Indirect Signs of Adenomyosis on MRI

1. Thickness of JZ:

   In T2W images, thickening of the JZ to 12 mm or more is a well-accepted criterion for diagnosing adenomyosis. A JZ thickness of less than 8 mm generally permits

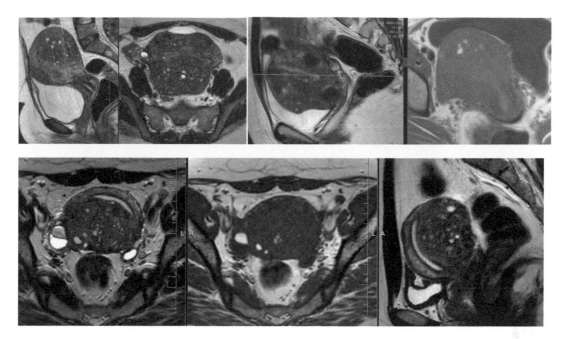

Figure 3.17 Magnetic resonance imaging (MRI) of the uterus of three different patients showing classic features of adenomyosis like globular enlargement of uterus, ill definition of junctional zone microcystic changes, and myometrium.

TABLE 3.4: **Points of differentiation between fibroids and adenomyomas**

Adenomyoma	Leiomyoma
Nodule with poorly defined edges	Well-defined nodule
Elliptical shape	Oval or rounded shape
Little mass effect	Mass effect proportionate to the volume
Absence of peripheral vessels	Presence of peripheral vessels
Hyperintense foci on T2- and T1-weighted images	Hypointense nodules on T2- and T1-weighted images

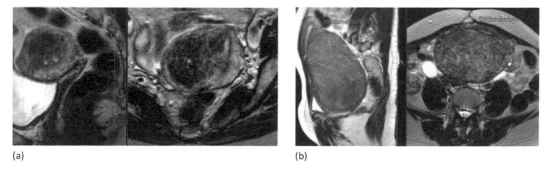

(a)   (b)

Figure 3.18 T2-weighted magnetic resonance imaging (MRI) of the uterus of two different patients in sagittal and axial planes showing differentiating features between (a) adenomyoma and (b) a fibroid as described in Table 3.4.

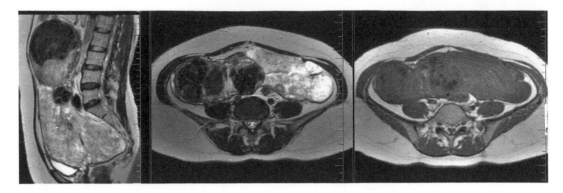

Figure 3.19 Magnetic resonance imaging (MRI) of the uterus in sagittal and axial planes showing coexistent fibroids and diffuse adenomyosis.

exclusion of the diagnosis. According to some authors, a JZ thickness between 8 and 12 mm can be diagnosed as adenomyosis but requires ancillary criteria.

2. JZ differential:

   It is calculated by measuring the difference between maximum and minimum thickness of JZ in anterior and posterior walls of the uterus. A JZ differential of more than 5 mm is a reliable indicator of diagnosis of adenomyosis.

3. Ratio of JZ and myometrial thickness:

   This is the ratio of maximal JZ thickness to myometrium. A thickness ratio over 40% allows a diagnosis of adenomyosis with a sensitivity of 64% and a specificity of 92%.

4. A blurred interface of JZ with the outer myometrium.

5. Hyperintense linear striations radiating from the endometrium toward the myometrium.

6. Globally enlarged uterus.

Diagnosing Leiomyosarcoma or Possible Sarcomatous Transformation of a Fibroid

There are findings on MRI that can suggest sarcomatous changes in presumed fibroid uterus. Table 3.5 describes these changes that may raise suspicion of such changes in various sequences.

Differentiate a Subserosal Fibroid from an Ovarian Tumor

A mass that is homogenously low-signal intensity on T2 is likely to be a leiomyoma, and the only ovarian tumors that could mimic this appearance are ovarian fibroma and Brenner tumor and also benign lesions. But avid dynamic contrast enhancement of fibroids can be a differentiating feature in case of doubt.

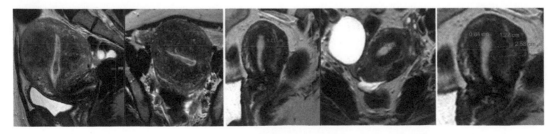

Figure 3.20 Magnetic resonance imaging (MRI) of the uterus of three different patients showing indirect signs of adenomyosis as mentioned above.

TABLE 3.5: Suspicious changes in magnetic resonance imaging (MRI) suggestive of sarcomatous change

Features of leiomyosarcoma on MRI

Feature	Finding
Margins	Ill-defined, infiltrating, often solitary
Shape	Irregular
On T1-weighted images	Heterogeneous, hyperintense areas (resulting from areas of hemorrhage)
On T2-weightged images	Heterogeneous, hyperintense areas (resulting from areas of cystic necrosis)
Enhancement on gadolinium contrast-enhanced images	Heterogeneous (caused by hemorrhage and necrosis)
Diffusion-weighted imaging (DWI) and comparison with apparent diffusion coefficient (ADC) map	Hyperintense on DWI, corresponding Hypointensity on ADC maps U.S.—to be consistent confirming restricted diffusion

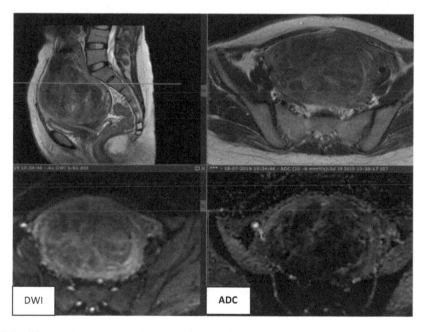

Figure 3.21   Magnetic resonance imaging (MRI) of the uterus and pelvis of a patient with leiomyosarcoma showing most of the features described in Table 3.5.

REFERENCES

Malcolm G. Munro, Hilary O.D. Critchley, Michael S. Broder, Ian S. Fraser. FIGO classification system (PALM-COEIN) for causes of abnormal uterine bleeding in non-gravid women of reproductive age. (2011) International Journal of Gynecology & Obstetrics. 113 (1): 3.

Schwartz LB, Panageas E, Lange R, Rizzo J, Comite F, McCarthy S. Female pelvis: impact of MR imaging on treatment decisions and net cost analysis. Radiology 1994;192(1):55–60.

Dähnert W. Radiology Review Manual. Lippincott Williams & Wilkins. (2011) ISBN:1609139437.

American College of Obstetricians and Gynecologists Committee on Practice Bulletins - Gynecology. ACOG practice bulletin no. 128. Diagnosis of abnormal uterine bleeding in reproductive-aged women. *Obstet Gynecol*. 2012 120;1:197–206.

Sudderuddin S, Helbren E, Telesca M, Williamson R, Rockall A (2014) MRI appearances of benign uterine disease. Clin Radiol 69(11):1095–1104.

4 Fibroid and Infertility

When to Suggest Myomectomy?

Aarti Deenadayal Tolani, Kadambari, Hema Desai,
Suhasini Donthi, and Mamata Deenadayal

CONTENTS

INTRODUCTION

Uterine fibroids are the most common benign neoplasms of the myometrium and are composed of smooth muscles and connective tissue. They are common in reproductive-age women and have a significant impact on quality of life, affecting fertility and pregnancy outcomes. Twenty to fifty percent of women are estimated to have fibroids, and the incidence increases with age until menopause. Although it is accepted that submucosal fibroids are of clinical significance, the effect of intramural and subserosal fibroids and the benefit of their surgical removal remains debatable. This chapter will review current evidence on the association of fibroids and infertility and assess the impact of surgical management of fibroids on fertility outcomes. Myomectomy for submucosal fibroids and for intramural fibroids more than 2 cm distorting the endometrial contour will likely have improvement in fertility outcome. The relative effect of multiple or different-sized fibroids on fertility outcome is uncertain, as is the relative usefulness of myomectomy in these situations. Medical management of fibroids delays conception and is not recommended for the management of infertility associated with fibroids.

ETIOPATHOGENESIS

Leiomyomas, often called fibroids or simple myomas, are benign monoclonal tumors arising from the smooth muscle cells of the myometrium. Two distinct processes that contribute to the development of fibroid are transformation of normal myocytes into abnormal myocytes and growth of abnormal myocytes into tumors. There are three cell populations in leiomyomas: well differentiated, intermediate differentiation, and fibroid stem cells. Tumor growth depends on the relative population of these cells.

Fibroids are classified depending on their location in the uterus relative to the submucous and subserosal layer. The International Federation of Gynecology and Obstetrics (FIGO) (Chapter 2, Figure 2.3) classification of myomas is widely followed because it offers a broad distribution of the location. It also includes the European Society for Gynaecological Endoscopy classification of submucous fibroids.

The incidence of fibroid as evaluated by ultrasound varies from 25 to 60% depending on race and ethnicity and is highest in women of African descent. Early-onset menarche, nulliparity, caffeine and alcohol consumption, and obesity increase the risk. Genetics and epigenetic factors, including steroid hormones, growth factors, cytokines, and chemokines, are all implicated in the development and growth of fibroids.

CLINICAL PRESENTATION

Fibroid symptomatology varies depending on location, size, and number. Abnormal uterine bleeding, pelvic pain, pressure, and reproductive dysfunction are common. However, the majority of fibroids are asymptomatic. Since the focus of this chapter is on infertility, the association of fibroids with infertility will be dealt with in detail.

IMPACT OF FIBROIDS ON FERTILITY

Infertility is a multifactorial entity; hence, fibroids being sole cause, is difficult to substantiate. Careful evaluation of the couple is necessary before undertaking any treatment, especially surgical procedures, in order to avoid the harm of unnecessary interventions. Depending on the location of the fibroids, various mechanisms have been proposed as a cause for infertility and pregnancy losses.

Mechanisms of Infertility in Fibroids

Physical Factors

Distortion of the endometrial cavity may compromise implantation potential. Sperm transportation can be altered by an enlarged and deformed uterus. Cervical displacement will hinder sperm passage into the cervical canal. Deviations of the tubal ostia and alteration of the tubo-ovarian relationship may also be contributing factors.

Effect on Uterine Peristalsis

Fibroids induce a chronic inflammatory reaction in the uterus. As a result, there may be an increase of cytokines, chemokines, neurotensives, neuropepides, and oxytocine modulators in the capsule, all of which increase uterine peristalsis. Yoshino et al. demonstrated an increase in uterine peristalsis, defined as more than two movements in 3 min in the periovulatory period in cases of intramural fibroids [1]. They also reported a low pregnancy rate in such women with an improvement fertility rate followed by myomectomy.

Molecular Impact

Disturbances in the endometrial expression of cytokines are an important factor in decreasing uterine receptivity. Intramural fibroid-derived transforming growth factor beta 3 (TGFβ-3) impairs the activity of bone morphogenetic protein 2 (BMP2). This results in decreases in interleukin 1 (IL-1) and leukemia inhibitory factor (LIF), leading to defective decidualization and implantation [2].

Genetic Alterations

HOXA10 (homeobox protein) gene expression is important in influencing the endometrial receptivity by altering target genes such as integrin beta 3 and EMX2. HOXA10 gene expression is reduced in submucous myomas not only on the overlaying endometrium but throughout the endometrial cavity [3].

Impact of Fibroids on Reproductive Outcome

Available evidence shows a 21% reduction in live birth rates following in vitro fertilization (IVF) in women with non-cavity-distorting intramural fibroids, as compared with controls. The presence of fibroids at baseline scan reduced IVF implantation and live birth rates by 18% (95% confidence interval [CI] 2–31%) and 27% (95% CI 4–44%), respectively.

A meta-analysis of 19 observational studies comprising 6087 IVF cycles showed a significant decrease in the live birth (relative risk [RR] = 0.79, 95% CI 0.70–0.88, $P < 0.0001$) and clinical pregnancy (RR = 0.85, 95% CI 0.77–0.94, $P = 0.002$) rates in women with non-cavity-distorting intramural fibroids, compared with those without fibroids, following IVF treatment. The presence of non-cavity-distorting intramural fibroids is associated with adverse pregnancy outcomes in women undergoing IVF treatment.

The impact of a fibroid on reproductive outcome depends on the location of the fibroid. The effect is highest in submucosal fibroids and least in subserosal fibroids.

Submucosal Fibroids

The presence of submucosal fibroids exerts a detrimental effect on reproductive outcome (Figure 4.1a,b). As per the current evidence based on systemic reviews and meta-analysis by Pritts et al. (2009), the presence of submucosal fibroids was associated with lower implantation (RR 0.28, CI 0.10–0.72) and pregnancy (RR 0.30, CI 0.13–0.70) rates in patients undergoing assisted reproductive technology [4].

Intramural Fibroids

The effect of intramural fibroids (Figures 4.2a,b) is still controversial. Fibroids influence female fertility and the pregnancy outcome according to their location, size, and number. Systemic reviews and meta-analysis by Pritts et al. (2009)

TABLE 4.1: Fibroids decrease the fertility chances and pregnancy outcome [11–15]

Serial number	Adverse outcome	Risk ratio with fibroid
1	Risk of spontaneous abortion	1.6–7.8
2	Preterm labor	1.0–4.0
3	Malpresentation	1.5–4.0
4	Placenta previa	1.8–3.9
5	Placental abruption	0.5–16.5
6	Postpartum hemorrhage	1.6–4.0
7	Retained placenta	2.0–2.7

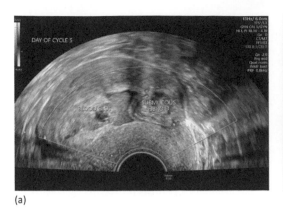

(a)

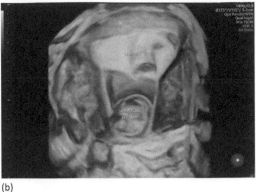

(b)

Figure 4.1   (a) Two-dimensional ultrasound image of submucous myoma. (b) Type 0 three-dimensional transvaginal ultrasound image of submucous myoma.

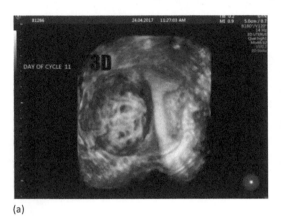

(a)

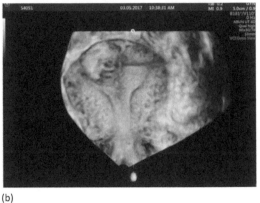

(b)

Figure 4.2   (a) Three-dimensional picture of intramural fibroid not impinging the junctional zone. (b) Three-dimensional ultrasound scan showing fibroid impinging the junctional zone (Type 2 submucous).

demonstrated that intramural fibroids were associated with decreased implantation, clinical pregnancy, and ongoing pregnancy [4]. The findings were reinforced by the meta-analysis by Sunkara et al. on the effect of intramural fibroids in IVF [5]. The impact of the size of the intramural fibroid was assessed by Yan et al., who reported a deleterious effect of type 3 intramural fibroid of more than 2.85 cm [6] (Figures 4.3–4.6).

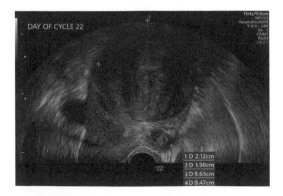

Figure 4.3   Two-dimensional ultrasound image of large intramural fibroid.

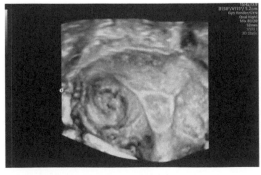

Figure 4.4   Three-dimensional ultrasound image of large intramural fibroid.

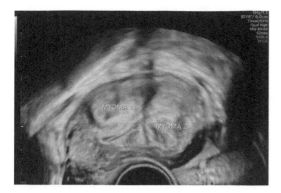

Figure 4.5 Intramural fibroid close to the endometrial cavity.

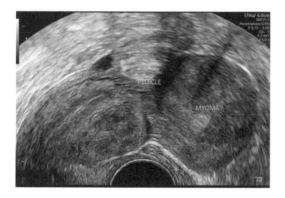

Figure 4.6 Pedunculated myoma.

Subserosal Fibroids

There is no evidence that subserosal fibroids of FIGO type 5–7 have any negative effect on fertility.

MANAGEMENT OF WOMEN WITH FIBROIDS AND INFERTILITY

Women with symptomatic fibroids have to be managed as per the clinical presentation. An infertile couple should undergo a detailed evaluation to rule out other causes of infertility. The assessment should include the following:

1. Ovarian reserve assessment and ovulation

2. Male factor evaluation

3. Tubal patency tests like hysterosalpingography or hysterosalpingo contrast sonography or at myomectomy

Overall probability of conception depends on various factors. The most important are age and other comorbidity factors, fibroid size, location, and number.

Fibroid Evaluation
Pelvic Examination

A thorough pelvic examination is essential for assessment of the fibroids and is to be confirmed by imaging technology.

Imaging of Fibroids
Ultrasound

Transvaginal sonography (TVS) has high sensitivity (95–100%) for detecting myomas in uterine size less than 10 weeks' size. TVS should be supplemented by transabdominal sonography in women with large and multiple fibroids (Figures 4.7, 4.8, and 4.9).

3D Ultrasound

Three-dimensional ultrasound has a useful role in assessing the endometrial junctional zone and localization of fibroids (Figure 4.2b). It can be especially useful in assessing the intramural fibroids abutting the endometrium (Figure 4.4).

Three-dimensional ultrasound is very good for volume measurement of uterine leiomyomas and vascularity assessment by using vascularity index or vascularity volume display [7]. A 3D reconstruction gives a clear picture

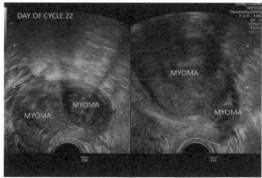

Figure 4.7 Multiple fibroids.

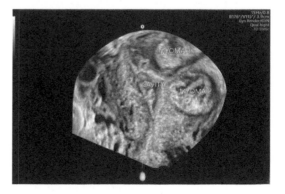

Figure 4.8 Multiple fibroids.

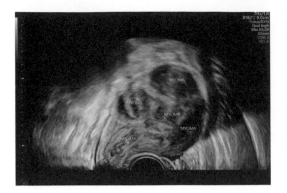

Figure 4.9   Multiple fibroids.

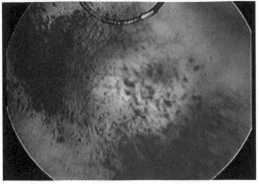

Figure 4.10   Submucous myoma on hysteroscopy.

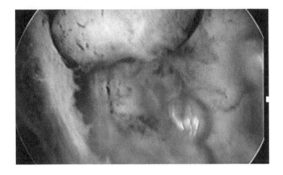

Figure 4.11   Submucous myoma hysteroscopic resection.

regarding the outer contour of the uterus, shape of uterine cavity, junctional zone, relation of myometrial pathologies to the endometrium, and serosa. In addition to the multiplanar mode, the volume data may be used for a multi-slice mode, rendered display mode, thick slice mode, or other modes (e.g., invert mode). In patients with a distorted endometrium on 2D ultrasound, 3D hysterosonography may readily demonstrate submucosal leiomyomas, help distinguish a pseudopolyp or an endometrial polyp, and allow accurate assessment of intra-uterine abnormalities [7, 8]. Minimally invasive surgical approaches such as hysteroscopy and laparoscopy have become the standard of care.

Saline Infusion Sonography (Sonohysterography)

Another modality that can add informa-tive value and complement the traditional sonographic evaluation is 2D and 3D sono-hysterography. In patients with a distorted endometrium on 2D US, 3D hysterosonog-raphy may readily demonstrate submucosal leiomyomas, help distinguish a pseudopolyp or an endometrial polyp, and allow accurate assessment of intrauterine abnormalities [9]. A 3D TVS can be combined with saline instil-lation into the uterine cavity to complement diagnostic hysteroscopy for the assessment of a submucosal leiomyoma (Figures 4.10 and 4.11). Three-dimensional saline contrast sonohys-terography may provide even more informa-tion than conventional 3D TVS in this respect [7, 8]. It improves the characterization of extent of protrusion into the endometrial cavity by submucous myoma.

Diagnosis by Hysteroscopy

Hysteroscopy performed in an office set-ting helps identify and classify the intracav-ity fibroid into type 0 or type 1. But depth of

penetration cannot be made out. STEPW (size, topography, extension, penetration, wall) clas-sification by Lasmar et al. can be used plan hysteroscopic management of fibroids [10].

Magnetic Resonance Imaging

Magnetic resonance imaging (MRI) is the best modality to visualize the size and location of all uterine myomas and differentiate between fibroids, adenomyosis, and leiomyosarcomas. MRI is especially beneficial in delineating intramural fibroids and their association with submucosal layer. However, MRI is expensive and availability is limited in low-resource settings.

Treatment Options

Treatment options are mainly medical and surgical. Medical treatments delay the time to conception and hence are not preferred for infer-tility patients. They are used mainly in large mucous myomas to reduce the size prior to sur-gery. Gonadotropin-releasing hormone (GnRH) analogues are the mainstay of treatment.

Hysteroscopic Myomectomy

Submucous myomas are optimally treated by hysteroscopy. Mechanical instruments such as scissors or loop electrocautery (thermal loops and vaporization), laser fibers or intrauterine morcellators are the various techniques available. Resectoscopic slicing is the most popular method. Type 0 and type 1 myomas can be easily resected. Type 2 myomas with more than 50% extension into the myometrium may require a two-step approach. Preoperative GnRH agonist may also be used in large or type 2 myomas. Type 2–5 myomas may require resection under laparoscopy guidance (Figure 4.11).

Laparoscopic Myomectomy

Laparoscopic myomectomy is indicated in all type 3 (and above) lesions. Large type 2 fibroids may also require laparoscopic approach (Figures 4.12–4.14).

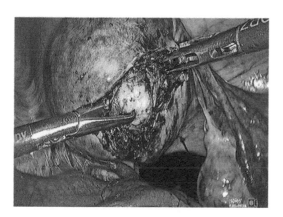

Figure 4.12 Deep intramuscular myoma dissection on laparoscopy.

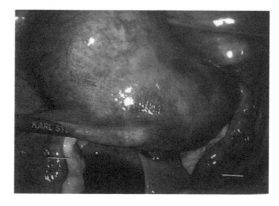

Figure 4.13 Laparoscopic picture of large anterior wall subserous fibroid.

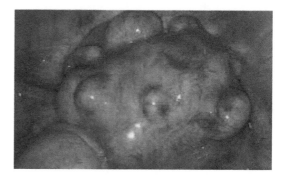

Figure 4.14 Multiple myomas on laparoscopy.

Laparoscopic-Assisted Myomectomy

Laparoscopic-assisted myomectomy is useful in dealing with large myomas. The advantages of laparoscopic myomectomy include fast recovery, fewer postoperative adhesions, and less pain.

Robotic-Assisted Laparoscopic Myomectomy

More recently, robotic-assisted myomectomy is being performed in some centers. Short-term outcomes are comparable to those of laparoscopies.

Myomectomy by Laparotomy

The choice between laparoscopy and laparotomy for myomectomy depends mainly on the size and number of fibroids. The deciding factors are skill of the surgeon and availability of equipment. Alternative non surgical approaches such as uterine artery embolization and non-invasive high-frequency MRI-guided focused ultrasound have not been adequately evaluated for fertility preservation.

CONCLUSION

Fibroids are common benign tumors in the reproductive age group and frequently co-present with infertility. Submucous myomas have a deleterious effect on fertility and pregnancy outcome. They not only exert their effect by mechanical disruption of the endometrial cavity but also have a global effect on the endometrium through a signaling effect and therefore have to be resected. Intramural myomas abutting the endometrial lining have an adverse impact on fertility outcome and hence have to be excised. Three-dimensional ultrasound is an important tool in mapping the intramural myomas and is comparable to MRI.

Large intramural myomas also need to be operated. Subserosal myomas have no effect on pregnancy outcome and they have to be managed if symptomatic. Clinical judgment and proper evaluation of the fibroids are the most important aspects of management.

REFERENCES

1. Yoshino O, Nishii O, Osuga Y, Asada H, Okuda S, Orisaka M, et al. Myomectomy decreases abnormal uterine peristalsis and increases pregnancy rate. *J Minim Invasive Gynecol.* 2012;19(1):63–67.

2. Doherty LF, Taylor HS. Leiomyoma-derived transforming growth factor-β impairs bone morphogenetic protein-2-mediated endometrial receptivity. *Fertil Steril.* 2015;103(3):845–852.

3. Du H, Taylor HS. The role of hox genes in female reproductive tract development, adult function, and fertility. *Cold Spring Harb Perspect Med.* 2015;6(1):a023002.

4. Pritts EA, Parker WH, Olive DL. Fibroids and infertility: an updated systematic review of the evidence. *Fertil Steril.* 2009;91(4):1215–1223.

5. Sunkara SK, Khairy M, El-Toukhy T, Khalaf Y, Coomarasamy A. The effect of intramural fibroids without uterine cavity involvement on the outcome of IVF treatment: a systematic review and meta-analysis. *Hum Reprod.* 2010;25(2):418–429.

6. Yan L, Yu Q, Zhang YN, Guo Z, Li Z, Niu J, Ma J. Effect of type 3 intramural fibroids on in vitro fertilization–intracytoplasmic sperm injection outcomes: a retrospective cohort study. *Fertil Steril.* 2018;109(5):817–822.e2.

7. Makris N, Kalmantis K, Skartados N, Papadimitriou A, Mantzaris G, Antsaklis A.

Three-dimensional hysterosonography versus hysteroscopy for the detection of intracavitary uterine abnormalities. *Int J Gynaecol Obstet.* 2007;97:6–9.

8. Muniz CJ, Fleischer AC, Donnelly EF, Mazer MJ. Three-dimensional color Doppler sonography and uterine artery arteriography of fibroids. *J Ultrasound Med.* 2002;21:129–133.

9. Yang T, Pandya A, Marcal L, Bude RO, Platt JF, Bedi DG, et al. Sonohysterography: principles, technique and role in diagnosis of endometrial pathology. *World J Radiol.* 2013;5:81–87.

10. Lasmar RB, Lasmar BP, Celeste RK, da Rosa DB, Depes Dde B, Lopes RG. A new system to classify submucous myomas: a Brazilian multicenter study. *J Minim Invasive Gynecol.* 2012;19(5):575–580.

11. Olive D, Pritts E. Fibroids and reproduction. *Semin Reprod Med.* 2010;28:218–227.

12. Exacoustòs C, Rosati P. Ultrasound diagnosis of uterine myomas and complications in pregnancy. *Obstet Gynecol.* 1993;82:97–101.

13. Klatsky P, Tran N, Caughey A, Fujimoto VY. Fibroids and reproductive outcomes: a systematic literature review from conception to delivery. *Am J Obstet Gynecol.* 2008;198: 357–366.

14. Vergani P, Locatelli A, Ghidini A, Andreani M, Sala F, Pezzullo JC, et al. Large uterine leiomyomas and risk of cesarean delivery. *Obstet Gynecol.* 2007;109:410–414.

15. Rice J, Kay H, Mahony B. The clinical significance of uterine leiomyomas in pregnancy. *Am J Obstet Gynecol.* 1989;160:1212–1216.

5 Surgical Treatment of Fibroids

Ibrahim Alkatout and Liselotte Mettler

CONTENTS

INTRODUCTION

One of the many treatment possibilities for myomas, considering all laparoscopic surgical, medical, or interventional techniques, is total laparoscopic hysterectomy (TLH) or subtotal laparoscopic hysterectomy (SLH). As SLH is a much less invasive procedure, a good number of patients with myomas can consider a subtotal approach. However, only TLH can offer 100% protection from new fibroid formation and avoid later sarcoma formation, uncontrolled bleedings, cervical and endometrial cancer, or any other problems arising from the uterus.

In spite of numerous theories, the etiology of fibroid formation remains unclear. While a genetic disposition must be given, as Africans have a much higher frequency of multiple myomas than Caucasians, certain up- and down-regulations in the genes of patients with or without myomas have been described. However, as yet, no clear guidelines for the prevention of fibroids are available. Hereditary leiomyomatosis and renal cell carcinoma syndrome are rare syndromes involving fibroids. Individuals with the gene that leads to both fibroids and skin leiomyomas have an increased risk of developing a rare case of kidney cell cancer (papillary renal cell carcinoma).

Understanding which genes are involved in fibroids does not automatically tell us why fibroids develop or how to control them. From our understanding of fibroid behavior, we would guess that genes involved in estrogen or progesterone production, metabolism, or action are involved. Unfortunately, science is seldom that straightforward. Most guesses regarding these "candidate genes" turn out to be wrong, and much research is still required to find out how these genes lead to disease. There are also small variations, called polymorphisms, in genes that may play a role in influencing the risk of fibroids. Both polymorphisms and mutations are changes in the sequence of genes, but the difference is in the degree of change. A mutation makes a major change in the gene that leads to a change in the protein the gene is coding for. For example, it can change the amino acid from alanine to glycine or cause the protein to be prematurely cut off.

MICROSCOPIC FACTS AND FIBROID VIABILITY

Fibroids are composed primarily of smooth muscle cells. The uterus, stomach, and bladder are all organs made of smooth muscle. Smooth muscle cells are arranged so that the organ can stretch instead of being arranged in rigid units, like the cells in skeletal muscle in arms and legs, that are designed to "pull" in a particular direction. In women with fibroids, tissue from the endometrium typically looks normal under the microscope. Sometimes, however, in submucosal fibroids, there is an unusual type of uterine lining that does not have the normal glandular structure. The presence of this abnormality, called aglandular functionalis (functional endometrium with no glands), in women having bleeding disorders is sometimes a clinical clue for their doctors to look more closely for a submucosal fibroid (Patterson-Keels et al. 1994). A second pattern of endometrium, termed chronic endometritis, can also suggest that there may be a submucosal fibroid, although this pattern can also be associated with other problems, such as retained products of conception and various infections of the uterus. Hysterectomy is not the only solution for treating fibroids; distinctions in size, position, and appearance have to be taken into account when deciding upon the best treatment option. If we understand these issues, we may be able to tell why some women have severe bleeding and other women with a similarly sized fibroid have no problem.

COSTS OF FIBROIDS

In fact, accurately capturing all of the costs attributable to uterine fibroids will help us move toward more (and more effective) innovative therapies. When deciding whether to launch a new concept, companies typically look at the amount currently spent for other treatments. The economics of fibroids has been discussed chiefly in terms of the health-care costs of hysterectomy. This in itself is a huge amount of money. According to a 2006 estimate, in the United States, more than $2 billion is spent every year on hospitalization costs due to uterine fibroids alone (Flynn et al. 2006). Additionally, one study estimates that the health-care costs due to uterine fibroids are more than $4600 per woman per year (Hartmann et al. 2006).

However, when you incorporate all the costs of fibroids, the way of treatment becomes even more significant. Let us consider what costs arise:

- The costs of myomectomy, uterine artery embolization (UAE), and other minimally invasive therapies

- The costs of birth control pills and other hormonal treatments to control bleeding

- The costs of tampons, pads, and adult diapers that many women require to contain the bleeding

- The costs of alternative and complementary therapies

- The cost of doing nothing (for many women, this means missing work or working less productively during their period)

REASONS FOR HYSTERECTOMIES IN PATIENTS WITH FIBROIDS

Why should a patient have a hysterectomy today when so many alterative treatment possibilities are given? First, up to a certain size of the enlarged uterus, laparoscopic subtotal hysterectomy completely solves the problem, and if women want to eliminate every risk of recurrent fibroids, hysterectomy is their only choice. Hysterectomy also solves coexisting problems, such as adenomyosis, endometriosis and endometrial polyps, or cervical dysplasia, and there is no danger of ever leaving a sarcoma or carcinoma behind.

REVIEW OF ALL UTERINE-PRESERVING TREATMENT POSSIBILITIES FOR FIBROIDS

The surgical treatment of fibroids can be differentiated between less invasive and more invasive surgical techniques. Time and type of treatment have to be chosen individually and are dependent on the patient and the treating gynecologist (Table 5.1).

Expectant Management

Wait-and-see is a possibility if patients are asymptomatic, decline medical or surgical treatment, or have contraindications to any kind of treatment. However, existing data describe the possibility that fibroids shrink substantially either by optimizing endocrinological disorders, such as hypothyroidism, or during the postpartum period (Peddada et al. 2008; Laughlin, Hartmann, and Baird 2011).

To pursue the idea of expectant management, the pelvic mass must definitely be classified as a fibroid and differentiated from an ovarian mass. The complete blood count should be normal, especially in patients with severe symptoms, such as menorrhagia or hypermenorrhea. Women must also be informed that the risk of miscarriage, premature labor and delivery, abnormal fetal position, and placental abruption is increased during pregnancies with uterine fibroids (Zaima and Ash 2011).

Medical Therapy

The benefit of medical treatment in the management of women with symptomatic fibroids is still difficult to prove. Medical therapy can provide adequate symptom relief, especially in cases where hypermenorrhea is the leading problem. The benefit of symptom improvement decreases in long-term treatment periods and so more than 50% undergo surgery within 2 years (Marjoribanks, Lethaby, and Farquhar 2006).

Nevertheless, there has been a shift in traditional thinking that medical treatment of fibroids is based solely on the manipulation of steroid hormones. A deeper analysis and understanding of specific genes or pathways associated with leiomyomatosis may open new possibilities for prevention and medical treatment (Al-Hendy et al. 2004).

Primarily as a preoperative treatment to decrease heavy bleeding in patients with fibroids, hormonal treatment with selective progesterone modulators, such as ulipristal acetate 5 to 10 mg daily, has become widely used within the last 2 years (Donnez et al. 2012, 2014, 2015).

Alternative Treatment Methods

If the patient does not want to undergo surgery or there are contraindications to surgery, there are alternative procedures:

TABLE 5.1: Treatment options for uterine fibroids

Conservative	Alternative	Surgical						
		Myomectomy				Hysterectomy		
		Hysteroscopic	Laparoscopic	Abdominal	Robotic assisted	Vaginal	Laparoscopic	Abdominal
Expectant treatment	Uterine artery Embolization							
Medical therapy	High-intensity focused ultrasound						■ Supracervical	
■ Hormonal	Miscellaneous methods (myoma coagulation, myolysis)						■ Total	
■ GnRH agonist								
■ Ulipristal acetate								

UAE: This minimally invasive therapeutic option allows an occlusion of the specific arteries supplying blood to the fibroids. A catheter is introduced via the femoral artery under local anesthesia, and particles are injected to block the blood flow to the fibroid. This can be an effective treatment option if the uterus should not be removed, surgery is contraindicated, and family planning is completed. It results in myoma shrinkage of up to 46%. Nevertheless, there is still a significant rate of postinterventional complications (Edwards et al. 2007; van der Kooij et al. 2011).

Magnetic resonance–guided focused ultrasound: This is a more recent treatment method for uterine fibroids in premenopausal women. Again, the patients should have completed their family planning. In this non-invasive thermal ablative technique, multiple waves of ultrasound energy are converged on a small volume of tissue, resulting in maximal thermal destruction. The limiting factors are size, vascularity, and access (Kim et al. 2011; Funaki, Fukunishi, and Sawada 2009).

Uterine-Preserving Surgical Treatment of Fibroids

The surgical removal of fibroids is still the main pillar in the treatment of leiomyomas. Hysterectomy is the only definitive solution and can be performed as supracervical or total hysterectomy. Myomectomies performed by hysteroscopy, conventional laparoscopy, or laparoscopy with robotic assistance and by the open or vaginal approach are alternative surgical methods.

Indications for surgical therapy of uterine fibroids are the following:

1. Abnormal uterine bleeding disorders (hypermenorrhea, dysmenorrhea, menorrhagia, and metrorrhagia)

2. Bulk-related symptoms

3. Primary or secondary infertility and recurrent pregnancy loss

Counseling and Informed Consent

Patients undergoing an operative procedure have to be informed of the risks and potential complications as well as alternative operating methods. Counseling before surgery should include discussion of the entry technique and the associated risks: injury of the bowel, urinary tract, blood vessels, omentum, and other surrounding organs and (at a later date) wound infection, adhesion-associated pain, and hernia formation.

Counseling needs to integrate the individual risk dependent on the body mass index of the patient. Depending on the medical history, it is important to consider anatomical malformations, number of vaginal births, midline abdominal incisions, a history of peritonitis, or inflammatory bowel disease (RCoOa 2008).

Myomectomy

Myomectomy is a surgical treatment option for women who have not completed their family or who wish to retain their uterus for any other reasons. The enucleation of fibroids by any method is an effective therapy for bleeding disorders or displacement pressure in the pelvis. Nevertheless, the risk of recurrence remains after myomectomy. Furthermore, if any other pathologies might be causative or only co-causative for the symptoms (such as adenomyosis uteri), these problems will persist (Wallach and Vlahos 2004). Complications arising at myoma enucleations and pregnancy-related complications have been investigated extensively. All operating possibilities, especially laparoscopic versus laparotomic but recently also laparoscopic versus robotic-assisted myomectomy, have been evaluated. Uterine rupture or uterine dehiscence is rare and occurs in less than 1% of laparoscopic cases and even less seldom in robotic-assisted and laparotomic cases. Careful patient selection and secure preparation and suture techniques appear to be the most important variables for myomectomy in women of reproductive age (Kim et al. 2013; Lonnerfors and Persson 2011). Uteri with multiple fibroids have an increased number of uterine arterioles and venules. Therefore, myomectomy can lead to significant blood loss and corresponding arrangements should be made (Mettler et al. 2012b).

Hysteroscopic Myomectomy

Submucosal fibroids have their origin in myometrial cells underneath the endometrium and represent about 15 to 20% of all fibroids. Before the establishment of hysteroscopy as a minimally invasive and effective treatment method, these myomas were removed by hysterotomy or even hysterectomy. Increased surgical training, improvement of technology, and the widespread use of hysteroscopic myomectomy have made it a safe, fast, effective, and inexpensive method of fibroid resection while preserving the uterus (Di Spiezio Sardo et al. 2008).

Patient selection concentrates on intracavitary submucous and some intramural fibroids. More than 50% of the fibroid circumference needs to be protruding into the uterine cavity. Deep myometrial leiomyomas require advanced operative skills and have an increased risk for perioperative complications and incomplete resection. The depth of myometrial penetration correlates with the volume of distension fluid absorbed (Emanuel et al. 1997; Wamsteker, Emanuel, and de Kruif 1993). Few data are available on the myoma size that prevents the use of the hysteroscopic approach. The European Society of Hysteroscopy suggests limiting the myoma size to 4 cm, but the few existing data report a significant increase of complications in fibroids that are more than 3 cm. Surgical skills determine the size and number of myomas that can be resected (Hart, Molnar, and Magos 1999).

Prior to hysteroscopy, knowledge of the patient's medical history (e.g., history of cesarean section) or any other reason to expect an anatomical disorder is important. A vaginal ultrasound scan must be performed to precisely determine the uterus location and size and all cervical and uterine pathologies (Mettler et al. 2011). If available and feasible, fluid hysterosonography should be performed to better differentiate the relationship of leiomyoma to the endometrial cavity and the myometrium. No prophylactic antibiotic is required to prevent infection of the surgical site.

The first step is the dilation of the cervical channel with Hegar dilators up to Hegar 9. The most commonly used instrument for fibroid resection is the monopolar or bipolar wire loop. With a monopolar device, the fluid medium must be nonelectrolytic; with a bipolar device, the fluid medium is isotonic (Varma et al. 2009). A continuous flow allows the clearance of blood out of the uterine cavity to improve visualization. Furthermore, the resected pieces can be retracted. Nevertheless, the surface of the myoma and the time needed for resection increase the risk of excessive fluid absorption (Loffer et al. 2000).

The resectoscope is inserted through the cervix into the uterine cavity, and after distension with fluid, the uterine cavity is carefully inspected. The monopolar resectoscope requires a cutting current of 60 to 120 watts. Bipolar resectoscopes offer the possibility of simultaneous cut and coagulation. The wire loop passes easily through the tissue. The incision starts at the highest point of the myoma. Only in pedunculated fibroids might the incision cut the peduncle first. The loop is then moved toward the surgeon by using the spring mechanism and simultaneously the entire resectoscope is gently pulled backward. The wire loop must be in view of the surgeon during the whole procedure. This motion is repeated until the whole myoma has been resected and the surrounding myometrium (depth) and endometrium (side) can be differentiated. All resected specimen is sent to the pathologist. In cases of heavy bleeding and reduced vision, the endometrium and the cutting surface have to be reinspected. These areas can be desiccated with the coagulating current.

The resected area will be recovered by the surrounding endometrium during the following weeks. The complication rate is low (0.8–2.6%) (Loffer et al. 2000; Jansen et al. 2000). Complications that can occur, especially after extensive resection, are uterine perforation or excessive fluid absorption. Absorption of distension fluid might result in hyponatremia or volume overload (Propst et al. 2000). The recurrence rate is about 20% in a follow-up period of more than 3 years (Hart, Molnar, and Magos 1999).

Laparoscopic Myomectomy

With the improvement of laparoscopic techniques and skills, myomectomy can be performed laparoscopically in most women. The laparoscopic approach is usually used for intramural or subserosal fibroids. The main advantage over abdominal myomectomy is decreased morbidity and a shorter recovery period. Nevertheless, laparoscopic myomectomy is limited by surgical expertise and especially laparoscopic suturing skills (Parker and Rodi 1994; Lefebvre et al. 2003). Selection criteria for laparoscopic myomectomy are location, size, and number of fibroids. Nevertheless, these characteristics are variable in relation to surgical expertise. Preoperative imaging is performed by vaginal ultrasound to assess the precise features of the leiomyomas (Alkatout et al. 2011a; Dueholm et al. 2002; Mettler et al. 2011, 2012b).

Laparoscopic myomectomy starts with the usual placement of ports and trocars. After placement of the initial port in the umbilicus or higher up in the midline, depending on the size of the fibroids, two or three ancillary trocars are placed in the lower abdomen about 2 cm medial of each iliac crest and possibly in the midline (Mettler et al. 2012b; Alkatout et al. 2012; Alkatout et al. 2011b). Myomectomy can lead to severe bleeding that will complicate the procedure because of reduced vision. Vessel bleeding is controlled by bipolar electrosurgical power tools. Intraoperative bleeding can be reduced by using vasopressin or other vasoconstrictors. Vasopressin is diluted (e.g., 20 units in 100 mL of saline) and injected into the planned uterine incision site. Vasopressin constricts the smooth muscle in the walls of capillaries, small arterioles, and venules. Nevertheless, owing to side effects, the surgeon should pull back the plunger of the syringe before insertion to check that the needle is not inserted intravascularly (Kongnyuy and Wiysonge 2011; Zhao et al.

2010; Tinelli et al. 2013). Alternatively, misoprostol can be administered vaginally to reduce blood loss about 1 hour before surgery (Celik and Sapmaz 2003).

The uterine incision is preferably made vertically as this allows a more ergonomic suturing of the defect. The incision is performed with a monopolar hook directly over the fibroid and carried through deeply until the entire myoma tissue has been reached (Figures 5.1–5.6).

After exposure of the myoma, it is grasped with a tenaculum or sharp forceps and traction and countertraction are applied. The removal of the myoma can easily be performed with blunt and sharp dissecting devices. Capsular vessels should be coagulated before complete removal of the myoma as coagulation becomes more difficult if traction is unsuccessful and bipolar coagulation occurs in the remaining myometrium wall. Subsequent to removal, the myoma is morcellated with an electromechanical device under direct vision and at a safe distance to all structures, such as the small bowel, to avoid inadvertent injury. The myoma tissue is removed and sent for pathologic evaluation. The uterine defect is closed with delayed absorbable sutures in one or two layers, depending on the

depth of the myometrial defect. It is important that the suture start at the deepest point to avoid any cavity that might lead to a weak uterine wall. Furthermore, we tie the knot extracorporeally so that it can be pushed into the deep layers with full strength (Figure 5.7).

Alternatively, barbed sutures, such as V-Loc, can be used to tighten the tissue or a third ancillary trocar can be inserted to hold the suture tight. The security of the uterine closure has bearing on the risk of uterine rupture in subsequent pregnancy. Different kinds of adhesion prevention barriers can be applied (Mettler, Schollmeyer, and Alkatout 2012a; Mettler et al. 2013b; Tulandi, Murray, and Guralnick 1993). Women should wait at least 4 to 6 months before attempting to conceive (Tsuji et al. 2006).

Abdominal Myomectomy

Abdominal or open myomectomy has its origin in the early 1900s as a uterus-preserving procedure. Today, it is performed mostly for women with intramural or subserosal myomas and less frequently for submucosal localization. Since the introduction of endoscopic procedures, the indication for abdominal myomectomy has become rare. It becomes an option if hysteroscopic or

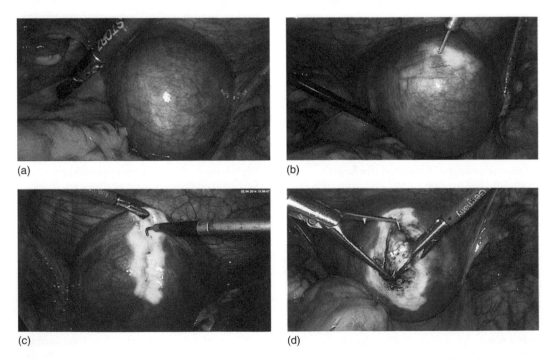

(a) (b)

(c) (d)

Figure 5.1 Laparoscopic myoma enucleation. (a) Situs of a fundal/anterior wall fibroid. (b) Prophylactic hemostasis with 1:100 diluted vasopressin solution (gylcilpressin) in separate wells. The injection intends to separate the pseudocapsule from the fibroid and reduces bleedings. (c) Bipolar superficial coagulation of the longitudinal incision strip and opening of the uterine wall with the monopolar hook or needle till the fibroid surface. (d) Grasping of the fibroid and beginning of the enucleation. The pseudocapsule remains within the uterine wall and is pushed off bluntly.

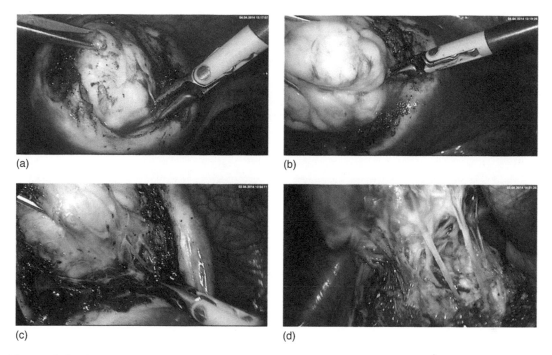

Figure 5.2 Laparoscopic myoma enucleation. (a) Traction of the fibroid with a tenaculum and blunt delineation from the capsule. (b) Focal bipolar coagulation of basic vessels. (c) Continuous enucleation of the fibroid under traction and specific coagulation of capsule fibers containing vessels. (d) Magnification of remaining capsule fibers to be coagulated and cut.

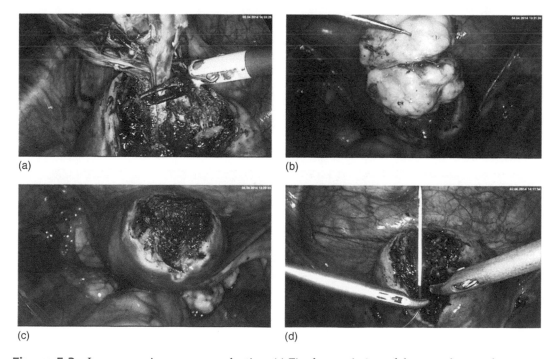

Figure 5.3 Laparoscopic myoma enucleation. (a) Final coagulation of the capsule vessels. (b) Double belly fibroid after complete enucleation. (c) Minimal coagulation of bleeding vessels under suction and irrigation. (d) Approximation of wound edges with either straight or round, sharp needle and a monofilar late-absorbable suture.

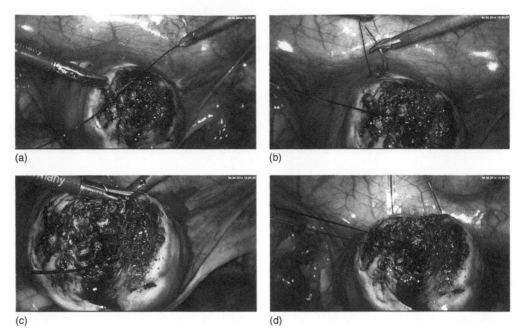

Figure 5.4 Laparoscopic reconstruction of myoma bed. (a) Advantage of round needle stitch. The wound angle is elevated safely and completely by elevating it with a Manhes forceps. Deeper layers of the myometrium can be grasped more easily using a round needle. (b) Needle exit and simplified regrasping with the right needle holder. (c) Final stitch to invert the knot. (d) Extirpation of the needle and completion of the extracorporeal knot and preparation to push down the extracorporeal knot.

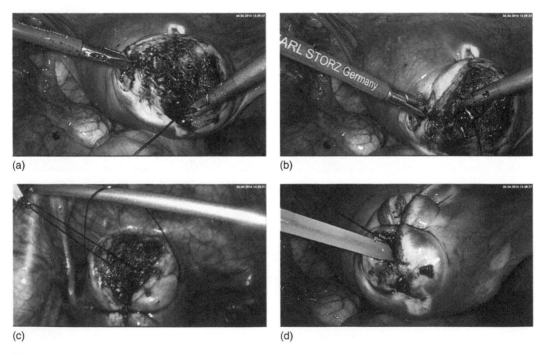

Figure 5.5 Laparoscopic reconstruction of myoma bed. (a) Second single stitch starting as deep as possible in the uterine wound. (b) Exiting of the needle on the left wound margin (just next to the Manhes forceps). (c) Completion of the stitch and preparation of the extracorporeal von Leffern knot. The needle holder elevates the thread to avoid tearing of the uterine wall while pulling through the monofilar thread (PDS). (d) The extracorporeal knot is pushed down with a plastic push-rod and deposited deep in the wound minimizing the external suture part.

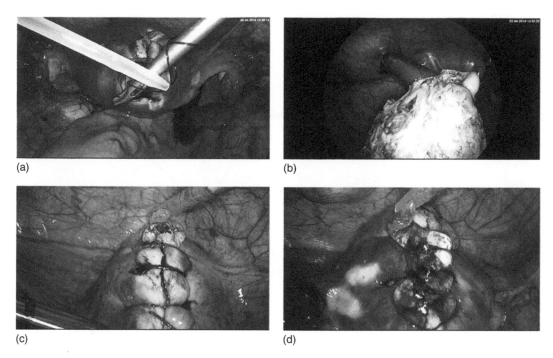

Figure 5.6 Laparoscopic morcellation and final appearance. (a) Intracorporeal safety knot of the knot performed extracorporeally. (b) Morcellation of the fibroid with the Rotocut morcellator (Storz) in an apple-peeling manner. (c) Final situs showing the extracorporeal sutures to adapt the uterine wound edges. (d) Application of Hyalo Barrier (Nordic Pharma) for adhesion prevention.

laparoscopic myomectomy is not feasible or if a laparotomy is required for any other reason. The indication to exclude uterine sarcomas has to be taken very strictly; however, uterine sarcoma is a very rare malignancy and the rate of sarcoma after clinical diagnosis of myoma is very low. The risk of severe complications in association with open surgery is higher than with hysteroscopic or laparoscopic moymectomy. Prophylactic antibiotics should be given for any abdominal fibroid operation (D'Angelo and Prat 2009; Mukhopadhaya, De Silva, and Manyonda 2008). After the Pfannenstil incision, either a vertical or transverse uterine incision is performed (Discepola et al. 2007). The myoma enucleation is performed by traction on the myometrial edges (e.g., with Allis clamps). After exposure of the fibroid, it can be extirpated. The pseudocapsule is typically dissected bluntly. The uterine defects are closed with sutures in several layers to reapproximate the tissue and achieve hemostasis without excessive bipolar coagulation.

Robotic Myomectomy

Robot-assisted laparoscopic myomectomy is a relatively new approach. The advantages of robotic surgery are three-dimensional imaging and mechanical improvement, including 7 degrees of freedom for each instrument, stabilization of the instruments within the surgical field, and improved ergonomics for the surgeon. Technical difficulties are decreased as suturing is easier than during conventional laparoscopy; however, there are few data comparing robot-assisted with conventional laparoscopic myomectomy (Pundir et al. 2013; Barakat et al. 2011; Mettler et al. 2013a). The advantages over abdominal myomectomy are decreased blood loss and shorter recovery time. Nevertheless, operation duration and operating costs are much higher than for conventional procedures. Furthermore, robotic devices are large and bulky. Robotic surgery is limited by the lack of tactile feedback, and additional team training is necessary to minimize the risk of mechanical failure (Schollmeyer et al. 2011). To date, no advantage over conventional laparoscopy could be demonstrated regarding blood loss or operative duration. A more secure myometrial closure has not yet been proven (Barakat et al. 2011). In obese patients, robot-assisted surgery might be beneficial (George, Eisenstein, and Wegienka 2009).

Hysterectomy as Treatment for Myomas

As fibroids are also the most common indication for hysterectomy (30% of hysterectomies in white women and 50% of hysterectomies in black women), a specific focus in this chapter

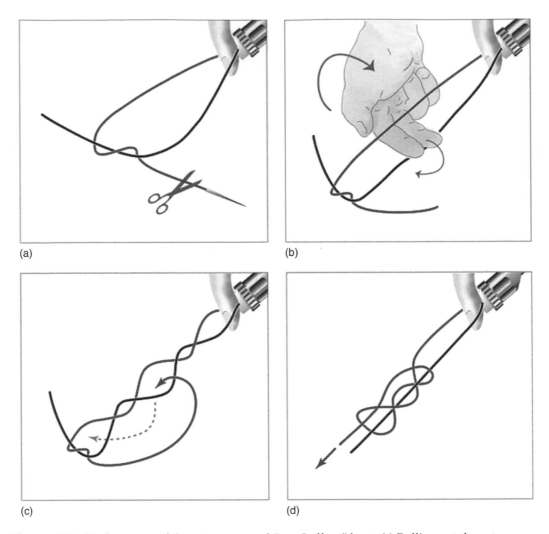

Figure 5.7 Performance of the extracorporeal "von Leffern" knot. (a) Pulling out the suture, removing the needle, half hitch. (b) Holding the knot with the left hand and reaching over with the right hand. (c) Grasping the short end from below and leading it back, exiting before the half hitch. (d) Turning back the knot. Holding the straight suture and tightening the knot.

is given to hysterectomies. The decision for a hysterectomy in a multifibroid uterus depends on the wish of the patient, her health status, whether childbearing has been completed, and the combined decision with the doctor. Only if the patient has metrorrhagia does the disorder need to be examined preoperatively in more detail as this may be a sign of endometrial cancer or sarcoma. Nevertheless, the combined evaluation of magnetic resonance imaging and tumor markers preoperatively leads to a more specific diagnosis of rapidly growing uterine masses or adnexas in the case of a leiomyomatous uterus or adnexal tumors. Only in cases where malignancy is not suspected is a simple TLH or SLH recommended; otherwise,

an oncological approach has to be selected. Hysterectomy such as TLH and SLH is recommended for the following indications:

■ Acute hemorrhage with nonresponse to other therapies

■ Completion of family and current or increased future risk of other diseases, such as cervical intraepithelial neoplasia or endometrial hyperplasia, or an increased risk of uterine or ovarian cancer. A precondition for the indication for hysterectomy is that these risks can be eliminated or decreased by hysterectomy

■ Failure of previous treatment

■ Completion of family and significant symptoms (e.g., multiple fibroids or adenomyosis) and the desire for a definitive solution

The main advantage of hysterectomy over all other therapeutic possibilities is the definitive solution in eliminating all existing symptoms and the risk of recurrence. Nevertheless, the advantage of a definitive solution that allows freedom from future problems can be an obstacle if family planning has not been completed or the patient has a personal inhibition against the removal of the central genital female organ (Falcone and Parker 2013). These issues must be discussed with the patient before the decision for a hysterectomy is taken. Furthermore, for a solitary submucous, subserous, pedunculated, or intramural myoma, the complication rate of a hysterectomy has to be compared with the complication rate of a myomectomy. The operational risks have to be compared with the operational risks of hysteroscopy, laparoscopic fibroid enucleation, or conservative management. With the advances in cervical cancer screening, the prevention of future cervical or uterine pathologies is no longer a relevant indication for hysterectomy. The decision must be tailored to meet the needs of each individual patient.

Laparoscopic hysterectomy was introduced in 1989 with the aim of reducing the morbidity and mortality of abdominal hysterectomy to the level reached with vaginal hysterectomy. Laparoscopic assistance for vaginal hysterectomy can be an advantage if there is a need for adhesiolysis, a need to treat endometriosis simultaneously, or a need to treat large leiomyomas and to ensure an easier and safer adnexectomy. If feasible, vaginal hysterectomy allows a more rapid and less painful recovery than open or laparoscopic surgery and is much less expensive (Garry et al. 2004).

SHOULD OVARIES OR FALLOPIAN TUBES (OR BOTH) BE REMOVED OR LEFT IN PLACE AT HYSTERECTOMY?

Ovaries

Generally, the ovaries are not removed when a hysterectomy is performed for uterine fibroids. Removing the uterus alone will cure the bleeding and the size-related symptoms caused by the fibroids. When fibroids are treated, it is not necessary to remove the ovaries or fallopian tubes as is sometimes the case when treating other diseases, such as endometriosis or gynecologic cancers.

However, more recent research suggests that although after menopause the ovaries produce little estradiol (the major estrogen in premenopausal women), they produce a tremendous amount of androgens (usually thought of as male hormones) (Adashi 1994). It is thought that these androgens may be important in maintaining mood and sex drive (Shifren 2004; Buster et al. 2005; Nyunt et al. 2005). In addition, the risks of hormone replacement have become clearer, and many women choose to use hormones following menopause (Manson et al. 2003; Anderson et al. 2004). Most women are aware of the research from the Women's Health Initiative demonstrating significant complications with postmenopausal hormone replacement therapy. However, it is not widely known that the risks are lower for women without a uterus, who are able to take estrogen alone (Anderson et al. 2004). The association of premature loss of ovarian function and the increasing risk of heart disease has also been investigated (Parker et al. 2005).

Given all of these factors, there are good reasons to retain the ovaries if possible. The major reason to remove them at the time of fibroid surgery is if the woman has a high risk of ovarian cancer.

Fallopian Tubes

According to research presented at the Annual Clinical Meeting of the American College of Obstetricians and Gynecologists in 2013, bilateral salpingectomy at hysterectomy, with preservation of the ovaries, is considered a safe way of potentially reducing the development of ovarian serous carcinoma, the most common type of ovarian cancer. Increasing evidence points toward the fallopian tubes as the origin of this type of cancer. Removing the fallopian tubes does not cause the onset of menopause, as does the removal of the ovaries.

Prophylactic removal of the fallopian tubes during hysterectomy or sterilization would rule out any subsequent tubal pathology, such as hydrosalpinx, which is observed in up to 30% of women after hysterectomy. Moreover, this intervention is likely to offer considerable protection against later tumor development even if the ovaries are retained. Thus, we recommend that any hysterectomy be combined with salpingectomy. Women undergoing hysterectomy with retained fallopian tubes or sterilization have at least double the risk of subsequent salpingectomy. Therefore, removal of the fallopian tubes at hysterectomy should be recommended (Dietl, Wischhusen, and Hausler 2011; Guldberg et al. 2013).

CONCLUSION

Treatment options for uterine leiomyomas vary. The choice of treatment should be made on an individual basis while taking into account the following factors: the patient's level of suffering due to bleeding disorders or displacement-caused pain, the status of family planning, and the patient's preferences regarding the different treatment options.

In *asymptomatic women*, expectant management except for hydronephrosis caused by displacement or hysteroscopically resectable submucous fibroids in women who pursue pregnancy is suggested.

In *postmenopausal women* without hormonal therapy, fibroids usually shrink and become asymptomatic. Therefore, expectant management is the method of choice. However, sarcoma should be excluded if a new or enlarging pelvic mass occurs in a postmenopausal woman. Surgical treatment is the option of choice if the leiomyomas are symptomatic. If there are contraindications to operative procedures or hysterectomy is declined by the patient for personal reasons, any of the alternative treatment options (medical, embolization, or guided ultrasound) can be considered.

In *premenopausal women*, appropriate submucosal leiomyomas should be resected hysteroscopically if the women wish to preserve their childbearing potential or they are symptomatic (e.g., bleeding and miscarriage) or both. Intramural and subserosal leiomyomas in women who wish to preserve their fertility can be removed laparoscopically. Nevertheless, an appropriate surgical technique and advanced laparoscopic skills are necessary. If this cannot be guaranteed, abdominal myomectomy has to be recommended or the patient has to be referred to a laparoscopic center to maximize the possibility and safety of pregnancy after uterine reconstruction. The risk of uterine rupture in pregnancy following myomectomy needs to be discussed with the patient.

Robotic assistance makes laparoscopic suturing easier and offers surgery with three-dimensional vision; however, costs are still high. Further developments in robotic assistance, including force feedback, will receive more of our attention in the future.

For *women who have completed their family planning*, hysterectomy is the definitive procedure for relief of symptoms and prevention of recurrence of fibroid-related problems. With increasing experience in laparoscopic hysterectomies, the risk of side effects has become manageable. In relation to the compliance and individuality of the patient, a suitable solution can be either laparoscopic supracervical or total laparoscopic hysterectomy.

REFERENCES

Adashi, E. Y. 1994. The climacteric ovary as a functional gonadotropin-driven androgen-producing gland. *Fertil Steril* 62 (1):20–27.

Al-Hendy, A., E. J. Lee, H. Q. Wang, and J. A. Copland. 2004. Gene therapy of uterine leiomyomas: adenovirus-mediated expression of dominant negative estrogen receptor inhibits tumor growth in nude mice. *Am J Obstet Gynecol* 191 (5):1621–1631.

Alkatout, I., B. Bojahr, L. Dittmann, V. Warneke, L. Mettler, W. Jonat, and T. Schollmeyer. 2011a. Precarious preoperative diagnostics and hints for the laparoscopic excision of uterine adenomatoid tumors: two exemplary cases and literature review. *Fertil Steril* 95 (3):1119.e5–1119.e8.

Alkatout, I., T. Schollmeyer, N. A. Hawaldar, N. Sharma, and L. Mettler. 2012. Principles and safety measures of electrosurgery in laparoscopy. *JSLS* 16 (1):130–139.

Alkatout, I., C. Stuhlmann-Laeisz, L. Mettler, W. Jonat, and T. Schollmeyer. 2011b. Organ-preserving management of ovarian pregnancies by laparoscopic approach. *Fertil Steril* 95 (8):2467–70.e1–2.

Anderson, G. L., M. Limacher, A. R. Assaf, T. Bassford, S. A. Beresford, H. Black, et al. 2004. Effects of conjugated equine estrogen in postmenopausal women with hysterectomy: the Women's Health Initiative randomized controlled trial. *JAMA* 291 (14):1701–1712.

Barakat, E. E., M. A. Bedaiwy, S. Zimberg, B. Nutter, M. Nosseir, and T. Falcone. 2011. Robotic-assisted, laparoscopic, and abdominal myomectomy: a comparison of surgical outcomes. *Obstet Gynecol* 117 (2 Pt 1): 256–265.

Buster, J. E., S. A. Kingsberg, O. Aguirre, C. Brown, J. G. Breaux, A. Buch, et al. 2005. Testosterone patch for low sexual desire in surgically menopausal women: a randomized trial. *Obstet Gynecol* 105 (5 Pt 1):944–952.

Celik, H., and E. Sapmaz. 2003. Use of a single preoperative dose of misoprostol is efficacious for patients who undergo abdominal myomectomy. *Fertil Steril* 79 (5):1207–1210.

D'Angelo, E., and J. Prat. 2009. Uterine sarcomas: a review. *Gynecol Oncol* 116 (1):131–139.

Di Spiezio Sardo, A., I. Mazzon, S. Bramante, S. Bettocchi, G. Bifulco, M. Guida, and C. Nappi. 2008. Hysteroscopic myomectomy: a comprehensive review of surgical techniques. *Hum Reprod Update* 14 (2):101–119.

Dietl, J., J. Wischhusen, and S. F. Hausler. 2011. The post-reproductive Fallopian tube: better removed? *Hum Reprod* 26 (11):2918–2924.

Discepola, F., D. A. Valenti, C. Reinhold, and T. Tulandi. 2007. Analysis of arterial blood vessels surrounding the myoma: relevance to myomectomy. *Obstet Gynecol* 110 (6):1301–1303.

Donnez, J., R. Hudecek, O. Donnez, D. Matule, H. J. Arhendt, J. Zatik, Z. Kasilovskiene, M. C. Dumitrascu,

H. Fernandez, D. H. Barlow, P. Bouchard, B. C. Fauser, E. Bestel, P. Terrill, I. Osterloh, and E. Loumaye. 2015. Efficacy and safety of repeated use of ulipristal acetate in uterine fibroids. *Fertil Steril* 103 (2):519–527.e3.

Donnez, J., T. F. Tatarchuk, P. Bouchard, L. Puscasiu, N. F. Zakharenko, T. Ivanova, G. Ugocsai, M. Mara, M. P. Jilla, E. Bestel, P. Terrill, I. Osterloh, and E. Loumaye. 2012. Ulipristal acetate versus placebo for fibroid treatment before surgery. *N Engl J Med* 366 (5):409–420.

Donnez, J., F. Vazquez, J. Tomaszewski, K. Nouri, P. Bouchard, B. C. Fauser, D. H. Barlow, S. Palacios, O. Donnez, E. Bestel, I. Osterloh, and E. Loumaye. 2014. Long-term treatment of uterine fibroids with ulipristal acetate. *Fertil Steril* 101 (6):1565–73.e1–18.

Dueholm, M., E. Lundorf, E. S. Hansen, S. Ledertoug, and F. Olesen. 2002. Accuracy of magnetic resonance imaging and transvaginal ultrasonography in the diagnosis, mapping, and measurement of uterine myomas. *Am J Obstet Gynecol* 186 (3):409–415.

Edwards, R. D., J. G. Moss, M. A. Lumsden, O. Wu, L. S. Murray, S. Twaddle, and G. D. Murray. 2007. Uterine-artery embolization versus surgery for symptomatic uterine fibroids. *N Engl J Med* 356 (4):360–370.

Emanuel, M. H., A. Hart, K. Wamsteker, and F. Lammes. 1997. An analysis of fluid loss during transcervical resection of submucous myomas. *Fertil Steril* 68 (5):881–886.

Falcone, T., and W. H. Parker. 2013. Surgical management of leiomyomas for fertility or uterine preservation. *Obstet Gynecol* 121 (4):856–868.

Flynn, M., M. Jamison, S. Datta, and E. Myers. 2006. Health care resource use for uterine fibroid tumors in the United States. *Am J Obstet Gynecol* 195 (4):955–964.

Funaki, K., H. Fukunishi, and K. Sawada. 2009. Clinical outcomes of magnetic resonance-guided focused ultrasound surgery for uterine myomas: 24-month follow-up. *Ultrasound Obstet Gynecol* 34 (5):584–589.

Garry, R., J. Fountain, J. Brown, A. Manca, S. Mason, M. Sculpher, V. Napp, S. Bridgman, J. Gray, and R. Lilford. 2004. EVALUATE hysterectomy trial: a multicentre randomised trial comparing abdominal, vaginal and laparoscopic methods of hysterectomy. *Health Technol Assess* 8 (26):1–154.

George, A., D. Eisenstein, and G. Wegienka. 2009. Analysis of the impact of body mass index on the surgical outcomes after robot-assisted laparoscopic myomectomy. *J Minim Invasive Gynecol* 16 (6):730–733.

Guldberg, R., S. Wehberg, C. W. Skovlund, O. Mogensen, and O. Lidegaard. 2013. Salpingectomy as standard at hysterectomy? A Danish cohort study, 1977–2010. *BMJ Open* 3 (6):e002845.

Hart, R., B. G. Molnar, and A. Magos. 1999. Long term follow up of hysteroscopic myomectomy assessed by survival analysis. *Br J Obstet Gynaecol* 106 (7):700–705.

Hartmann, K. E., H. Birnbaum, R. Ben-Hamadi, E. Q. Wu, M. H. Farrell, J. Spalding, and P. Stang. 2006. Annual costs associated with diagnosis of uterine leiomyomata. *Obstet Gynecol* 108 (4):930–937.

Jansen, F. W., C. B. Vredevoogd, K. van Ulzen, J. Hermans, J. B. Trimbos, and T. C. Trimbos-Kemper. 2000. Complications of hysteroscopy: a prospective, multicenter study. *Obstet Gynecol* 96 (2):266–270.

Kim, H. S., J. H. Baik, L. D. Pham, and M. A. Jacobs. 2011. MR-guided high-intensity focused ultrasound treatment for symptomatic uterine leiomyomata: long-term outcomes. *Acad Radiol* 18 (8):970–976.

Kim, M. S., Y. K. Uhm, J. Y. Kim, B. C. Jee, and Y. B. Kim. 2013. Obstetric outcomes after uterine myomectomy: laparoscopic versus laparotomic approach. *Obstet Gynecol Sci* 56 (6):375–381.

Kongnyuy, E. J., and C. S. Wiysonge. 2011. Interventions to reduce haemorrhage during myomectomy for fibroids. *Cochrane Database Syst Rev* (11):CD005355.

Laughlin, S. K., K. E. Hartmann, and D. D. Baird. 2011. Postpartum factors and natural fibroid regression. *Am J Obstet Gynecol* 204 (6):496.e1–6.

Lefebvre, G., G. Vilos, C. Allaire, J. Jeffrey, J. Arneja, C. Birch, M. Fortier, and M. S. Wagner. 2003. The management of uterine leiomyomas. *J Obstet Gynaecol Can* 25 (5):396–418; quiz 419–22.

Loffer, F. D., L. D. Bradley, A. I. Brill, P. G. Brooks, and J. M. Cooper. 2000. Hysteroscopic fluid monitoring guidelines. The ad hoc committee on hysteroscopic training guidelines of the American Association of Gynecologic Laparoscopists. *J Am Assoc Gynecol Laparosc* 7 (1):167–168.

Lonnerfors, C., and J. Persson. 2011. Pregnancy following robot-assisted laparoscopic myomectomy in women with deep intramural myomas. *Acta Obstet Gynecol Scand* 90 (9):972–977.

Manson, J. E., J. Hsia, K. C. Johnson, J. E. Rossouw, A. R. Assaf, N. L. Lasser, M. Trevisan, H. R. Black, S. R. Heckbert, R. Detrano, O. L. Strickland, N. D. Wong, J. R. Crouse, E. Stein, and M. Cushman. 2003. Estrogen plus progestin and the risk of coronary heart disease. *N Engl J Med* 349 (6):523–534.

Marjoribanks, J., A. Lethaby, and C. Farquhar. 2006. Surgery versus medical therapy for heavy menstrual bleeding. *Cochrane Database Syst Rev* (2):CD003855.

Mettler, L., L. Clevin, A. Ternamian, S. Puntambekar, T. Schollmeyer, and I. Alkatout. 2013a. The past, present and future of minimally invasive endoscopy in gynecology: a review and speculative outlook. *Minim Invasive Ther Allied Technol* 22 (4):210–226.

Mettler, L., W. Sammur, I. Alkatout, and T. Schollmeyer. 2011. Imaging in gynecologic surgery. *Womens Health (Lond Engl)* 7 (2):239–248; quiz 249–50.

Mettler, L., W. Sammur, T. Schollmeyer, and I. Alkatout. 2013b. Cross-linked sodium hyaluronate, an anti-adhesion barrier gel in gynaecological endoscopic surgery. *Minim Invasive Ther Allied Technol* 22 (5):260–265.

Mettler, L., T. Schollmeyer, and I. Alkatout. 2012a. Adhesions during and after surgical procedures, their prevention and impact on women's health. *Womens Health (Lond Engl)* 8 (5):495–498.

Mettler, L., T. Schollmeyer, A. Tinelli, A. Malvasi, and I. Alkatout. 2012b. Complications of uterine fibroids and their management, surgical management of fibroids, laparoscopy and hysteroscopy versus hysterectomy, haemorrhage, adhesions, and complications. *Obstet Gynecol Int* 2012:791248.

Mukhopadhaya, N., C. De Silva, and I. T. Manyonda. 2008. Conventional myomectomy. *Best Pract Res Clin Obstet Gynaecol* 22 (4):677–705.

Nyunt, A., G. Stephen, J. Gibbin, L. Durgan, A. M. Fielding, M. Wheeler, and D. E. Price. 2005. Androgen status in healthy premenopausal women with loss of libido. *J Sex Marital Ther* 31 (1):73–80.

Parker, W. H., M. S. Broder, Z. Liu, D. Shoupe, C. Farquhar, and J. S. Berek. 2005. Ovarian conservation at the time of hysterectomy for benign disease. *Obstet Gynecol* 106 (2):219–226.

Parker, W. H., and I. A. Rodi. 1994. Patient selection for laparoscopic myomectomy. *J Am Assoc Gynecol Laparosc* 2 (1):23–26.

Patterson-Keels, L. M., S. M. Selvaggi, H. K. Haefner, and J. F. Randolph, Jr. 1994. Morphologic assessment of endometrium overlying submucosal leiomyomas. *J Reprod Med* 39 (8):579–584.

Peddada, S. D., S. K. Laughlin, K. Miner, J. P. Guyon, K. Haneke, H. L. Vahdat, R. C. Semelka, A. Kowalik, D. Armao, B. Davis, and D. D. Baird. 2008. Growth of uterine leiomyomata among premenopausal black and white women. *Proc Natl Acad Sci U S A* 105 (50):19887–19892.

Propst, A. M., R. F. Liberman, B. L. Harlow, and E. S. Ginsburg. 2000. Complications of hysteroscopic surgery: predicting patients at risk. *Obstet Gynecol* 96 (4):517–520.

Pundir, J., V. Pundir, R. Walavalkar, K. Omanwa, G. Lancaster, and S. Kayani. 2013. Robotic-assisted laparoscopic vs abdominal and laparoscopic myomectomy: systematic review and meta-analysis. *J Minim Invasive Gynecol* 20 (3):335–345.

RCoOa, Gynaecologists. 2008. Preventing entry-related gynaecological laparoscopic injuries. *RCOG Green-top Guideline* 49:1–10.

Schollmeyer, T., L. Mettler, W. Jonat, and I. Alkatout. 2011. Roboterchirurgie in der Gynäkologie. *Der Gynäkologe* 44 (3):196–201.

Shifren, J. L. 2004. The role of androgens in female sexual dysfunction. *Mayo Clin Proc* 79 (4 Suppl):S19–S24.

Tinelli, A., L. Mettler, A. Malvasi, B. Hurst, W. Catherino, O. A. Mynbaev, M. Guido, I. Alkatout, and T. Schollmeyer. 2013. Impact of surgical approach on blood loss during intracapsular myomectomy. *Minim Invasive Ther Allied Technol* 23 (2):87–95.

Tsuji, S., K. Takahashi, I. Imaoka, K. Sugimura, K. Miyazaki, and Y. Noda. 2006. MRI evaluation of the uterine structure after myomectomy. *Gynecol Obstet Invest* 61 (2):106–110.

Tulandi, T., C. Murray, and M. Guralnick. 1993. Adhesion formation and reproductive outcome after myomectomy and second-look laparoscopy. *Obstet Gynecol* 82 (2):213–215.

van der Kooij, S. M., S. Bipat, W. J. Hehenkamp, W. M. Ankum, and J. A. Reekers. 2011. Uterine artery embolization versus surgery in the treatment of symptomatic fibroids: a systematic review and metaanalysis. *Am J Obstet Gynecol* 205 (4):317.e1–317.18.

Varma, R., H. Soneja, T. J. Clark, and J. K. Gupta. 2009. Hysteroscopic myomectomy for menorrhagia using Versascope bipolar system: efficacy and prognostic factors at a minimum of one year follow up. *Eur J Obstet Gynecol Reprod Biol* 142 (2):154–159.

Wallach, E. E., and N. F. Vlahos. 2004. Uterine myomas: an overview of development, clinical features, and management. *Obstet Gynecol* 104 (2):393–406.

Wamsteker, K., M. H. Emanuel, and J. H. de Kruif. 1993. Transcervical hysteroscopic resection of submucous fibroids for abnormal uterine bleeding: results regarding the degree of intramural extension. *Obstet Gynecol* 82 (5):736–740.

Zaima, A., and A. Ash. 2011. Fibroid in pregnancy: characteristics, complications, and management. *Postgrad Med J* 87 (1034):819–828.

Zhao, F., Y. Jiao, Z. Guo, R. Hou, and M. Wang. 2010. Evaluation of loop ligation of larger myoma pseudocapsule combined with vasopressin on laparoscopic myomectomy. *Fertil Steril* 95 (2):762–766.

6 Reducing Intraoperative Blood Loss in Myomectomy

Better to Prepare and Prevent than Repair and Repent

Sunita R. Tandulwadkar, Manish Y. Machave, and Abhishek Chandavarkar

CONTENTS

INTRODUCTION

Myomectomy is the surgical treatment option of choice for women who wish to either preserve their fertility potential or simply wish to conserve their uterus. A myomectomy can be performed by a laparotomy or endoscopy (laparoscopy or hysteroscopy).

Laparoscopic myomectomy has smaller incisions as compared to large incision of laparotomy, consequently there is less postoperative pain, shorter hospital stay, and faster recovery. However, large and multiple fibroids are more difficult to excise by laparoscopy. The choice of surgical approach depends on the number, size, location, and type of fibroids and in particular on the expertise of the surgeon and his or her team.

Myomatous uteri have an increased number of arterioles and venules, and myomectomy may involve significant blood loss [1]. However, studies show that with comparable uterine size, the blood loss is similar whether hysterectomy or myomectomy is performed [2]. The average volumes of blood loss are 200–800 mL during abdominal myomectomy (performed via laparotomy, also referred to as open myomectomy) [2] and 80–250 mL for laparoscopic myomectomy [3]. Surgical hemorrhage may result in anemia, hypovolemia, and coagulation abnormalities.

Controlling blood loss during myomectomy continues to be a challenge faced by endoscopic surgeons. Multiple options have been described and promoted over the years to achieve this goal. Despite the application of even the best technique, excessive bleeding can be encountered and further options are needed in controlling blood loss during surgery. This chapter intends to discuss the various options with respect to their mechanism of action, effectiveness, and evidence supporting their use. Although the individual surgeon always has his or her favorite method, it shall be prudent here to throw some light on the comparative efficacies of individual methods.

CLASSIFICATION SYSTEM

Which route to choose when deciding to do a myomectomy is the first decision to make. The age-old classification of submucous, intramural, and subserous does not help in deciding the route of the surgery. Categorization or classification of submucous leiomyomas can be useful when considering therapeutic options, including the surgical approach. The most widely used system categorizes the leiomyomas into three subtypes according to the proportion of the lesion's diameter that is within the myometrium, usually as determined by saline infusion sonography or hysteroscopy (Table 6.1).

The FIGO (International Federation of Gynecology and Obstetrics) system (Refer Figure 2.3) classifies fibroids similar to ESGE but adds a number of other categories, including type 3 lesions that abut the endometrium without distorting the endometrial cavity. In addition, this system allows categorization of the relationship of the leiomyoma outer boundary with the uterine serosa, a relationship that is important when evaluating women for resectoscopic surgery. Thus, a European Society

TABLE 6.1: European Society of Gynecological Endoscopy: Classification of submucous myomas

Type O
  Entirely within endometrial cavity
  No myometrial extension (pedunculated)

Type I
  <50% myometrial extension (sessile)
  <90° angle of myoma surface to uterine wall

Type II
  ≥50% myometrial extension (sessile)
  ≥90° angle of myoma surface to uterine wall

of Gynecological Endoscopy (ESGE) type 2 leiomyoma that reaches the serosa is considered to be a type 2–5 lesion and therefore is not a candidate for resectoscopic surgery.

APPROACHES TO REDUCE BLOOD LOSS

These can broadly be divided into preoperative and intraoperative approaches. Preoperatively, patients can be administered gonadotropin-releasing hormone (GnRH) analogues or aromatase inhibitors in an attempt to shrink the myoma(s) and potentially decrease blood loss. The effectiveness of this has been questioned secondary to the potential loss of the surgical plane and consequently increased difficulty in completing the surgery. Newer agents under current investigation include selective progesterone receptor modulators.

Intraoperative options can be further categorized as chemical and mechanical. Chemical options include intravenous administration of medications (oxytocin, tranexamic acid, injection of normal saline, or a vasoconstrictive agent such as vasopressin) into the subcapsular layer of the myoma. Mechanical options include application of a tourniquet at the level of the uterine artery insertion into the uterus, ligating/clipping/coagulating the uterine arteries, or temporary clamping of the uterine arteries (Table 6.2).

PREOPERATIVE APPROACHES

Myomectomy has potential risks of complications. To reduce these risks, medical pretreatment can be applied to reduce fibroid size and thereby potentially decrease intraoperative blood loss, the need for blood transfusion, and emergency hysterectomy.

Gonadotropin-Releasing Hormone Analogues

A Cochrane review showed significant improvement with GnRH agonist over placebo or no treatment in preoperative hemoglobin and hematocrit and in reduction of uterine and myoma volumes [4]. Compared with no treatment prior to hysterectomy, GnRH agonists reduce intraoperative bleeding and operative time, increase postoperative hemoglobin and hematocrit values, and decrease postoperative complications and length of hospital stay.

Use of GnRH increase the proportion of hysterectomies performed vaginally rather than abdominally. The need for vertical incisions during hysterectomy is reduced when GnRH is used preoperatively as compared to the cases when it was not used [4]. In a 2001 systematic review and meta-analysis, when GnRH agonists were used prior to myomectomy, intraoperative bleeding and rates of vertical incisions were also reduced while postoperative hemoglobin was slightly increased.

However, patients who received GnRH agonists were more likely to have a recurrence of fibroids at 6 months after myomectomy compared with no treatment. No differences were seen in rates of postoperative complications. No differences were seen in rates of blood transfusion for either type of surgery. A 2011 systematic review of GnRH agonist showed no reduction in operative time but did show decreased intraoperative blood loss [5].

However, there is controversy over the ability to dissect myomas from surrounding myometrium after exposure to GnRH agonist. A double-blind, placebo-controlled trial of GnRH agonist prior to hysteroscopic myomectomy found no differences in the number of complete fibroid resections, operative times, or amount of fluid absorbed [6].

Ulipristal Acetate

The two randomized controlled trials mentioned previously have shown the effectiveness of 3 months' treatment to correct anemia and reduce uterine fibroid size [7, 8]. There were no surgical parameters reported in these studies, and surgical experience is variable.

INTRAOPERATIVE APPROACHES

A number of intraoperative adjuncts have been used in an effort to reduce blood

TABLE 6.2: Approaches to reduce blood loss

Preoperative	Intraoperative	
	Chemical	Surgical steps
Gonadotropin-releasing hormone analogues	Oxytocin	1. Temporary uterine occlusion
	Vasopressin	2. Remaining in correct intracapsular plane
Aromatase inhibitors	Normal saline	3. Compression of myoma bed after enucleation or taking box suture
Selective progesterone	Tranexamic acid	
Receptor modulators		4. Immediate suturing with obliteration of dead space

loss and improve surgical outcomes in leiomyoma surgery.

Misoprostol

Misoprostol is a prostaglandin E1 analogue that reduces uterine blood flow, increases myometrial contractions, and has the potential to reduce blood loss during uterine surgery [9]. The evidence for misoprostol as an adjunct for myomectomy is limited and conflicting. However, even a single dose of misoprostol is efficacious in patients undergoing abdominal myomectomy. Placebo-controlled randomized studies have shown that a single dose of misoprostol 400 µg given vaginally 1 h prior or rectally 30 min prior to abdominal myomectomy resulted in a statistically significant reduction in operative time [10], blood loss, postoperative hemoglobin drop, and need for postoperative blood transfusion. No differences were observed in length of hospital stay [10]. In one randomized trial, no benefit was observed in the use of misoprostol alone for abdominal myomectomy, but misoprostol 400 µg by rectum combined with intravenous oxytocin (10 U/h) in women undergoing laparoscopically assisted vaginal hysterectomy found significant improvements in operative outcomes compared with placebo [11].

The role of misoprostol for cervical priming before operative hysteroscopy has also been reported, although not all patients in that study had fibroids as the indication for surgery [12]. The authors found that in the misoprostol group there was less need for surgical dilation, shorter time for cervical dilation to Hegar 9, shorter operative time, and fewer occurrences of cervical lacerations than the placebo group. Though not statistically significant, fewer instances of false passages (1.4% vs. 6.3%) and perforations (0% vs. 2.5%) were observed [12].

Oxytocin

Although recent evidence suggests the presence of oxytocin receptors in uterine myomas, the evidence for its use to reduce blood loss is somewhat conflicting. For myomectomy, a systematic review of two randomized trials that compared intraoperative oxytocin against placebo for operative outcomes at myomectomy did not suggest a benefit for operative bleeding, although the pooled numbers may be difficult to interpret because of the significant heterogeneity between the two trials [13].

Vasopressin

Vasopressin is a naturally occurring hormone that can cause vascular spasm and uterine muscle contraction and hence has the potential to prevent bleeding during uterine surgery [14].

As there have been several reports of cardiovascular collapse following intramyometrial injection of vasopressin, caution should be taken to ensure proper dilution and clear communication with the anesthesiologist [15].

A retrospective comparison of prospectively collected data of 150 patients who underwent laparoscopic myomectomy was conducted [16]. They were divided into two groups: 50 were treated without any vasoconstrictive agent, and 100 were treated with intraoperative intramyometrial injection of dilute vasopressin (20 IU/100 mL normal saline). The blood loss was significantly lower in the group that used vasopressin as compared with the one that did not use anything. This study shows that vasopressin is effective in reducing blood loss during laparoscopic myomectomy [16].

What dose should be administered for adequate hemostasis? Conventionally, 0.1 U/mL is infiltrated at the pseudocapsule by most surgeons. A randomized multicenter clinical trial tried to address this issue [17]. Patients undergoing conventional laparoscopic or robot-assisted laparoscopic myomectomy were randomly assigned to receive 200 mL of diluted vasopressin solution (20 U in 400 mL normal saline) or 30 mL of concentrated vasopressin solution (20 U in 60 mL normal saline). The trial concluded that higher-volume administration of vasopressin does not reduce blood loss [17].

Two trials compared vasopressin with tourniquets in myomectomy. In one trial, dilute vasopressin (20 U in 20 mL saline injected prior to uterine incision) had effects comparable to those of mechanical vascular occlusion (Penrose drain tourniquet and vascular clamps at the infundibulopelvic ligament) with respect to blood loss, postoperative morbidity, and transfusion requirements [18]. In contrast, another study reported less blood loss in the vasopressin group (20 U in 20 mL) than in the tourniquet group (512.7 ± 400 mL, $P = 0.036$) [19]. However, no statistically significant differences were seen in the hemoglobin drop, number of transfusions, intraoperative blood pressure, or highest postoperative pulse and temperature [19].

A 2011 study compared intraoperative bleeding during laparoscopic myomectomy using dilute vasopressin (6 U in 20 mL) with Roeder knot loop ligation at the base of the fibroid with use of vasopressin alone and with placebo [19]. Blood loss in the placebo (mean ± standard deviation, 363.7 ± 147.8 mL) and vasopressin-only (224.4 ± 131.2 mL) groups was significantly reduced by the addition of loop ligation at the base of the myoma (58.7 ± 27.5 mL) [19].

Bupivacaine and Epinephrine

In one study on laparoscopic myomectomy, the use of bupivacaine (50 mL of 0.25%) and epinephrine (0.5 mL of 1 mg/mL) was significantly more effective than placebo in reducing intraoperative bleeding, total operative time, myoma enucleation time, and subjective surgical difficulty as measured on a 1–10 visual analogue scale [20]. The analgesic requirement was also reduced in the bupivacaine group ($P < 0.05$ for all comparisons). No differences in blood pressure or heart rate were observed [20].

Antifibrinolytics

Tranexamic acid is a synthetic derivative of lysine with antifibrinolytic activity and has been used to reduce blood loss and the need for blood transfusion in surgical procedures. However, only one trial has studied its effect during abdominal myomectomy using intravenous tranexamic acid (10 mg/kg patient body weight to a maximum of 1 g) given 15 min before skin incision versus placebo [21]. The trial did show average reduced blood loss of 243 mL but did not reach the authors' level of clinical significance (250 mL) [21].

Gelatin–Thrombin Matrix

Gelatin–thrombin matrix is a hemostatic sealant with bovine-derived gelatin and thrombin components. In contrast to fibrin glue, gelatin–thrombin matrix is hydrophilic and adheres well to wet tissue. When applied to tissue, the large concentration of thrombin and gelatin can result in rapid hemostasis, which may be useful in gynecologic surgery.

In a randomized prospective trial, 50 women with uterine fibroids with a uterine size greater than 16 weeks' gestation were included. Half the women received the FloSeal gelatin–thrombin matrix (FloSeal Matrix; Baxter, Deerfield, IL, USA) at the site of the uterine bleeding via a single-barrel syringe and a special applicator tip. The control group received isotonic sodium chloride solution. Postoperative blood losses were about 25 mL for the FloSeal group and 250 mL in the other group. This study suggests the ability of gelatin–thrombin matrix to reduce blood loss when applied immediately and directly to the bleeding uterine site before closure of the hysterotomy incision [22].

Intraoperative Uterine Artery Occlusion

Another option is to perform uterine artery occlusion (UAO) by laparoscopy at the time of

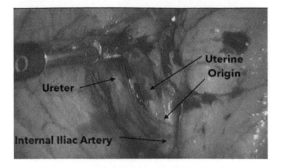

Figure 6.1 The anatomy of the uterine artery in relation to internal iliac artery where the uterine artery occlusion is performed.

myomectomy, although the benefit seems controversial. In one study comparing laparoscopic myomectomy with or without UAO, blood loss did not differ significantly and operating time was slightly longer when UAO was performed [23] (Figure 6.1).

Jin et al. evaluated for the optimal hemostatic technique for laparoscopic myomectomy by comparing temporary uterine artery blockage alone or combined with blockage of the utero-ovarian vessels [24]. Two hundred patients were randomly divided into three groups. All women received 6 U of vasopressin into the myometrium before myomectomy. One group underwent temporary bilateral UAO and myomectomy while another group underwent temporary ligation of both bilateral uterine artery and utero-ovarian vessel occlusion. The blood loss was significantly lower in the group with both bilateral uterine artery and utero-ovarian vessel occlusion ($P < 0.001$) [24].

RECOMMENDATIONS

- Anemia should be corrected prior to proceeding with elective surgery.
- Selective progesterone receptor modulators and gonadotropin-releasing hormone analogues are effective at correcting anemia and should be considered preoperatively in patients with anemia.
- Use of vasopressin, bupivacaine and epinephrine, misoprostol, pericervical tourniquet, or gelatin–thrombin matrix reduces blood loss at myomectomy and should be considered.

PRACTICAL TIPS & TRICKS

Whether hysteroscopy or laparoscopy, myomectomy surgery should always be planned in a postmenstrual phase.

Hysteroscopic Myomectomy

- In case of a large submucous myoma or multiple submucous myomas, preoperative use of GnRH may help by reducing the size and making it relatively avascular.
- Speed is an important factor during resection of the myoma. Meticulous input and output chart during hysteroscopic myomectomy will prevent fluid over load related complications.

Laparoscopic Myomectomy

- Tranexamic acid, misoprostol, or oxytocin preoperatively should be used as options to prevent blood loss.
- Intramyometrial vasopressin is the mainstay for laparoscopic myomectomies. A dilution of 20 U in 200 mL of normal saline is recommended. In view of the cardiac side effects associated with vasopressin, aspiration prior to every injection is recommended. The use of Pisat's VVIN needle (visual vasopressin injection needle) for increasing the safety of vasopressin works on the principle of a transparent tip which can visualize aspiration of blood and prevent inadvertent injection into vessels. Spinal needles to inject vasopressin into the myometrium can also be used.
- If the use of vasopressin is considered risky, clipping of uterine artery at its origin is extremely useful technique. (e.g., severe hypertension and cardiac disorders). It is also useful for large and multiple fibroids in association with vasopressin or by itself.
- Horizontal or vertical incision for myomectomy depends on the individual surgeon's preferences (whether he or she prefers ipsilateral or contralateral suturing), the position of the myoma, and number of myomas that can be removed from one incision in case of multiple myomas.
- Remaining in the proper intracapsular plane at the time of enucleation avoids opening of large vessels.

- After enucleation of the fibroid, a horizontal mattress or a box stitch at the base of the myoma or compression of the myoma bed is an excellent tool for immediate control of bleeding.
- Energy sources should be avoided as far as possible but in cases where arterial bleeding is encountered, bipolar energy sources to coagulate the bleeders are essential.
- The use of barbed sutures in layers is useful to increase the speed of suturing, obliteration of dead space, and prevention of blood loss.

REFERENCES

1. Sampson JA. The blood supply of uterine myomata. *Surg Gynecol Obstet.* 1912;14:215.

2. Iverson RE Jr, Chelmow D, Strohbehn K, Waldman L, Evantash EG. Relative morbidity of abdominal hysterectomy and myomectomy for management of uterine leiomyomas. *Obstet Gynecol.* 1996;88:415.

3. Sinha R, Hegde A, Mahajan C, Dubey N, Sundaram M. Laparoscopic myomectomy: do size, number, and location of the myomas form limiting factors for laparoscopic myomectomy? *J Minim Invasive Gynecol.* 2008;15:292.

4. Lethaby A, Vollenhoven B, Sowter M. Preoperative GnRH analogue therapy before hysterectomy or myomectomy for uterine fibroids. *Cochrane Database Syst Rev.* 2001;(2):CD000547.

5. Chen I, Motan T, Kiddoo D. Gonadotropin-releasing hormone agonist in laparoscopic myomectomy: systematic review and meta-analysis of randomized controlled trials. *J Minim Invasive Gynecol.* 2011;18:303–309.

6. Mavrelos D, Ben-Nagi J, Davies A, Lee C, Salim R, Jurkovic D. The value of pre-operative treatment with GnRH analogues in women with submucous fibroids: a double-blind, placebo-controlled randomized trial. *Hum Reprod.* 2010;25:2264–2269.

7. Donnez J, Tomaszewski J, Vazquez F, Bouchard P, Lemieszczuk B, Baro F, et al. Ulipristal acetate versus leuprolide acetate for uterine fibroids. *N Engl J Med.* 2012;366:421–432.

8. Donnez J, Vazquez F, Tomaszewski J, Nouri K, Bouchard P, Fauser B, et al. PEARL III and PEARL III Extension Study Group. Long-term treatment of uterine fibroids with ulipristal acetate*. *Fertil Steril.* 2014;101(6):1565–1573.

9. Chang FW, Yu MH, Ku CH, Chen CH, Wu GJ, Liu JY. Effect of uterotonics on intra-operative blood loss during laparoscopy assisted vaginal hysterectomy: a randomised controlled trial. *BJOG*. 2006;113:47–52.

10. Celik H, Sapmaz E. Use of a single preoperative dose of misoprostol is efficacious for patients who undergo abdominal myomectomy. *Fertil Steril*. 2003;79:1207–1210.

11. Frederick S, Frederick J, Fletcher H, Reid M, Hardie M, Gardner W. A trial comparing the use of rectal misoprostol plus perivascular vasopressin with perivascular vasopressin alone to decrease myometrial bleeding at the time of abdominal myomectomy. *Fertil Steril*. 2013;100:1044–1049.

12. Preutthipan S, Herabutya Y. Vaginal misoprostol for cervical priming before operative hysteroscopy: a randomized controlled trial. *Obstet Gynecol*. 2000;96:890–894.

13. Cesen-Cummings K, Houston KD, Copland JA, Moorman VJ, Walker CL, Davis BJ. Uterine leiomyomas express myometrial contractile-associated proteins involved in pregnancy-related hormone signaling. *J Soc Gynecol Invest*. 2003;10:11–20.

14. Wang CJ, Yuen LT, Yen CF, Lee CL, Soong YK. A simplified method to decrease operative blood loss in laparoscopic-assisted vaginal hysterectomy for the large uterus. *J Am Assoc Gynecol Laparosc*. 2004;11:370–373.

15. Kongnyuy EJ, Wiysonge CS. Interventions to reduce haemorrhage during myomectomy for fibroids. *Cochrane Database Syst Rev*. 2011;(11):CD005355.

16. Protopapas A, Giannoulis G, Chatzipapas I, Athanasiou S, Grigoriadis T, Kathopoulis N, et al. Vasopressin during laparoscopic myomectomy: does it really extend its limits? *J Minim Invasive Gynecol*. 2019;26(3):441–449. doi: 10.1016/j.jmig.2018.05.011. Epub 2018 May 18.

17. Cohen SL, Senapati S, Gargiulo AR, Srouji SS, Tu FF, Solnik J, et al. Dilute versus concentrated vasopressin administration during laparoscopic myomectomy: a randomised controlled trial. *BJOG*. 2017;124(2):262–268. doi: 10.1111/1471-0528.14179. Epub 2016 Jun 30.

18. Fletcher H, Frederick J, Hardie M, Simeon D. A randomized comparison of vasopressin and tourniquet as hemostatic agents during myomectomy. *Obstet Gynecol*. 1996;87:1014–1018.

19. Zhao F, Jiao Y, Guo Z, Hou R, Wang M. Evaluation of loop ligation of larger myoma pseudocapsule combined with vasopressin on laparoscopic myomectomy. *Fertil Steril*. 2011;95:762–766.

20. Zullo F, Palomba S, Corea D, Pellicano M, Russo T, Falbo A, et al. Bupivacaine plus epinephrine for laparoscopic myomectomy: a randomized placebo-controlled trial. *Obstet Gynecol*. 2004;104:243–249.

21. Caglar GS, Tasci Y, Kayikcioglu F, Haberal A. Intravenous tranexamic acid use in myomectomy: a prospective randomized double-blind placebo controlled study. *Eur J Obstet Gynecol Reprod Biol*. 2008;137:227–231.

22. Raga F, Sanz-Cortes M, Bonilla F, Casañ EM, Bonilla-Musoles F. Reducing blood loss at myomectomy with use of a gelatin-thrombin matrix hemostatic sealant. *Fertility Steril*. 2009; 92(1):356–360. doi: 10.1016/j.fertnstert.2008.04.038.

23. Bae JH, Chong GO, Seong WJ, Hong DG, Lee YS. Benefit of uterine artery ligation in laparoscopic myomectomy. *Fertil Steril*. 2011;95:775–778.

24. Jin L, Ji L, Shao M, Hu M. Laparoscopic myomectomy with temporary bilateral uterine artery and utero-ovarian vessels occlusion compared with traditional surgery for uterine fibroids: blood loss and recurrence. *Gynecol Obstet Invest*. 2019;84(6):548–554. doi: 10.1159/000499494.

7 Hysteroscopic Myomectomy

Resection Techniques and Safety

Sergio Haimovich

CONTENTS

Myomas or leiomyomas are benign monoclonal tumors in the uterine wall and are usually asymptomatic. The symptoms of heavy menstrual bleeding (HMB), infertility, and recurrent pregnancy loss occur largely as a result of lesions that distort the endometrial cavity that are adjacent to the endometrium and consequently referred to as submucous (SM) leiomyomas. SM myomas represent only 5 to 10% of all myomas.

The surgical approach to the SM myomas depends on different factors such as size, intramural component, situation in the uterine cavity, and size of the cavity. According to the FIGO (International Federation of Gynecology and Obstetrics) classification (Figure 7.1), SM myomas are type 0, 1, or 2 depending on the grade of penetration into the uterine cavity.

Lasmar et al. [1] developed a new classification for evaluating the viability and degree of difficulty of hysteroscopic myomectomy: the STEPW (size, topography, extension, penetration, and wall) (Figure 7.2). This classification not only considers the degree of penetration of the myoma into the myometrium but also adds parameters such as the distance of the base of the myoma from the uterine wall, the size of the nodule (in centimeters), and the topography of the uterine cavity. Each parameter receives a score, and the total sum of them indicates the myoma group.

A major advantage of the STEPW classification is its ability to group the SM fibroids by score, identifying a group in which 100% of the myomectomies will be complete and another group in which some incomplete myomectomies will occur. This will permit the surgeon to plan and better prepare for the surgery and even to better inform the patient prior to consenting to the procedure.

In order to estimate the grade of difficulty of the hysteroscopic approach, there is another factor to include: the relation between the cavity size (container) and the myoma (content) or what we call the "ratio factor." In Figure 7.3, the myoma is the same size in both cavities but the surgical difficulty in the small nulliparous uterus is higher than in the big multiparous one.

SURGICAL TECHNIQUES FOR HYSTEROSCOPIC MYOMECTOMY

The hysteroscopic myomectomy technique depends on a number of factors, including the desire for future fertility; the size, number, and location of the SM leiomyomas; and (particularly with type 2 lesions) the distance between the myoma and the serosa.

We need to know whether the lesions are lying entirely or mostly in the uterine cavity or have a major intramural component. In this case, should the myometrial free margin still be considered a limiting factor? Some authors think that should be a limit [2] and a one-step hysteroscopic myomectomy may be performed to remove deeply infiltrating SM myomas when

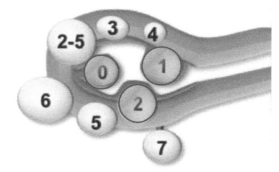

SM- Submucosal	0	Pedunculated Intracavitary
	1	<50% Intramural
	2	≥50% Intramural

Figure 7.1 International Federation of Gynecology and Obstetrics (FIGO) classification of submucous myomas.

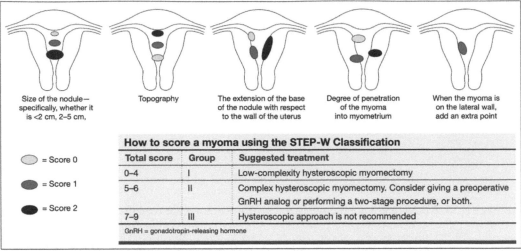

Size of the nodule— specifically, whether it is <2 cm, 2–5 cm,

Topography

The extension of the base of the nodule with respect to the wall of the uterus

Degree of penetration of the myoma into myometrium

When the myoma is on the lateral wall, add an extra point

◯ = Score 0

⬤ = Score 1

⬤ = Score 2

How to score a myoma using the STEP-W Classification

Total score	Group	Suggested treatment
0–4	I	Low-complexity hysteroscopic myomectomy
5–6	II	Complex hysteroscopic myomectomy. Consider giving a preoperative GnRH analog or performing a two-stage procedure, or both.
7–9	III	Hysteroscopic approach is not recommended

GnRH = gonadotropin-releasing hormone

A score of 4 or less is desired for low-complexity hysteroscopic myomectomy.

Figure 7.2 Lasmar's STEPW (size, topography, extension, penetration, and wall) classification of submucous (SM) myomas.

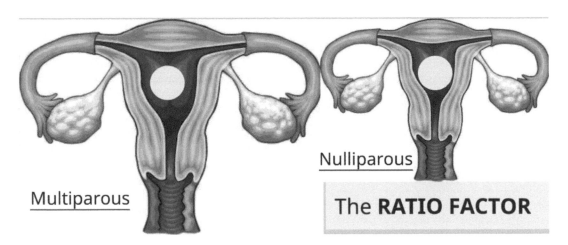

Multiparous

Nulliparous

The **RATIO FACTOR**

Figure 7.3 The "ratio factor."

myometrial thickness at the implantation site is more than 5 mm.

But is this fact a real limitation? Another study [3] evaluated the feasibility of the hysteroscopic resection of type 2 SM fibroids regardless of the myometrial free margin separating them from the serosa. In this work, the authors reported the dynamic changes the margin undergoes after the various phases of resection. During the hysteroscopic myomectomy, ultrasound evaluation of the myometrial free margin was measured before and after each phase of the procedure. The authors found that the myometrial free margin increases progressively with each step of the procedure, probably leading to an increasing margin of safety.

The most frequent technique is resection but there now exist a growing number of other hysteroscopic techniques for dissection, vaporization, or morcellation and excision of SM myomas. There are three basic methods for removing leiomyomas under hysteroscopic direction: morcellation, cutting with an electrosurgical loop, and vaporization.

The procedure can be performed depending on the technique and the fibroid, in both the operating room (OR) and the office setting.

SM myomas (types 0, 1, and 2) up to 4 to 5 cm in diameter can be removed under hysteroscopic direction by experienced surgeons, whereas larger and multiple myomas are best removed abdominally. Type 2 myomas are more likely to require a multistage procedure.

Resectoscopy

By far the most common hysteroscopic technique has been transcervical resectoscopic myomectomy (TCRM) with a modified urologic resectoscope, first reported in 1976 [4]. The operating hysteroscope (resectoscope) is the instrument that allows the performance of an SM myomectomy under direct and constant visual control. It includes a straightforward telescope (0°) or a slightly fore-oblique 12 to 30° telescope with an outer diameter of 3 to 4 mm and internal and external sheaths of 24 to 27 Fr outer diameter that provide a constant inflow and outflow of distension fluid for generating a continuous and efficient lavage system of the uterine cavity.

The resectoscope with a radiofrequency electrosurgical generator and a loop electrode is needed. The electrosurgical system can be monopolar or bipolar. The use of monopolar electrodes requires nonconducting distending solution (sorbitol 5% or glycine 1.5%).

The use of a bipolar set of instruments would be much safer. With bipolar, the current will only have to pass through the tissue with which the thermal loop comes into contact, thus minimizing the danger deriving from the random passage through the corporeal structures. An intrauterine bipolar diathermy allows the use of an electrolitic uterine distension medium such as normal saline.

Loop electrosurgical resection is performed with the electrode activated with low-voltage ("cutting") current to allow the repetitive creation of "strips" of myoma; the "chips" of tissue can be removed one at a time manually with the cutting loop without current. Alternatively, the chips can be left in place until they obstruct visualization of the uterine cavity for later removal.

The removal of type 0 and most type 1 lesions is generally straightforward, but for deep type 1 and type 2 lesions, more than one surgical stage is sometimes needed.

The trend during the last decade is to pass from OR to office procedures. New devices such as new bipolar mini-resectoscopes of 15 Fr (Karl Storz, Tuttlingen, Germany) and 16 Fr (Tontarra Medizintechnik GmbH, Wurmlingen, Germany) appeared, making it possible to perform myomectomy of small fibroids in an office setting.

Morcellation or Tissue Removal System

The hysteroscopic tissue removal system (TRS) for the treatment of SM myomas is usually applied with the patient under general or spinal anesthesia, typically as a day-case procedure. A specially designed TRS is introduced via the hysteroscope and used to cut and simultaneously aspirate the leiomyoma tissue. The aspirated tissue can be collected for histological analysis. Currently, there are three different kinds of hysteroscopic TRS:

Truclear (Medtronic): The first to be approved by the US Food and Drug Administration (2005). The Truclear 8.0 has a diameter of 8 mm and is introduced into the uterine cavity with a 9-mm rigid sheath. The Truclear 5.0 hysteroscopy system incorporates a 2.9-mm rotatory-style blade through a 5-mm, 0° hysteroscope.

MyoSure (Hologic) 19 Fr or 6.25 mm. MyoSure is introduced into the uterus through a 6- or 7-mm, 0°, continuous flow hysteroscope.

Biggati Shaver (Karl Storz) in both 19 Fr and 24 Fr.

These devices have a short learning curve and work in a fast way to reduce the myoma volume. Their main limitation is the difficulty in cases of deep myomas for extracting the intramural portion.

In a 2017 review on the use of hysteroscopic TRS, the authors conclude that" "Despite the limitations in the number and type of studies, our overview allows us to confirm a good feasibility of hysteroscopic TRS use for type 0 and type 1 SMs and, similarly to what happens for 'classic' resectoscopic myomectomy, a more difficult procedure for type 2 SM" [5].

Enucleation

The enucleation of a myoma is based on finding the right "cleavage plane," like in an open or laparoscopic myomectomy. The cleavage plane is the space between the fibroid and the adjacent myometrial tissue, also called the "myoma pseudocapsule" (Figure 7.4). This space contains a proper vascular network; there is no true vascular pedicle. The myoma is anchored to a space named pseudocapsule by connectival bridges (Figure 7.5). Inside this space, there are different elements such as smooth muscle cells similar to the myometrium, neuropeptides, and angiogenesis factors; this ultrastructural feature suggests that when fibroids are being removed, their pseudocapsules should be preserved as much as possible in order to preserve the myometrium [6, 7]. Depending on the myoma type, there are myomectomy techniques that respect this important cleavage plane, such as those that enucleate the myoma.

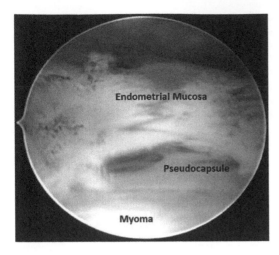

Figure 7.4 The pseudocapsule between the endometrium and the myoma.

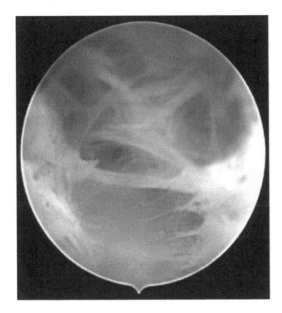

Figure 7.5 Connective tissue bridges inside the pseudocapsule.

The "cold loop" technique described by Mazzon [8] is characterized by a sequence of three different operating steps:

1. *Excision of the intracavitary component of the fibroid*: This is carried out with the usual technique of resectoscope slicing. This action must stop at the level of the plane of the endometrial surface so that the identification of the passage between the fibroid and the adjacent myometrial tissue is not impaired (cleavage plane).

2. *Enucleation of the intramural component of the fibroid*: Once the cleavage plane is identified, the usual cutting loop of the resectoscope is substituted by a suitable blunt dissection cold loop (mechanical loops of Mazzon; Karl Storz). Usually the rectangular loop is used first. This loop, once inserted into the plane between the fibroid and myometrium, is used in a mechanical way along the surface of the fibroid (usually clearly recognizable by its smooth, white, and compact surface), thus bringing about its progressive blunt dissection from the myometrial wall. Then the single-tooth loop is used to hook and lacerate the slender connective bridges that join the fibroid and the adjacent myometrium. During the entire phase of enucleation, electric energy must not be used in the thickness of the wall, and the loop must be used "cold" or in a mechanical way.

3. *Excision of the intramural component*: At the end of the enucleation phase, the intramural part of the fibroid is totally dislocated inside the uterine cavity. At this point, it can be completely and safety excised by means of the usual progressive excision using an angled cutting loop.

Based on the myoma's pseudocapsule, Bettocchi et al. (2009) published the OPPIuM (office preparation of partially intramural myomas) technique [9] to facilitate the subsequent scheduled resectoscopic myomectomy. The procedure consists of an incision of the endometrial mucosa and the pseudsocapsule covering the myoma aimed at facilitating protrusion of the intramural portion of the myoma into the uterine cavity as a preliminary step for in-patient resectoscopic surgery after two menstrual cycles. At follow-up hysteroscopy, the conversion of myomas with partially intramural development into totally or prevalently intracavitary ones was observed in 55 (93.2%) out of 59 patients.

Based on the results of Bettocchi et al., we developed a new two-step technique for G2 and deep G1 fibroids; both steps were in an office setting without anesthesia [10].

The first step was the same as the technique of Bettocchi et al., and the second step for excision of the myoma was performed 4 weeks later using the same hysteroscope and setup (pressure, flow, and suction) as those used for the first office procedure. The myoma was excised by means of diode laser or a mechanical instrumentation technique (scissors and grasping forceps). In those patients in whom extraction of the myoma was not possible because of the size of the mass, a biopsy was taken, the myoma was left free in the uterine cavity, and an ultra-sound check-up was performed 2 months later to assess the presence or absence of myoma remnants. In 100% of the cases, the cavity was empty [11].

Success of surgery was significantly associated with size, location, and women's parity. All myomas less than 18 mm were successfully enucleated as compared with 85% of 19 to 30 mm and 0% of more than 30 mm ($P < 0.001$).

At the second step of office hysteroscopy, the conversion of myoma with partially intramural development into totally (G0) or mainly (<50%) (G1) intracavitary ones was observed in 95.3% (41/43) of cases.

With this technique, preserving the integrity of adjacent fibers avoids disruption of the uterine wall and ensures a successful outcome, especially in young women who desire future childbearing. In case of type 0 pedunculated myomas, after a tissue sample for histology was taken, the pedicle was cut and surgery finished.

Hysteroscopic Myolysis

Myolysis was introduced in the late 1980s in Europe as a conservative treatment for uterine fibroids. Myolysis refers to the destruction of uterine fibroids by focused energy. The technique uses energy to shrink fibroids and destroy their blood supply. These techniques can be performed laparoscopically or transvaginally under ultrasound guidance and recently with direct vision by hysteroscopy.

In our case, we perform myolysis by laser-induced interstitial thermotherapy with diode laser.

The especially designed laser fiber works through the 5-Fr working canal of the 4.3-mm Bettocchi® Hysteroscope (Karl Storz). This laser applies a wavelength of 1470 nm that has affinity to both water (cut/vaporize) and hemoglobin (coagulate). So, even if the vaporization of the myoma is not complete, the vascularity is compromised.

The myolysis procedure was performed by office hysteroscopy without anesthesia. We included 64 patients with SM myomas (type 0, 1, and 2) between 25 and 63 mm (34 mm).

The laser fiber was introduced inside the fibroid, leaving just a 1-mm insertion hole on the endometrium. The energy application time was between 3 and 16 min depending on the myoma volume and the energy (watts) applied. All of the included cases had HMB.

A follow-up ultrasound was performed between 1 and 2 months after the procedure, and a second-look hysteroscopy was performed after 2 months. The mass reduction was 60 to 100% (myoma disappearance), and the mean

volume reduction was 72%. All of the patients reported an improvement in bleeding pattern immediately after the procedure. There were no complications and it was well tolerated by the patients. We have probed the feasibility of this new technique that is differentiated from other techniques not only by the results but especially by the fact that it is performed in an office setting without anesthesia. We believe that it is going to be a prevailing technique for the treatment of SM myomas, breaking the limits of the size.

MYOMA G0 (SESSILE OR PEDUNCULATED)

With this myoma type, all of the techniques achieve complete surgery. The only limitation for this technique is the technical access to the myoma's pedicle. There are no limits regarding the myoma's size. The rest of the techniques extract all the fibroid mass from the cavity, and surgery time will depend on the volume.

The traditional resectoscopy (bipolar or monopolar) is the slowest; surgery time is shorter with morcellator and vaporization. In case of small fibroids (up to 20 mm), it is possible to achieve excision with office hysteroscopy techniques.

There is no indication for "cold loop."

In terms of safety, there is a risk of excessive fluid absorption, or even thermal burns, with the use of monopolar resectoscopy in long surgery. In all the techniques that require cervical dilatation, there is a probability of perforation or false routes. In G0-type surgery, the risk of adhesions or bleeding is very low. The subjacent myometrium, as well as the fertility, is preserved with all of the different procedures. All of the office setting procedures have a lower cost compared with those that are performed in the OR, even on an outpatient basis.

MYOMA G1 OR G2

It is in these myoma types where the differences among the procedures are best appreciated. Some of the risk remains equal for the different techniques, such as perforation or false route whenever dilatation is required. Again, the size together with the proportion of the intramural portion will be the determinant factors of risk in each technique.

Resectoscopy with Monopolar Energy

This technique will achieve successful surgery in a one-step procedure in most G1-type myomas and some of the G2-type myomas. In cases of deep fibroids, there is an increased risk of uterine wall injury, depending on the distance to the serosa, and a second procedure will be necessary in order to extract the intramural portion. The risk of excessive fluid absorption (that will limit the operation time) and thermal burns also exists together with bleeding. The resectoscopy technique is also responsible for the adjacent myometrium injury, and there is increased risk of adhesions and associated fertility problems. This is always performed in the OR and anesthesia is needed.

Resectoscopy with Bipolar Energy

The risks are the same as with monopolar with one exception: the possibility of using a saline solution as distension media decreases the risk of excessive fluid absorption. For that reason, it is slowly changing the monopolar system in the hysteroscopy units and probably will become the gold standard because there is no need to learn a new procedure; the bipolar just improves the existing one.

"Cold Loop"

This technique can be performed with a monopolar or bipolar resectoscope with the risk associated described before. The advantage of this procedure is that it preserves the integrity of the subjacent myometrium with a low risk of adherences and posterior fertility is preserved.

Because it is based on converting a G2 or G1 myoma into a G0, there is almost no risk of uterine wall injury and most procedures can achieve the fibroid enucleation in just a one-step operation, increasing the percentage of surgery success. Learning the technique is required.

Vaporization

Resectoscope with monopolar vaporizing electrodes, with this device the myoma is vaporized for achieving a reduction in the fibroid's volume, to facilitate the posterior extraction with the resectoscope. Because the fibroid volume is vaporized, the probability of surgery success in a one-step procedure is increased and surgery time is reduced. Owing to the high potency of the laser (120–300 W), the surgeon must be very careful because of the risk of uterine wall perforation and the possibility of bowel injury.

The Nd:yAG (neodymium-doped yttrium aluminum garnet) laser is not in use.

The diode laser is similar to the monopolar vaporizing electrodes with the advantage that the former can be used with saline solution; it is a quick way to reduce the myoma's volume. In some cases, it can be performed in an office setting thanks to the 6.3-mm diameter. None of the vaporization techniques preserves the integrity of the myometrium subjacent. It requires experience with the procedure.

Morcellator or TRS

The major advantages are the ease of removal of tissue fragments through the instrument and the use of saline solution instead of electrolyte-free solutions used in monopolar high-frequency resectoscopy. It seems that the technique is easier to learn than resectoscopy. van Dongen et al. [12] conducted a randomized controlled trial to compare conventional resectoscopy and hysteroscopic morcellation among residents in training. The mean operating times for resectosocpy and morcellation were 17.0 min (95% confidence interval [CI] 14.1–17.9, standard deviation [SD] 8.4) and 10.6 min (95% CI 7.3–14.0, SD 9.5), respectively ($P = 0.008$). Subjective surgeon and trainer scores for convenience of technique on a visual analogue scale were in favor of the morcellator.

Regarding the integrity of the myometrium, it is not clear that this procedure preserves it. More experience is needed in order to determine the effect on post-surgery adhesions and in the fertility after procedure.

Laser

The two-step procedure with diode laser is performed as an office setting procedure with a 4.3-mm hysteroscope. It achieved enucleation in 92% of the myomas up to 30 mm. There is no need for a dilation of the cervical canal, with a reduction in the risk of perforation, saline solution as distension media without risk of excessive fluid absorption. This technique uses the cleavage plane for the myoma enucleation and preserves the integrity of the subjacent myometrium. There are no adhesions post-surgery and it preserves fertility.

It requires experience with the technique and is limited to those patients who tolerate the procedure without anesthesia.

Given the published evidence, it is understandable that the perfect hysteroscopic myomectomy technique does not exist. Each procedure has advantages and disadvantages, and it is up to the surgeon to choose the best technique in a given case, and the choice must be based on lowering risk and improving long-term results. If we follow these principles, we will be in a position to say we are using the best hysteroscopy myomectomy technique.

REFERENCES

1. Lasmar RB, Lasmar BP, Celeste RK, da Rosa DB, de Batista Depes D, Lopes RGC. A new system to classify submucous myomas: a Brazilian multicenter study. *J Minim Invasive Gynecol*. 2012;19(5):575–580. doi: 10.1016/j.jmig.2012.03.026. Epub 2012 Jul 20.

2. Yang JH, Lin BL. Changes in myometrial thickness during hysteroscopic resection of deeply invasive submucous myomas. *J Am Assoc Gynecol Laparosc*. 2001;8(4):501–505.

3. Casadio P, Youssef AM, Spagnolo E, Rizzo MA, Talamo MR, De Angelis D, et al. Should the myometrial free margin still be considered a limiting factor for hysteroscopic resection of submucous fibroids? A possible answer to an old question. *Fertil Steril*. 2011;95:1764–1768.

4. Neuwirth RS, Amin HK. Excision of submucous fibroids with hysteroscopic control. *Am J Obstet Gynecol*. 1976;126:95–99.

5. Vitale SG, Sapia F, Rapisarda AMC, Valenti G, Santangelo F, Rossetti D, et al. Hysteroscopic morcellation of submucous myomas: a systematic review. *Biomed Res Int*. 2017;2017:6848250. doi: 10.1155/2017/6848250. Epub 2017 Aug 29.

6. Malvasi A, Cavallotti C, Morroni M, Lorenzi T, Dell'Edera D, Nicolardi G, et al.. Uterine fibroid pseudocapsule studied by transmission electron microscopy. *Eur J Obstet Gynecol Reprod Biol*. 2012;162:187–191.

7. Malvasi A, Tinelli A, Rahimi S, D'Agnese G, Rotoni C, Dell'Edera D, et al. A three-dimensional morphological reconstruction of uterine leiomyoma pseudocapsule vasculature by the Allen-Cahn mathematical model. *Biomed Pharmacother*. 2011;65:359–363.

8. Mazzon I. Nuova tecnica per la miometomia isteroscopica: enucleazione con ansa fredda. In: Cittadini E, Perino A, Angiolillio M, Minelli L, editors. *Testo-Atlante di Chirurgia Endoscopica Ginecologica*. Palermo: COFESE Ed; 1995, cap XXXIIIb.

9. Bettocchi S, Di Spiezio SA, Ceci O, Nappi L, Guida M, Greco E, et al. A new hysteroscopic technique for the preparation of partially intramural myomas in office setting (OPPIuM technique): a pilot study. *J Minim Invasive Gynecol*. 2009;16:748–754.

10. Haimovich S, Mancebo G, Alameda F, Agramunt S, Solé JM, Hernandez JL, et al. Feasibility of a new two-step procedure for office hysteroscopic resection of submucous myomas: results of a pilot study. *Eur J Obstet Gynecol Reprod Biol*. 2013;168(2):191–194.

11. Haimovich S, López-Yarto M, Ávila JU, Tascón AS, Hernández JL, Collado RC. Office hysteroscopic laser enucleation of submucous myomas without mass extraction: a case series study. *Biomed Res Int*. 2015:5. Article ID 905204. doi: 10.1155/2015/905204.

12. Van Dongen H, Emanuel MH, Wolterbeek R, Trimbos JB, Jansen FW. Hysteroscopic morcellator for removal of intrauterine polyps and myomas: a randomized controlled pilot study among residents in training. *J Minim Invasive Gynecol*. 2008;15:466–471.

8 Laparoscopic-Assisted Myomectomy

Rooma Sinha, Bana Rupa, and Neha Singh

CONTENTS

INTRODUCTION

Large fibroids pose certain challenges during minimal access myomectomy. Limited visualization with decreased space can lead to an increased incidence of conversion to open procedures during the laparoscopic surgery. Laparoscopic-assisted surgery is an excellent approach to tackle large fibroids during myomectomy. It not only helps us to do the myomectomy but also helps to quickly extract the fibroid by manual morcellation. This technique may aid an intact retrieval of a large specimen to avoid morcellation when there is a concern for malignancy. It can provide a suitable method to reconstruct the uterus by using the open surgery techniques and instruments, thus providing multilayer complete closure of hysterotomy without leaving any dead space. The uterine reconstruction is carried out intracorporeally without extracting the uterus from the abdominal cavity. This technique can give the benefits of minimal access surgery to many more patients, even in the hands of surgeons who otherwise would have resorted to open myomectomy. Hence, it bridges the gap between open myomectomy and minimal access myomectomy. The need for a large and likely a vertical midline incision can be avoided, thus reducing the morbidity associated with the traditional open approach. There is no denying the fact that, when compared with abdominal myomectomy, laparoscopic myomectomy has the advantages of shorter hospitalization, faster recovery, fewer adhesions, less blood loss, and better cosmetic results.

The first hand-assisted laparoscopic hysterectomy was documented in 1999 by Pelosi and Pelosi [1]. They reported a 3050-g fibroid uterus that was removed by this technique. A fibroid uterus of this size occupies most of the abdominal cavity. With one 10-cm laparoscopic incision and a 7.5-cm transverse suprapubic incision, the hysterectomy was successfully performed in 150 min, blood loss was 220 mL, and the patient was discharged on the second day. In 1994, Nezhat et al. [2] reported the technique of laparoscopic-assisted myomectomy. Smith et al. [3], in a study published in 2019, reported factors that predict prolonged length of stay. The factors that predict long postoperative stay were body mass index of at least 30.1 kg/m^2, preoperative blood transfusion, removal of at least five fibroids, and operative time greater than 120 min [3]. Thus, it is imperative to plan the approach of myomectomy on the basis of the clinical situation and surgical expertise. This is done to ensure that the total operative time is around 2 to 3 hours.

When to Choose a Patient for Laparoscopic-Assisted Myomectomy

The laparoscopic-assisted approach is best suited for a difficult myomectomy with an enlarged uterus that poses a significant risk of intraoperative conversion to laparotomy (Figure 8.1). Patients with a large fibroid uterus that occupies the whole of the pelvic cavity and obstructs the surgical field can be offered laparoscopic-assisted myomectomy. On preoperative evaluation, any fibroid that is larger than 10 cm^2 or multiple (more than five) fibroids are suitable candidates. The ability to palpate the uterus and identify all fibroids is another potential advantage of the laparoscopic-assisted approach. A decision to use this approach is often made during the preoperative evaluation on the basis of significantly enlarged uterine size. Preoperative magnetic resonance imaging is what we usually do to decide whether the laparoscopic-assisted myomectomy technique should be carried out in a particular case (Figure 8.2). It can be also made in the operating room after the initial survey by the laparoscope. The effort is to reduce operative time and associated morbidity.

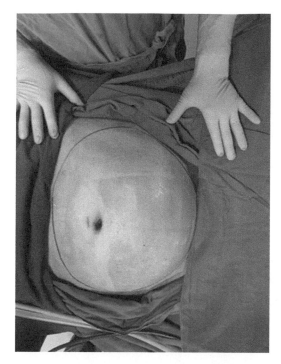

Figure 8.1 28-week size fibroid occupying the whole abdominal cavity for myomectomy.

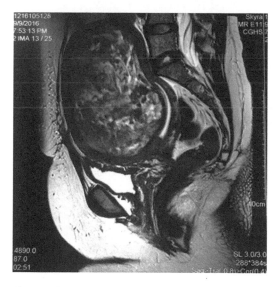

Figure 8.2 Magnetic resonance imaging depicting a large anterior wall fibroid.

LAPAROSCOPIC-ASSISTED MYOMECTOMY

Our Technique

We describe stepwise the technique for laparoscopic-assisted myomectomy.

After induction of general endotracheal anesthesia, the patient is placed in a low dorsal

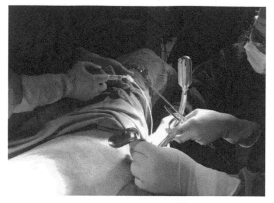

Figure 8.3 RUMI manipulator being introduced into the uterine cavity.

lithotomy position. A Foley catheter is inserted in the bladder. A uterine manipulator is placed in the uterine cavity (Figure 8.3). The surgical team can choose to use any manipulator that they are comfortable with. A 10-mm primary port is placed in the midline about 8–10 cm above the upper border of the uterus. On a surface anatomy, one palm breath above the upper part of the uterus is usually sufficient space to plan the laparoscopic port for telescope. When the pneumoperitoneum is achieved, this distance becomes 10 cm or more. Next, two 5-mm ports are inserted on the left side of the patient as we operate standing on the left side of the patient. The lower left port is placed almost at the level of the uterine fundus. The upper left port position is then selected 6–8 cm above the previous port so that the manipulation angle between instruments in the two left side ports is between 30 and 60° (Figure 8.4a,b). After insertion of the trocar, the uterus is infiltrated with dilute vasopressin to minimize blood loss. We prefer to use 20 U of vasopressin in 200 mL of saline and inject the diluted solution after confirming that the needle tip is not aspirating blood. Before the start of the hysterotomy, an initial survey is made to evaluate the position of the tubes and ovaries on both sides. Distortion in an extremely large uterus can alter the anatomy significantly. This is carried out to avoid inadvertent injury to the tubes and ovaries while performing hysterotomy and enucleation.

Once the ports are secured, we use a harmonic scalpel through the ipsilateral 5-mm port on the left side of the patient to make a hysterotomy incision (Figure 8.5a). Hysterotomy is performed with the right hand while the left hand, through the second ipsilateral port, uses the myoma screw to stabilize

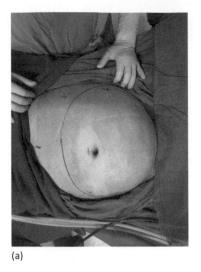
(a)

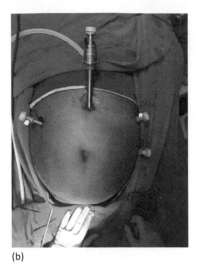
(b)

Figure 8.4 (a) Surface anatomy of the ports and (b) The picture showing the location of the ports after insertion. The blue ports are 5mm ports.

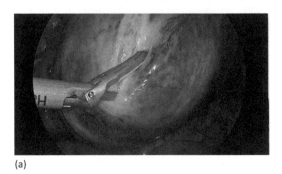
(a)

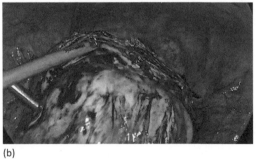
(b)

Figure 8.5 (a) Hysterotomy incision using the harmonic scalpel. (b) Enucleation in progress with the help of myoma screw and harmonic scalpel.

the fibroid. We prefer a vertical hysterotomy incision as it is easier to suture in this particular technique. Then an incision is made on the maximum setting of the harmonic scalpel, and an effort is made to reach up to the pseudocapsule. The length of the hysterotomy incision should be according to the size of the fibroid. Often, the surgeon struggles at the enucleation if either the correct plane is not reached or the incision length is not adequate. After the hysterotomy incision, the screw is inserted perpendicularly into the most prominent part of fibroid. The surgeon holds the knob of the myoma screw in her left hand and holds the harmonic scalpel or the aspirator/irrigator probe in the right hand to provide traction and countertraction against the myometrium through the ipsilateral ports. This facilitates the identification of tissue planes and can also wash the blood from the surgical site. The

aspirator/irrigator is used to bluntly dissect the fibroid at the capsule level. The harmonic scalpel blade is used at the capsule level to exert gentle pressure, as well as to facilitate cutting and coagulation along the pseudo-capsule. The harmonic scalpel performs two functions at this point. It helps to dissect the fibroid from the capsule. It can be used to cut the fibers if the capsule is adherent deeply as one dissects. The harmonic scalpel can also be used to give blunt traction, and the counter-traction is carried out with the myoma screw (Figure 8.5a,b).

Once removed, the fibroid is placed in the posterior cul-de-sac or in the right paracolic gutter. If there are multiple fibroids, they are enucleated one by one. However, at this point, one must decide the method used to account for all the fibroids as well as to keep them safely for easy extraction. In our practice, we use one of

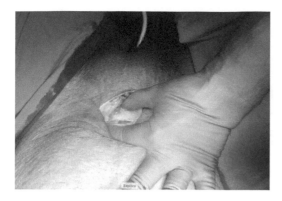

Figure 8.6 Suprapubic incision of 2–3 cm.

two methods. We either introduce a suture with a needle and thread all the fibroids together like a necklace and keep parking them in the right paracolic gutter. In the end of the procedure, this string of fibroids is introduced into a bag and extracted by morcellation. The other option in our surgical practice is to introduce a bag in the beginning and collect all the fibroids one by one as they are enucleated. The second option can be cumbersome as we already are dealing with reduced space in the pelvic cavity and a bag can take up the space and reduce vision.

After the enucleation is achieved, the next step is to make a 2- to 3-cm incision in the suprapubic area transversally (Figure 8.6). Once the suprapubic incision is made, we use small S-shaped curved retractors to retract the edges of the abdominal incision. The surgeon stands between the legs of the patient to do this part of the procedure, and the patient remains in the low lithotomy position (Figure 8.7). This suprapubic incision is now used to both morcellate and reconstruct the uterus. The morcellation is carried out by

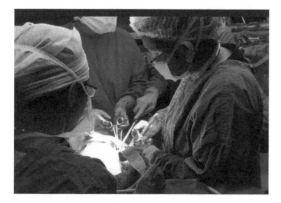

Figure 8.7 Position of the surgeon is between the legs of the patient for this part of the surgery.

cutting the fibroid serially into long strips by using a scalpel with a #11 blade.

Effort has to be made by the assistants to hold the abdominal wall up with the help of the retractors so that the bowel loops fall down and the uterus can be visualized through this small incision. The uterine reconstruction is carried out by identifying the edges of the hysterotomy incision and holding them with Allis forceps. This is carried out without attempting to extract the uterus outside the peritoneal cavity. With this technique without exteriororizing the uterus, we start reconstructing the uterus by intracorporeal suturing. The caudal end of the incision is identified, and multilayer closure of uterine defect is begun. Once this part of the defect is sutured, the uterus is moved caudally to expose the next part of the uterine incision into view through the small suprapubic incision. All suturing is carried out intracorporeally using open surgical instruments and 1/0 vicryl (Ethicon Polyglactin 910 with 1/2 circle taper point needle).

Approximation and hemostasis of the inner myometrial layers are carried out using interrupted sutures via an intracorporeal suture technique. The serosal layer is finally sutured by inverting the raw edges as in a baseball suture (Figure 8.8a–d). We close the suprapubic incision once the complete uterine reconstruction is achieved. The pneumoperitomeum is re-established and telescope is introduced for a final survey to irrigate the abdominal cavity and check for complete hemostasis (Figure 8.9). All trocars are removed under vision and ports closed (Figure 8.10). In the postoperative period, clear liquids are started in 4–6 h and solid food by 6–8 h. Recovery is quick and most patients are discharged in 24–48 hours after surgery.

DISCUSSION

The most important benefit of laparoscopic-assisted myomectomy is that one can offer minimal access surgery in situations that otherwise would have needed laparotomy. This technique is feasible and quick and does not require advanced levels of laparoscopic suturing skills. It also offers significantly faster extraction of fibroids without the use of mechanical electromorcellator. Pelosi et al. introduced hand-assisted laparoscopic surgery as a technique similar to what we have described in our technique [4]. Their approach includes the insertion of the surgeon's hand into the abdomen through a glove-sized incision at laparoscopy while preserving the pneumoperitoneum [4]. However, we make a smaller suprapubic incision and perform this part of the surgery

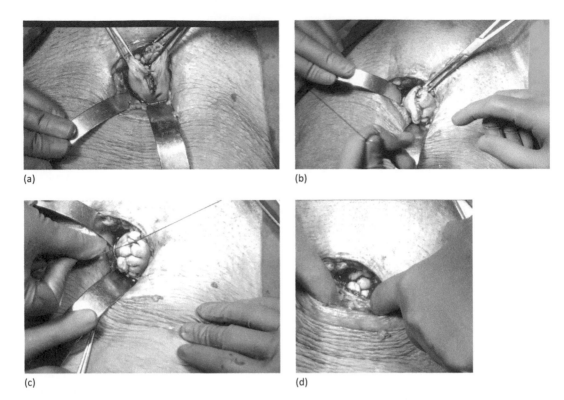

(a)

(b)

(c)

(d)

Figure 8.8 (a) Beginning of reconstruction form the caudal end of hysterotomy incision. (b) Rolling and exposing the uterine defect from caudal to cephalic end of the incision. (c) Completing the reconstruction in the whole length of hysterotomy incision. (d) View at the end of complete uterine reconstruction intracorporeally.

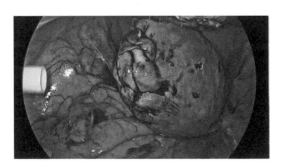

Figure 8.9 Final appearance of uterus on laparoscopic view after uterine reconstruction.

intracoporeally. Wu et al. describe a modified laparoscopic myomectomy technique that involved the insertion of two fingers into the vagina to elevate the uterus while one or two fingers of the other hand were inserted into the abdomen through a suprapubic incision to palpate for small fibroids, which did not distort the uterine contour [5]. This reduced the incidence of residual fibroids [5]. Some authors use the GelPort

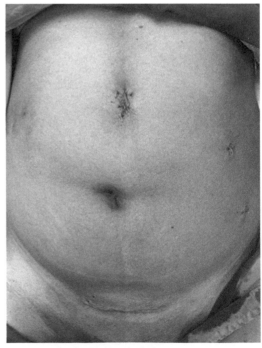

Figure 8.10 Final appearance of the ports after laparoscopic-assisted myomectomy.

TABLE 8.1: Data of last 50 cases that underwent laparoscopic-assisted myomectomy at Apollo Hospitals, Hyderabad, India

Clinical parameters	Average
Age, years	31.96
Body mass index	24.31
Median Clinical size of uterus, weeks	18.8
Median number of fibroids removed	2.38
Median volume of fibroids removed	895.37 cm³
Hemoglobin drop	2.27 gm/dL
Length of stay	2.52 days

Laparoscopic system for doing similar hand-assisted myomectomy.

We share the unpublished data from our unit at Apollo Hospitals of the last 50 cases that underwent laparoscopic-assisted myomectomy. Table 8.1 gives details of the various parameters of these 50 cases. The reason for choosing this method over laparoscopic myomectomy was large fibroid volume and to keep the operating time to less than 3 hours in these cases.

ADVANTAGES OF THIS APPROACH

1. It is a feasible and quick method of myomectomy for large and multiple fibroids.

2. Morcellation by knife can be achieved safely and swiftly by this method.

3. Uterine reconstruction is carried out in multiple layers with the aid of open surgical instruments. Suturing is simple and easy.

4. Recovery is similar to that of total laparoscopic myomectomy.

5. The approach avoids open myomectomy even in patients with large and multiple fibroids.

REFERENCES

1. Pelosi MA, Pelosi MA 3rd. Hand-assisted laparoscopy for complex hysterectomy. *J Am Assoc Gynecol Laparosc.* 1999;6(2):183–188.

2. Nezhat C, Nezhat F, Bess O, Nezhat CH, Mashiach R. Laparoscopically assisted myomectomy: a report of a new technique in 57 cases. *Int J Fertil Menopausal Stud.* 1994;39(1):39–44.

3. Smith CG, Davenport DL, Hoffman MR. Characteristics associated with prolonged length of stay after myomectomy for uterine myomas. *J Minim Invasive Gynecol.* 2019;26(7):1303–1310.

4. Pelosi MA, Pelosi MA 3rd, Eim J. Hand-assisted laparoscopy for megamyomectomy. A case report. *J Reprod Med.* 2000;45(6):519–525.

5. Wu J, Zhang Z-F, Xie Y-L, Jiang P-C, Chen L-P, Shi R-X. A novel modification of conventional laparoscopic myomectomy using manual assistance for multiple uterine myomas. *Eur J Obstet Gynecol Reprod Biol.* 2012;164(1):74–78.

9 Robot-Assisted Myomectomy

Arnold P. Advincula and Chetna Arora

CONTENTS

INTRODUCTION

Uterine leiomyomas are very common, occurring in up to 80% of reproductive-age women [1]. Over 50% of women with uterine leiomyomas are symptomatic, and the majority present with abnormal uterine bleeding, bulk symptoms from mass effect on surrounding structures, pelvic pain, recurrent pregnancy loss, and even infertility [2–4]. As a result, they are the single most common indication for hysterectomy and the source of a significant public health burden [2, 4].

Management of uterine leiomyomas can be organized into four different buckets: expectant, medical, interventional, and surgical. For those who remain asymptomatic, expectant management is advised as the risk of malignancy is low [5]. If the patient is symptomatic and an intervention is desired, the route of therapy should be individualized to the patient's age, symptom profile, and goals of treatment (i.e., fertility) in addition to regard for the size and location of the leiomyoma burden.

If medical therapy is desired, multiple options are available, both hormonal and nonhormonal. Ranges of medical treatment include nonsteroidal anti-inflammatory drugs, tranexamic acid, combined estrogen–progestin regimens, progestin-only methods, gonadotropin-releasing hormone agonists, and selective receptor modulators. Often, if the presenting complaints are primarily due to heavy menstrual bleeding, dysmenorrhea, or even pelvic pain, use of these interventions provides significant improvement [3, 6].

Alternatively, if the presenting complaint is due to bulk symptoms such as pelvic pressure, alterations in bowel or urinary function, recurrent pregnancy loss, infertility, or failed medical management, interventional or surgical therapy may be considered. If the intervention is tailored to the patient's clinical characteristics, several routes of therapy that include uterine artery embolization, magnetic resonance–guided high-intensity focused ultrasound, ultrasound-guided radiofrequency ablation, myomectomy, and hysterectomy can be considered [6, 7].

In this chapter, we will discuss the surgical approach to uterine leiomyomas via a robot-assisted laparoscopic myomectomy with the da Vinci Surgical System (Intuitive Surgical, Sunnyvale, CA, USA) in addition to current techniques in contained manual cold-knife tissue extraction.

ROBOT-ASSISTED LAPAROSCOPIC MYOMECTOMY

Several surgical approaches to a myomectomy include conventional laparoscopy, robot-assisted laparoscopy, operative hysteroscopy, and the traditional abdominal incision. Operative hysteroscopy is the gold-standard or preferred approach for submucosal leiomyomas under 3 cm with more than 50% intracavitary component (FIGO [International Federation of Gynecology and Obstetrics] 0 or 1 classification) [8]. Route is typically chosen on the basis of several factors such as (1) number of leiomyomas, (2) size of leiomyomas, (3) location of leiomyomas, (4) indication for surgery, (5) patient comorbidities, (6) patient preference, and importantly (7) surgical skill level. In patients desiring fertility preservation or simply a uterine-sparing procedure, myomectomy is the principal intervention [9]. In this chapter, we will focus on the robot-assisted laparoscopic route.

There are many benefits to a robotic-assisted laparoscopic approach compared with the alternative routes, including conventional laparoscopy. If the minimally invasive route is deemed feasible, robotic assistance is often chosen for more complex myomectomies because of the improved ergonomics, wristed instruments for more defined dissections, capacity for rapid suturing, and lack of need for an experienced assistant [10–14]. Benefits also include decreased blood loss, reduced postoperative pain, shorter recovery time, shorter hospital stay, and decreased perioperative complications [11–14]. Minimally invasive myomectomies is considered more technically challenging include those with multiple leiomyomas (due to multiple hysterotomy incisions requiring suturing), and difficult locations (i.e., posterior, cervical, and broad ligament) and those of a large size and depth that often are proximal to the endometrial cavity and require multiple layers of closure. No randomized controlled trials have directly compared conventional laparoscopy with the robotic approach, but in a large retrospective study of 575 patients, Barakat et al. demonstrated that the robotic approach was associated with a greater number of leiomyomas removed (compared with abdominal and laparoscopic routes) and a higher fibroid weight (compared with laparoscopy) [13]. The minimally invasive method should be considered first-line for patients unless the presence of an intramural myoma exceeds 10–12 cm or there are multiple leiomyomas (consensus at least four) that require several incisions based on varying locations within the uterus [15, 16]. While this is a recommendation, successful robotic approaches to extensive or large leiomyomas have been published, proving that experienced surgeons can safely perform this type of procedure despite the aforementioned recommendations [17–20].

KEY SURGICAL STEPS

The first, and arguably most critical, step to a robotic-assisted myomectomy is careful trocar placement individualized to the patient's pathology and abdominal topography. This should be governed by surgical history, clinical examination of leiomyoma burden, preoperative imaging, and surgeon's preference to optimize access [21]. These principles are applicable regardless of whether a Si or Xi da Vinci Surgical System is utilized. For patients with a surgically naïve abdomen and small leiomyoma(s), entry via the umbilicus is appropriate. With an intent to right-side-dock the robot, we first insufflate the abdomen with a Veress needle without an incision at the umbilicus and then place our 5/8-mm assistant port (the AirSeal device at our institution) in the right upper quadrant in the mid-clavicular line under direct visualization.

After the abdominal survey, we place the patient in a steep Trendelenburg position, observe the pathology, and place two lateral 8-mm telerobotic trocars parallel to the umbilicus on the right and left at the natural curvature of the abdomen where the rectus

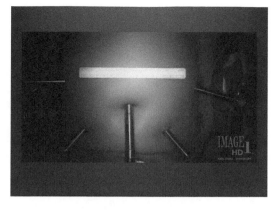

Figure 9.1 Trocar placement during robot-assisted laparoscopic myomectomy.

abdominis muscle tapers off. A third 8-mm telerobotic trocar is placed just to the left or right of the umbilical trocar site depending on which side the robot will be docked in order to incorporate the third operative arm (typically this is right-sided trocar placement given our preference for right-side docking). We then place a 12-mm trocar in the umbilicus for the scope since this will ultimately serve as the tissue extraction site (Figure 9.1). Rarely is a supraumbilical port necessary unless pathology is more than 20 weeks, significant adhesions are encountered, or the patient is markedly obese [22].

Another vital step when performing a robotic-assisted myomectomy is the use of a uterine manipulator. Leiomyomas can be difficult to remove if the location, such as the posterior fundus, precludes visualization or access. This becomes even more challenging when they compress surrounding structures such as the rectum or the pelvic side wall. Thus, there are multiple advantages to uterine manipulators. They improve visualization and exposure, provide traction–countertraction by means of an extra (or "fifth") arm, and push the pathology away from vital pelvic structures such as the ureters, major vasculature, and bowel [23–25]. In addition, inherent to the robotic approach is the increased autonomy gained; thus, this route can be further enhanced by the use of a static and hydraulic uterine manipulator, the ALLY Uterine Positioning System (Cooper Surgical, Trumball, CT, USA) (Figure 9.2a,b).

With the uterus now optimally visualized with the aid of a uterine manipulator, the leiomyomas are surveyed and subsequently enucleated. Careful surgical planning—for instance, with the aid of preoperative magnetic

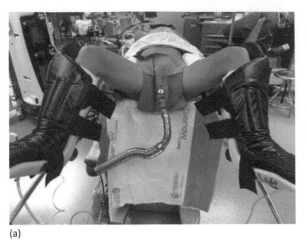
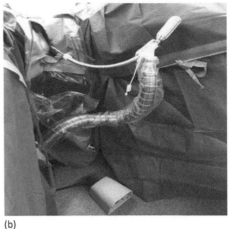

(a)   (b)

Figure 9.2   (a) Ally uterine positioning system mounted on operating room table prior to draping (Cooper Surgical, Trumball, CT, USA). (b) Ally uterine positioning system fully draped and holding advincula arch uterine manipulator with RUMI tip prior to placement in uterus (Cooper Surgical).

resonance imaging for mapping and also first tactfully addressing the bulkier leiomyomas— allows for a more systematic approach [21, 26] (Figure 9.3).

Before a strategic uterine incision is made, blood loss can be further minimized and

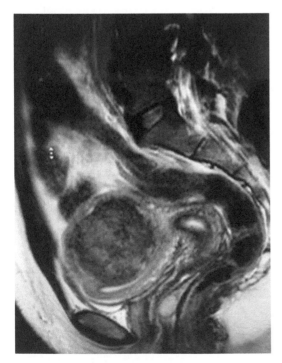

Figure 9.3   Pelvic magnetic resonance imaging T2-weighted sagittal view of posterior transmural fibroid.

visualization of the dissection planes optimized by injecting the leiomyoma with a dilute concentration of vasopressin directly into the pseudocapsule via a spinal needle traversing the abdominal wall [27–29]. Other options or synergistic ways of decreasing blood loss include the use of intravaginal prostaglandins, intravenous tranexamic acid, loop ligation of the myoma pseudocapsule, pericervical tourniquets, temporary or permanent occlusion of the bilateral uterine arteries, and oxytocin infusions in addition to the use of gelatin–thrombin matrices or cell salvage systems. The majority of these methods have been studied in open myomectomies with successful application in the laparoscopic realm [27, 30].

Once the desired hemostatic approach has been employed, the surgeon must thoughtfully dissect out the intramural leiomyoma by first incising the serosa and myometrium to the level of the pseudocapsule in one plane. Transverse incisions allow the surgeon to ergonomically close the hysterotomy, but awareness of the proximity to the uterine vessels is essential. Another benefit of robotics is the capacity to more feasibly adapt to the creation and subsequent rapid closure of oblique or vertical incisions where necessary. The instruments used to complete the enucleation are largely surgeon preference but can be accomplished with a variety of robotic devices such as the monopolar scissors and bipolar forceps [11, 20, 21]. Another significant advantage of the robotic technology is the use of the robotic tenaculum. When this is placed in the fourth arm, static and consistent tension can be more

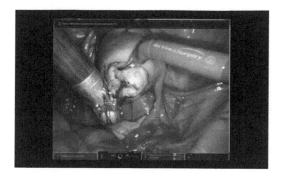

Figure 9.4 Endowrist tenaculum enucleating posterior intramural fibroid.

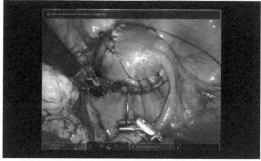

Figure 9.5 Barbed suture repair of hysterotomy defect.

fluidly applied while maintaining the ability to dissect and retract for oneself. Alternatively, this can be provided with a bedside assist using either a standard laparoscopic tenaculum or a corkscrew [21]. As with all routes, careful attention to the dissection planes allows the leiomyomas to be circumferentially enucleated and dissected from their fibrous attachments to the surrounding myometrium. When the number of incisions is intentionally minimized, blood loss is reduced from exposed myometrium, less serosa is disrupted (thus decreasing the formation of adhesions), and the overall integrity of the uterus can be maintained [21, 30] (Figure 9.4.).

The leiomyomas are then placed aside within the pelvis or strung onto a barbed suture to avoid loss within the abdomen while the uterine incisions are closed. Closure is mirrored from the traditional open technique as the same surgical principles apply. The hysterotomies are then rapidly sutured from the inside-out, and often a two- or three-layer closure is performed if the endometrium is not disturbed [31]. If there is concern for a breach in the endometrium, methylene blue can be injected directly into the uterine manipulator. If a defect in the endometrium is present, the methylene blue that distends the uterine cavity extrudes within the abdomen. Closure of this space can be carried out with a separate suture layer. As the majority of the blood loss is from disruption of the myometrium and uterine sinuses, hemostasis is obtained by swift closure with suture and occasional (but sparing) use of diathermy. The goal should be minimal use of energy in an effort to decrease myometrial necrosis and thus possible obstetric sequelae such as uterine rupture [32, 33]. The uterine incisions can be closed with either barbed or nonbarbed delayed absorbable monofilament sutures. The barbed suture contains small helically arranged hooks that grasp the tissue and

maintain tension. Barbed suture is the preference at our institution given that it allows a significantly shorter operating time and lower estimated blood loss and eliminates the need for surgical knots [34, 35]. Once the myometrial defect has been repaired, the serosa should already be largely approximated so that closure is off-tension and hemostatic. Closure of this layer eliminates raw tissue exposure, and imbrication techniques bury the suture, thus lessening possible foreign body reactions and adhesions [32] (Figure 9.5).

MORCELLATION/TISSUE EXTRACTION

Lastly, the leiomyomas are removed from the abdomen via the umbilicus without marked extension of the fascia or skin, thus maintaining a minimally invasive approach. Although the minimally invasive route has been proven to be associated with a lower mortality, fewer perioperative complications, quicker recovery, improved cosmesis, and an overall enhanced quality of life, tissue extraction of large leiomyomas can be difficult [36–38]. In April 2014, when the US Food and Drug Administration (FDA) issued a strong warning contraindicating the use of the power morcellator because of the fear of occult dissemination of an undiagnosed leioymyosarcoma, challenges in safe and efficient tissue extraction were created [39]. While the spreading of malignant cells is concerning, otherwise nonmalignant but sinister pathologies such as endometriosis or leiomyomatosis can occur from intraoperative dispersal as well. In addition, the device itself, though resulting in rapid removal of tissue, had complications of uncontained use, including damage to surrounding structures from the motorized blade in addition to the scattering of benign or malignant cells [40–42]. In the United States, both the American College of Obstetricians and Gynecologists and the American Association of Gynecologic Laparoscopists have taken heed to the FDA warning and have since made statements qualifying the use of the power morcellator in selected patients after thorough informed consent and consideration for preoperative endometrial cavity evaluation by means of either direct sampling or imaging [39]. Nonetheless, contained and manual methods for tissue extraction have been developed to allow for safe and continued minimally invasive approaches to myomectomy.

Several routes for tissue extraction have been successfully performed. When a posterior colpotomy is created, morcellation can be avoided entirely. Another option includes the extension of a trocar incision to a minilaparotomy and subsequent removal of smaller leiomyomas en bloc or with minimal and confined manual morcellation within an endoscopic bag. Although larger specimens prove to be more difficult, the option of contained in-bag hand morcellation improves the safety profile but also potentially increases operative time [43–45].

At our institution, we developed a reproducible technique to simply extract even the largest leiomyomas from the laparoscopic incisions carefully and efficiently. This published technique is called extracorporeal C-incision tissue extraction (or the ExCITE technique). It replicates the cutting principles of a power morcellator, but it is manual and contained within an endoscopic specimen bag [46].

The ExCITE technique has five key steps:

1. Specimen retrieval and containment

2. Self-retaining retractor placement

3. Creation of the C-incision

4. Tissue extraction

5. Fascial closure

In step 1 of the ExCITE technique, the myomas are placed within an endoscopic specimen retrieval bag. The incision at the level of the umbilicus (or the largest incision used during trocar placement) is extended approximately 2.5–3.5 cm. The bag's edges are then exteriorized and held in place.

Step 2 of the technique involves the placement of a self-retaining retractor within the bag. This placement not only allows for a wider exposure during tissue extraction but also holds the endoscopic specimen bag open and in place. Both the inner and outer rings should be fully deployed. Because an airtight seal is created at the extraction site, pneumoperitoneum can be maintained if desired, thereby elevating the contained specimen from critical structures such as the bowel.

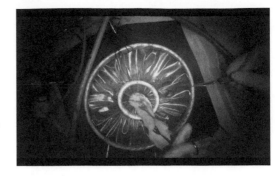

Figure 9.6 Extracorporeal C-incision tissue extraction (ExCITE) technique depicted.

Step 3 is the creation of the C-incision. First, grasp the specimen with a type of penetrating clamp (Lahey or single-tooth tenaculum unless the specimen is calcified or friable). With a #11 scalpel blade, a reverse C-incision is created with the clamp, providing upward traction in the nondominant hand and the scalpel, starting the incision from the nondominant side toward the dominant side. When the incisions are made wide, a specimen strip that can be efficiently removed will be created. A reciprocating sawing motion is preferred over single sweeping motions.

Step 4 is tissue extraction. With the basics of surgical traction–countertraction in mind, the strip of specimen being created is regrasped near the base with the penetrating clamp, allowing for the maintenance of tension. As the reciprocating sawing motions are continued, the tissue should progressively lengthen into one completely intact strip—similar to what one would see with a power morcellator (Figure 9.6).

Step 5 is standard fascial closure. The specimen bag, with the self-retaining retractor within it, is removed without contaminating the abdomen with either microscopic cells or gross tissue fragments.

CONCLUSION

Robotic-assisted laparoscopic myomectomy should be considered for the management of complex leiomyomas. This procedure is associated with proven success, even with large or multiple leiomyomas, especially when performed by experts in the field of minimally invasive gynecologic surgery. Regardless of the limitations sanctioned by the FDA's position on the power morcellator, many safe and efficient tissue extraction techniques have been developed that allow surgeons to continue to provide this route of surgery to the appropriate patients.

REFERENCES

1. Baird DD, Saldana TM, Shore DL, Hill MC, Schectman JM. A single baseline ultrasound assessment of fibroid presence and size is strongly predictive of future uterine procedure: 8-year follow-up of randomly sampled premenopausal women aged 35–49 years. *Hum Reprod.* 2015;30:2936–2944.

2. Stewart EA. Clinical practice. Uterine fibroids. *N Eng J Med.* 2015;372:1646–1655.

3. Haney AF. Clinical decision making regarding leiomyomata: what we need in the next millenium. *Environ Health Perspect.* 2000;108 Suppl 5:835–839.

4. Stewart EA, Laughlin-Tommaso SK, Catherino WH, Lalitkumar S, Gupta D, Vollenhoven B. Uterine fibroids. *Nat Rev Dis Primers.* 2016;2:16043.

5. Schwartz PE, Kelly MG. Malignant transformation of leiomyomas: myth or reality? *Obstet Gynecol Clin North Am.* 2006;33:183–198, xii.

6. De La Cruz MS, Buchanan EM. Uterine fibroids: diagnosis and treatment. *Am Fam Phys.* 2017;95:100–107.

7. Silberzweig JE, Powell DK, Matsumoto AH, Spies JB. Management of uterine fibroids: a focus on uterine-sparing interventional techniques. *Radiology.* 2016;280:675–692.

8. Munro MG, Critchley HO, Broder MS, Fraser IS. FIGO classification system (PALM-COEIN) for causes of abnormal uterine bleeding in nongravid women of reproductive age. *Int J Gynaecol Obstet.* 2011;113:3–13.

9. Flake GP, Andersen J, Dixon D. Etiology and pathogenesis of uterine leioleiomyomas: a review. *Environ Health Perspect.* 2003;111:1037–1054.

10. Kim S, Luu TH, Llarena N, Falcone T. Role of robotic surgery in treating fibroids and benign uterine mass. *Best Pract Res Clin Obstet Gynaecol.* 2017;45:48–59.

11. Gingold JA, Gueye NA, Falcone T. Minimally invasive approaches to myoma management. *J Minim Invasive Gynecol.* 2018;25:237–250.

12. Glaser LM, Friedman J, Tsai S, Chaudhari A, Milad M. Laparoscopic myomectomy and morcellation: a review of techniques, outcomes, and practice guidelines. *Best Pract Res Clin Obstet Gynaecol.* 2018;46:99–112.

13. Barakat EE, Bedaiwy MA, Zimberg S, Nutter B, Nosseir M, Falcone T. Robotic-assisted, laparoscopic, and abdominal myomectomy: a comparison of surgical outcomes. *Obstet Gynecol.* 2011;117:256–265.

14. Sinha R, Sanjay M, Rupa B, Kumari S. Robotic surgery in gynecology. *J Minim Access Surg.* 2015;11:50–59.

15. Donnez J, Dolmans MM. Uterine fibroid management: from the present to the future. *Human Reprod Update.* 2016;22:665–686.

16. Holub Z. [Laparoscopic myomectomy: indications and limits]. *Ceska Gynekologie.* 2007;72:64–68.

17. Moon HS, Jeong K, Lee SR. Robotic-assisted single incision myomectomy in large myoma cases. *Clin Exp Obstet Gynecol.* 2017;44:283–287.

18. Javadian P, Juusela A, Nezhat F. Robotic-assisted laparoscopic cervicovaginal myomectomy. *J Minim Invasive Gynecol.* 2018;26(1):31.

19. Kim H, Shim S, Hwang Y, et al. Is robotic-assisted laparoscopic myomectomy limited in multiple leiomyomas? a feasibility for ten or more leiomyomas. *Obstet Gynecol Sci.* 2018;61:135–141.

20. Gunnala V, Setton R, Pereira N, Huang JQ. Robotic-assisted myomectomy for large uterine leiomyomas: a single center experience. *Minim Invasive Surg.* 2016;2016:4905292.

21. Senapati S, Advincula AP. Surgical techniques: robotic-assisted laparoscopic myomectomy with the da Vinci surgical system. *J Robot Surg.* 2007;1:69–74.

22. Lambrou N, Diaz RE, Hinoul P, et al. Strategies to optimize the performance of robotic-assisted laparoscopic hysterectomy. *Facts Views Vis Obgyn.* 2014;6:133–142.

23. van den Haak L, Alleblas C, Nieboer TE, Rhemrev JP, Jansen FW. Efficacy and safety of uterine manipulators in laparoscopic surgery: a review. *Arch Gynecol Obstet.* 2015;292:1003–1011.

24. Janssen PF, Brolmann HA, Huirne JA. Causes and prevention of laparoscopic ureter injuries: an analysis of 31 cases during laparoscopic hysterectomy in the Netherlands. *Surg Endosc.* 2013;27:946–956.

25. Agdi M, Tulandi T. The benefits of intrauterine balloon: an intrauterine manipulator and balloon proved useful in myomectomy. Am J Obstet Gynecol. 2008;199:581.e1.

26. Laughlin-Tommaso SK, Stewart EA. Moving toward individualized medicine for uterine leioleiomyomas. *Obstet Gynecol.* 2018;132:961–971.

27. Hickman LC, Kotlyar A, Shue S, Falcone T. Hemostatic techniques for myomectomy: an evidence-based approach. *J Minim Invasive Gynecol.* 2016;23:497–504.

28. Lin XN, Zhang SY, Fang SH, Wang MZ, Lou HY. [Assessment of different homeostatic methods used in laparoscopic intramural myomectomy]. *Zhonghua yi xue za zhi.* 2008;88:905–908.

29. Cohen SL, Wang KC, Gargiulo AR, et al. Vasopressin administration during laparoscopic myomectomy: a randomized controlled trial. *J Minim Invasive Gynecol.* 2015;22:S39.

30. Gingold JA, Gueye NA, Falcone T. Minimally invasive approaches to myoma management. *J Minim Invasive Gynecol.* 2017.

31. Guarnaccia MM, Rein MS. Traditional surgical approaches to uterine fibroids: abdominal myomectomy and hysterectomy. *Clin Obstet Gynecol.* 2001;44:385–400.

32. Kim HS, Oh SY, Choi SJ, et al. Uterine rupture in pregnancies following myomectomy: A multicenter case series. *Obstet Gynecol Sci.* 2016;59:454–462.

33. Pistofidis G, Makrakis E, Balinakos P, Dimitriou E, Bardis N, Anaf V. Report of 7 uterine rupture cases after laparoscopic myomectomy: update of the literature. *J Minim Invasive Gynecol.* 2012;19:762–767.

34. Alessandri F, Remorgida V, Venturini PL, Ferrero S. Unidirectional barbed suture versus continuous suture with intracorporeal knots in laparoscopic myomectomy: a randomized study. *J Minim Invasive Gynecol.* 2010;17:725–729.

35. Tulandi T, Einarsson JI. The use of barbed suture for laparoscopic hysterectomy and myomectomy: a systematic review and meta-analysis. *J Minim Invasive Gynecol.* 2014;21:210–216.

36. Wright KN, Jonsdottir GM, Jorgensen S, Shah N, Einarsson JI. Costs and outcomes of abdominal, vaginal, laparoscopic and robotic hysterectomies. *JSLS.* 2012;16:519–524.

37. Stoica RA, Bistriceanu I, Sima R, Iordache N. Laparoscopic myomectomy. *J Med Life.* 2014;7:522–524.

38. Stentz NC, Cooney LG, Sammel M, Shah DK. Changes in myomectomy practice after the U.S. food and drug administration safety communication on power morcellation. *Obstet Gynecol.* 2017;129:1007–1013.

39. AAGL practice report: Morcellation during uterine tissue extraction. *J Minim Invasive Gynecol.* 2014;21:517–530.

40. Milad MP, Milad EA. Laparoscopic morcellator-related complications. *J Minim Invasive Gynecol.* 2014;21:486–491.

41. Milad MP, Sokol E. Laparoscopic morcellator-related injuries. *J Am Assoc Gynecol Laparosc.* 2003;10:383–385.

42. Wright JD, Tergas AI, Cui R, et al. Use of electric power morcellation and prevalence of underlying cancer in women who undergo myomectomy. *JAMA Oncol.* 2015;1:69–77.

43. Meurs E, Brito LG, Ajao MO, et al. Comparison of morcellation techniques at the time of laparoscopic hysterectomy and myomectomy. *J Minim Invasive Gynecol.* 2017;24:843–849.

44. Ghezzi F, Casarin J, De Francesco G, et al. Transvaginal contained tissue extraction after laparoscopic myomectomy: a cohort study. *BJOG.* 2017.

45. Frasca C, Degli Esposti E, Arena A, et al. Can in-bag manual morcellation represent an alternative to uncontained power morcellation in laparoscopic myomectomy? A randomized controlled rrial. *Gynecol Obstet Invest.* 2018;83:52–56.

46. Truong MD, Advincula AP. The extracorporeal C-incision tissue extraction (ExCITE) technique. *OBG Manag.* 2014;26(11):56.

10 Robotic Myomectomy

Tips and Tricks

Cela Vito, Braganti Francesca, and Malacarne Elisa

CONTENTS

Uterine myomas are the most common type of pelvic tumor in women; the lifetime risk is about 70–80% [1–3]. They arise in reproductive-age women and are asymptomatic in about 25% of cases [4]. Symptoms are related to their size and location and are represented by abnormal uterine bleeding or compression symptoms (abdominal pressure or pain and urinary or bowel symptoms) [5]. Uterine leiomyomas can also have a negative impact on fertility and be associated with obstetric adverse outcomes [6].

Conservative myomectomy represents a valid therapeutic choice in case of symptomatic myomas in women who wish to preserve the uterus and fertility [7]. Myomectomy can be performed by minimally invasive surgery, which offers several advantages compared with the open technique, including decreased postoperative pain and morbidity and shorter hospital stay [8–10]. However, the correct application of laparoscopic myomectomy is limited by the characteristic of the myomas and the surgical expertise, especially for laparoscopic suturing or when the myomas have an unfavorable location [11, 12].

For many years now, robotic-assisted laparoscopic myomectomy has been considered a safe and effective technique, especially for the removal of unfavorably located or even large myomas, because of increased technical difficulty compared with the laparoscopic procedure [13–17].

The most widely used robotic system is the da Vinci System. Since the 2005 approval of the US Food and Drug Administration (FDA) for gynecological surgery, the use of the da Vinci System (da Vinci Si and the most innovative system, da Vinci Xi) has become increasingly widespread thanks to its many advantages, like the comfortable working position for the surgeon, the more flexible movements made possible by 7° laparoscopic instruments, the use of three or four robotic arms, the three-dimensional optic, and the tremor filtering [18–20].

Numerous studies have compared the robotic technique with traditional laparoscopic myomectomy and open myomectomy. Even though no randomized trials are available, several retrospective and prospective studies demonstrated similar short-term outcomes [21, 22], a lower rate of postoperative complications, less blood loss, and a shorter hospital stay [23, 24] but longer surgical time [15].

These results must be interpreted with caution because of the heterogeneity of the disease: the use and the consequent outcomes of one technique over another can depend on many factors, such as size, localization, and number of myomas, and often the robotic approach was preferred in more complex cases [23, 24].

Determining whether a woman is a candidate for minimally invasive myomectomy depends upon the location, size, and number of leiomyomas. It is suitable for FIGO (International Federation of Gynecology and Obstetrics) type 3–7 leiomyomas and for hybrid leiomyomas [25].

Several authors have tried to outline parameters that limit the feasibility, safety, and success of the minimally invasive technique, but there are no standardized and universally accepted criteria. Although the number (fewer than four myomas) and the size (smaller than 12 cm) have been proposed as cutoffs, the safety and feasibility of the intervention are influenced mainly by the surgeon's expertise [26, 27].

Important factors regarding the locations of these tumors include the penetration into the myometrium and the location in relation to important structures; women with uterine fibroids located in anatomically challenging locations, such as the cervix or near uterine blood vessels, may be considered as appropriate candidates for robotic myomectomy. Furthermore, the lack of tactile feedback makes the removal of myomas with a submucosal component and the subsequent closure of the cavity more difficult; therefore, patients with intracavitary fibroids should not undergo robotic surgery [28, 29].

PATIENT AND TROCAR POSITIONING

The patient is positioned on the operating table in a low dorsal lithotomy position with the legs

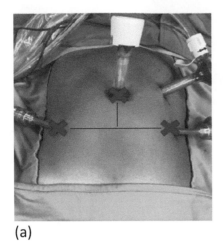
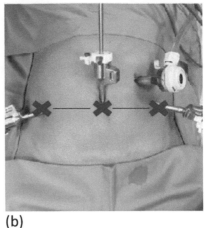

(a)   (b)

Figure 10.1 Trocar placement in robotic myomectomy with different robotic systems. (a) da Vinci Si Surgical System. (b) da Vinci Xi Surgical System.

supported by stirrups and the arms along the side of the body. The patient must be securely positioned on the operating table with the use of anti-skid material. The most used are underbody foam "egg crate" mattresses. Correct positioning of the body is essential to prevent nerve injuries and to improve surgery [30].

After general endotracheal anesthesia is induced, a vaginal examination is performed to evaluate uterus size, position, and mobility. A Foley catheter is then inserted into the bladder. A uterine manipulator is inserted into the uterus to improve the exposure of the myomas and their removal and to allow the instilling of dye to identify the opening of the endometrial cavity.

Pneumoperitoneum is established and can be achieved with a Veress needle in the umbilical area after the elevation of the anterior abdominal wall. Alternatively, an open technique (Hasson technique) for entering the abdomen under direct vision may be used if we suspect periumbilical adhesions or umbilical hernia [31].

When da Vinci Si is used, the surgical cart can be positioned between the patient's leg (central docking) or at 45° to the patient's leg stirrup (side docking). Side docking allows access to the vagina and perineum for the second assistant. When da Vinci Xi is used, the surgical cart is located lateral to the patient's bed and provides the surgeon with anatomical access from virtually any position, simplifying multiquadrant surgeries.

The multiport technique is the standard surgical approach, although myomectomy can be performed using a single-site approach.

For robotic myomectomy, four incisions are typically made:

- 12-mm (for da Vinci Si) or 8-mm (for da Vinci Xi) midline laparoscopic port for the optic. This can be at Umbilicus or supra umbilicus site depending on the size of the fibroid and the uterus, (at least 8–10 cm superior to the uterine fundus)

- 8-mm lateral abdominal-robotic port, two ports placed 8–10 cm lateral (left and right side) to the laparoscopic port, 1.5–2 cm below it for Si, or at the same level for Xi; if a fourth arm is used, it is placed 8–10 cm lateral to the previous one (either on the left or the right side, depending on the surgeon's needs) (Figure 10.1)

- 5- or 12-mm lateral upper abdominal-conventional accessory port (left or right side) for first assistant laparoscopic instruments.

The second assistant is located between the patient's legs to mobilize the uterus by using the uterine manipulator.

The patient is placed in the Trendelenburg position to increase the exposure of the operating field. Advanced smoke extraction systems can be used; allowing the surgeon to work with constant lower intra-abdominal pressures (<10 mm Hg) without compromising the exposure of the operating field.

SURGICAL TECHNIQUE

Perioperative hemorrhage is the main risk associated with conservative myomectomy. Bleeding can be prevented or decreased using several techniques based on two main principles: reduction of uterine blood flow (use of cervical "tourniquet," uterine artery ligation, or preoperative embolization) or use of uterotonic or vasoconstrictive agents (oxytocin, misoprostol or sulprostone, intramyometrial vasopressin, or epinephrine injection) [25]. Allogeneic blood transfusion can be avoided by using methods of intraoperative blood salvage and autologous blood transfusion.

Several therapies have been developed for the medical treatment of uterine fibroids, both as exclusive therapy and as preoperative ones. The potential benefits of preoperative medical treatment are to correct anemia before surgery and to decrease intraoperative blood loss and the possibility of reducing fibroid size. However, these agents could make removal of myomas more difficult and may increase the risk of persistent myomas [32]. The most used drugs are combined hormonal contraceptive, progestational agents, gonadotropin-releasing hormone agonists, and selective progesterone receptor modulators (ulipristal acetate) [25, 32, 33]. Athough, with increasing concerns regarding the safety of Ulipristal acetate, it is not recommended to be used for fibroid management.

Preoperative imaging with pelvic ultrasound or magnetic resonance imaging is essential to assess characteristics and location of the myomas.

For intramural myomas, a transverse myometrial incision, rather than a vertical incision, allows more ergonomic laparoscopic suturing of the uterine defect. A more oblique angle is useful for suturing anteriorly located leiomyomas [25].

The incision is made directly over the myoma and carried deeply until definite myoma tissue and the avascular plane just deep to the capsule of the myoma are noted. Before the hysterotomy, it is essential identify anatomical landmarks

such as ovaries, uterine vessels, or fallopian tubes to avoid any damage to them [29].

The removal of pedunculated and sessile subserosal leiomyomas is easier and requires only effective coagulation of the pedicle or of the base of the leiomyoma without requiring suturing of the uterine serosa in most cases.

A monopolar current with low intensity or an ultrasonic device should be preferred for the hysterotomy to limit necrosis, especially in women with a desire for future pregnancy. The enucleation of leiomyomas requires the use of grasping forceps to perform a good traction. This steady traction can be carried out with a robotic tenaculum or, failing that, with laparoscopic tenaculum forceps through the accessory port.

Hemostasis can be achieved though the use of bipolar coagulation forceps but without making excessive use of it so as to to limit necrosis and the subsequent risk of suture dehiscence. A good hemostasis indeed is due to not only tissues coagulation but also to a correct suturing.

Preservation of the endometrial cavity is essential, especially in women who desire pregnancy. Chromopertubation with methylene blue can be used to confirm the integrity of the endometrial cavity after myomectomy [25, 29].

The closure of uterine defects can be performed with absorbable sutures in one, two, or (rarely) three layers, depending on the depth of the myometrial defect. The surgeon can decide to carry out continuous running or interrupted sutures on the basis of his or her preference and the characteristics of the hysterotomy (Figure 10.2). A caliber 0 mono- or

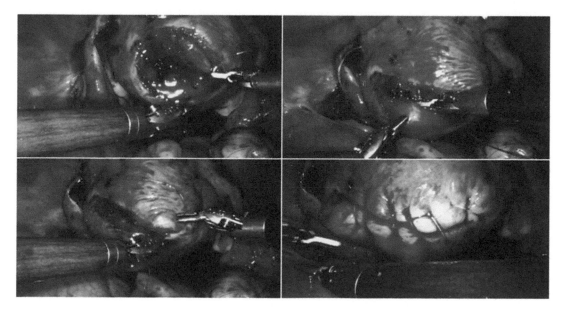

Figure 10.2 Photo sequence of a continuous two-layer suture.

multifilament suture is generally used for the myometrial closure, whereas the uterine serosa is preferentially closed with a caliber 2/0 monofilament suture [25]. If the endometrial cavity opens during the procedure, it must be sutured with a caliber 3/0 absorbable thread.

In recent years, the use of barbed suture has replaced conventional sutures as they allow reduced surgical times, intraoperative blood loss, and postoperative morbidity [34].

The security of the closure may impact the risk of uterine rupture in subsequent pregnancy. It has been shown that the robotic approach allows a greater number of layers than laparoscopic surgery and this could result in a better reconstruction of the uterus and consequently in better obstetric outcomes [35].

For large myomas that cannot be removed through the existing surgical ports, power morcellation is an option. In order to limit the dissemination of an occult malignant tissue, morcellation of myomas should take place within patented endobags, after the warning of the FDA in 2014. A protected in-bag power morcellation also limits the risk of visceral injury and parasitic leiomyomas [36].

If the surgeon does not want to use morcellation or if it is not available, he or she can enlarge the trocar incision or perform a minilaparotomy to remove myomas. Another option is their vaginal extraction by a posterior colpotomy if the vagina is easily accessible.

After the extraction of myomas, the robot can be undocked and moved away from the patient. The trocars are removed under direct visualization. Fascial closure is required for 12-mm port-site wounds. Skin closure is performed on the basis of the surgeon's preferences.

Conservative myomectomy is associated with a 1% increased risk of uterine rupture in subsequent pregnancy [37]. Women who undergo myomectomy with significant uterine disruption should wait several months before attempting to conceive; recommendations for the interval to conception range from 3 to 6 months [38]. The route of delivery during subsequent pregnancy depends on several factors: the perioperative conditions, the postoperative complications, the number of myomas removed, and the obstetric factors of the present pregnancy. Vaginal versus scheduled cesarean section involves shared decision making among the patient, the obstetrician, and the surgeon [25].

REFERENCES

1. Baird DD, Dunson DB, Hill MC, Cousins D, Schectman JM. High cumulative incidence of uterine leiomyoma in black and white women: ultrasound evidence. *Am J Obstet Gynecol.* 2003;188(1):100–107.

2. Buttram VC Jr., Reiter RC. Uterine leiomyomata: etiology, symptomatology, and management. *Fertil Steril.* 1981;36(4):433–445.

3. Serden SP, Brooks PG. Treatment of abnormal uterine bleeding with the gynecologic resectoscope. *J Reprod Med.* 1991;36(10):697–699.

4. Stewart, E.A., et al., Sustained relief of leiomyoma symptoms by using focused ultrasound surgery. *Obstet Gynecol*, 2007. 110(2 Pt 1):279–287.

5. Gupta, S., J. Jose, and I. Manyonda, Clinical presentation of fibroids. *Best Pract Res Clin Obstet Gynaecol*, 2008. 22(4):615–626.

6. Donnez, J. and P. Jadoul, What are the implications of myomas on fertility? *A need for a debate? Hum Reprod*, 2002. 17(6):1424–1430.

7. Palomba, S., et al., A multicenter randomized, controlled study comparing laparoscopic versus minilaparotomic myomectomy: reproductive outcomes. *Fertil Steril*, 2007. 88(4):933–941.

8. Jin, C., et al., Laparoscopic versus open myomectomy—a meta-analysis of randomized controlled trials. *Eur J Obstet Gynecol Reprod Biol*, 2009. 145(1):14–21.

9. Holzer, A., et al., Laparoscopic versus open myomectomy: a double-blind study to evaluate postoperative pain. *Anesth Analg*, 2006. 102(5):1480–1484.

10. Alessandri, F., et al., Randomized study of laparoscopic versus minilaparotomic myomectomy for uterine myomas. *J Minim Invasive Gynecol*, 2006. 13(2):92–97.

11. Parker, W.H. and I.A. Rodi, Patient selection for laparoscopic myomectomy. *J Am Assoc Gynecol Laparosc*, 1994. 2(1):23–26.

12. Liu, G., et al., The laparoscopic myomectomy: a survey of Canadian gynaecologists. *J Obstet Gynaecol Can*, 2010. 32(2): 139–148.

13. Advincula, A.P., et al., Robot-assisted laparoscopic myomectomy versus abdominal myomectomy: a comparison of short-term surgical outcomes and immediate costs. *J Minim Invasive Gynecol*, 2007. 14(6):698–705.

14. Advincula, A.P., et al., Preliminary experience with robot-assisted laparoscopic myomectomy. *J Am Assoc Gynecol Laparosc*, 2004. 11(4):511–518.

15. Nezhat, C., et al., Robotic-assisted laparoscopic myomectomy compared with standard laparoscopic myomectomy—a retrospective matched control study. *Fertil Steril*, 2009. 91(2):556–559.

16. Lonnerfors, C. and J. Persson, Robot-assisted laparoscopic myomectomy; a feasible technique for removal of unfavorably localized myomas. *Acta Obstet Gynecol Scand*, 2009. 88(9):994–9.

17. Gunnala, V., et al., Robot-assisted myomectomy for large uterine myomas: a single center experience. *Minim Invasive Surg*, 2016. 2016:4905292.

18. Advincula, A.P. and A. Song, The role of robotic surgery in gynecology. *Curr Opin Obstet Gynecol*, 2007. 19(4):331–336.

19. Advincula, A.P. and K. Wang, Evolving role and current state of robotics in minimally invasive gynecologic surgery. *J Minim Invasive Gynecol*, 2009. 16(3):291–301.

20. Shi, G., et al., WITHDRAWN: Robotic assisted surgery for gynaecological cancer. *Cochrane Database Syst Rev*, 2014(12):CD008640.

21. Bedient, C.E., et al., Comparison of robotic and laparoscopic myomectomy. *Am J Obstet Gynecol*, 2009. 201(6): 566 e1–5.

22. Gocmen, A., F. Sanlikan, and M.G. Ucar, Comparison of robotic-assisted laparoscopic myomectomy outcomes with laparoscopic myomectomy. *Arch Gynecol Obstet*, 2013. 287(1):91–96.

23. Barakat, E.E., et al., Robotic-assisted, laparoscopic, and abdominal myomectomy: a comparison of surgical outcomes. *Obstet Gynecol*, 2011. 117(2 Pt 1): 256–265.

24. Lonnerfors, C., Robot-assisted myomectomy. *Best Pract Res Clin Obstet Gynaecol*, 2018. 46:113–119.

25. Dubuisson, J., The current place of mini-invasive surgery in uterine leiomyoma management. *J Gynecol Obstet Hum Reprod*, 2019. 48(2):77–81.

26. Bean, E.M., et al., Laparoscopic myomectomy: a single-center retrospective review of 514 patients. *J Minim Invasive Gynecol*, 2017. 24(3):485–493.

27. Bhave Chittawar, P., et al., Minimally invasive surgical techniques versus open myomectomy for uterine fibroids. *Cochrane Database Syst Rev*, 2014(10):CD004638.

28. Dubuisson, J.B., et al., Laparoscopic myomectomy: predicting the risk of conversion to an open procedure. *Hum Reprod*, 2001. 16(8):1726–1731.

29. Arian, S.E., et al., Robot-assisted laparoscopic myomectomy: current status. *Robot Surg*, 2017. 4:7–18.

30. Barnett, J.C., et al., Laparoscopic positioning and nerve injuries. *J Minim Invasive Gynecol*, 2007. 14(5): 664–672; quiz 673.

31. Vilos, G.A., et al., No. 193-laparoscopic entry: a review of techniques, technologies, and complications. *J Obstet Gynaecol Can*, 2017. 39(7): e69–e84.

32. Ferrero, S., et al., Three-month treatment with uliprisal acetate prior to laparoscopic myomectomy of large uterine myomas: a retrospective study. *Eur J Obstet Gynecol Reprod Biol*, 2016. 205:43–47.

33. Lethaby, A., B. Vollenhoven, and M. Sowter, Pre-operative GnRH analogue therapy before hysterectomy or myomectomy for uterine fibroids. *Cochrane Database Syst Rev*, 2001(2):CD000547.

34. Gardella, B., et al., What is the role of barbed suture in laparoscopic myomectomy? A meta-analysis and pregnancy outcome evaluation. *Gynecol Obstet Invest*, 2018. 83(6):521–532.

35. Pluchino, N., et al., Comparison of the initial surgical experience with robotic and laparoscopic myomectomy. *Int J Med Robot*, 2014. 10(2):208–212.

36. Rimbach, S., et al., A new in-bag system to reduce the risk of tissue morcellation: development and experimental evaluation during laparoscopic hysterectomy. *Arch Gynecol Obstet*, 2015. 292(6):1311–1320.

37. Claeys, J., et al., The risk of uterine rupture after myomectomy: a systematic review of the literature and meta-analysis. *Gynecological Surgery*, 2014. 11(3):197–206.

38. Tsuji, S., et al., MRI evaluation of the uterine structure after myomectomy. *Gynecol Obstet Invest*, 2006. 61(2):106–110.

11 Cervical Fibroids

Techniques for Myomectomy and Hysterectomy

Nutan Jain and Shalini Singh

CONTENTS

INTRODUCTION

Cervical fibroids are smooth muscle benign tumors with varying amounts of fibrous connective tissues that arise from the cervix. They are classified as type 8 under the FIGO (International Federation of Gynecology and Obstetrics) classification and account for less than 5% of all cases [1]. Although fibroids are usually asymptomatic, symptoms depend on location, size, and number of fibroids. Cervical fibroids are classified as interstitial, supravaginal, and polypoidal [2]. Supravaginal fibroids can be interstitial or subperitoneal but rarely polyploidy. Interstitial fibroids may grow and expand such that the pelvic anatomy and ureter are distorted. Polypoidal fibroids are usually pedunculate and rarely sessile. Supravaginal leiomyoma is the commonest type [2] (Figure 11.1). Cervical myomas can attain a huge size so that intraoperatively a small uterus is seen resting on a huge fibroid giving a typical appearance of "Lantern on St. Paul's Dome" [3] (Figure 11.1). Such fibroids can have varying presentation depending on the anterior, posterior, or lateral location or protruded state. These fibroids can have excessive bleeding leading to anemia and fatigue, vaginal discharge, infection, interference with urination or defecation, dyspareunia, postcoital or intermenstrual bleeding, and subfertility [4].

The symptomatology of cervical myomas necessitates a thorough pelvic examination, including per speculum examination and even emergency management. They can be pedunculate myomas that gradually dilate the endocervical canal and protrude out of the cervical canal into the vagina [4, 5, 6]. Eventually, the surface can become ulcerated and infected if neglected [5]. Occasionally, the pedunculate

myomas twist, resulting in poor blood supply and necrosis. Sometimes, impacted myomas even mimic uterine inversion [6]. Large cervical myomas may compress the urethra or ureters, causing urinary complains as well. The urinary bladder is compressed because of the pressure effect of cervical fibroids, leading to urgency and frequency and even incontinence [5]. Acute urinary retention necessitates surgery because of rapidly growing myomas that compress the urethra and bladder neck against pubic symphysis, causing urinary retention [7]. Often, a large cervical myoma may get incarcerated in a cul-de-sac, wedging the cervix and obstructing urinary flow. Hence, the chances of urinary tract infections are high. An increase in intravesicular pressure due to compression by a

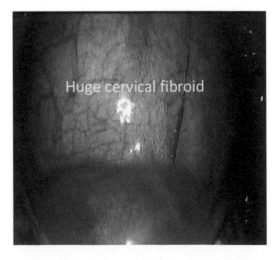

Figure 11.1 A huge anterior cervical fibroid.

cervical myoma can cause incontinence as well. Silent urethral compression against the pelvic wall can lead to infection, hydronephrosis, or renal parenchyma damage [5]. Constipation can aggravate because of pressure against the rectum [8–10]. Even the intestine can become entwined with pedunculated myomas, causing intermittent intestinal obstruction [5].

DIAGNOSIS

Clinical assessment must be carried out since per speculum and per vaginal examination can help in primary diagnosis. Diagnosis can be established in most cases with the use of imaging modalities, including transvaginal sonography, color doppler, computed tomography, and magnetic resonance imaging (MRI). On ultrasound, leiomyomas are hypoechoic. On MRI images, a myxoid component shows low signal intensity on the T1-weighted images and high signal intensity on the T2-weighted images. The triad of lactate dehydrogenase (LDH), color Doppler, and MRI is helpful in diagnosing sarcomatous changes in huge fibroids [11]. Preoperative intravenous urography, ureteric stenting, and intraureteric catheters can be required to trace ureters in case of cervical fibroids. As an innovation, the use of radioactive dye (indocyanine green, or ICG) and fluorescent imaging during surgery is also a preferred method to trace the ureters during surgery to prevent ureteric complications but it requires an advanced and dedicated system like Stryker 1588 or 1688. With the same concept, ureters can be traced with the use of ICG dye and using the Robotic DaVinci paltform.

PREOPERATIVE PREPARATIONS

The patient is investigated as for any other major surgery with all mandatory blood investigation and cross-match sample. The mechanical bowel preparations before surgery may not be required at all, but in case of large tumors or suspected adhesions, it is desirable to have a flat bowel, so it may be recommended. We keep the patient on a liquid diet for 2 days prior to surgery. Others may prefer to use Exelyte, Peglec, or Dulcolax with Gas-X for bowel preparation [12].

SURGICAL APPROACH

The laparoscopic approach is safer for any type of myomectomy, but treatment of cervical myoma remains crucial [13]. For safety in laparoscopic surgeries, it is essential to establish better techniques for different types of cervical myomas [14]. Surgical steps and techniques

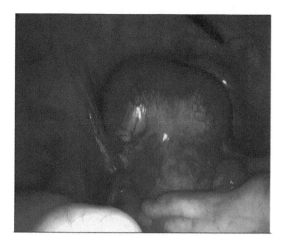

Figure 11.2 A large cervical fibroid with its anatomical relation to adjacent structures.

depend and differ on the basis of size, type, and location, either anterior or posterior, cervical or extracervical. As compared with other uterine myomas, cervical myomas are closer to the bladder, ureter, and rectum; hence, the approach needs to be modified depending on the organs in close proximity (Figure 11.2). Problems associated with these cases are difficult access to the operative field, difficulty in suturing the defects, excessive hemorrhage, and distorted anatomy in relation to the ureter and uterine artery or close proximity of major vessels and organs [4, 15]. The ureter and uterine artery may be in extracapsular relation to the fibroid; hence, this fact can turn a dangerous procedure into a relatively safe approach.

SURGICAL TECHNIQUE

Port placement is carried out in a usual preferred way at our center. We have found that the "Jain point" [16–19] can be beneficial as a first entry port in such a large myoma or in cases with previous surgeries, especially where Palmer's point entry has doubtful safety. The Jain point is a more lateral entry point located in the left paraumbilical region at the level of the umbilicus, in a straight line drawn vertically upward from a point 2.5 cm medial to the anterior superior iliac spine. With this technique, the 10-mm 30° telescope can be inserted supraumbilically higher up under the vision of a 5-mm telescope (Figure 11.18) according to the needs of the case.

Before surgery, a uterine manipulator is normally inserted through the cervix into the uterus; this may not be possible in cases of extracervical, vaginally protruding myoma. If a pedunculate myoma presents in the vagina, the first myomectomy can be carried out by hysteroscopic morcellation or resection [20]. Sometimes, the myoma is deeply impacted in the vagina and the manipulator cannot be inserted. In such cases, an alternative method to remove the fibroid is to make a Duhrssen's incision into the cervix and extend it to reach the myoma. Fibroid then can be removed and the manipulator can be inserted. Finally, the hysterectomy can be completed laparoscopically in a routine manner [21].

We usually begin the myomectomy by injecting large volumes of vasopressin (20 IU in 400 mL saline) into the myoma (Figure 11.3). Other methods include uterine artery ligation at the origin, vascular clips, and the "shoelace knot." In case of an anterior wall cervical fibroid, a transverse incision is made to dissect the uterovesical fold and perform blunt dissection of the bladder (Figures 11.3 and 11.4). For tackling the bladder, harmonic is a better option as it is an ultrasonic device and hence has less lateral thermal damage. During traction and enucleation with a laparoscopic myomectomy screw, the base of the wound is held with bipolar grasping forceps and simultaneous complete homeostasis is achieved along with dissection to avoid postenucleation difficulties due to retracted capillaries. Even harmonic ace can be used at the base with equally good results to achieve haemostatsis.

In the case of posterior myomas, a midline vertical incision can be given to avoid injuring the vessels and stay at a safe distance from the ureters [22]. Usually, after a large posterior wall myomectomy, the vertical midline incision tends to become transverse and hence

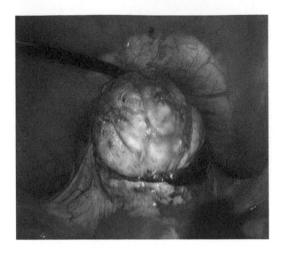

Figure 11.4 Myoma walking out of its bed through anterior incision.

can be sutured easily like any transverse incision and is easier for an ipsilateral suturing surgeon. The transverse incision is preferred as it helps in better hemostasis as the arcuate arteries lie parallel to incision. Another method to deal with posterior wall fibroids is using the principle of "Backyard theory" by keeping the incision anteriorly such that the ureters and uterine arteries lie safe posteriorly. (See details in Chapter 12 on broad ligament fibroid.)

Removal of Myoma

Enucleation of myoma can be carried out by using a myoma screw or tenaculum where the myoma easily walks out of its bed (Figure 11.4). After complete enucleation, cervical myoma can be removed by morcellation. If complete enucleation is difficult because of large size and deep location or limited pelvic space for traction, the myoma can be morcellated when it is still attached to the uterus [22]. The approach depends on the size and location of the myoma and the expertise or varied practices of different surgeons. Usually, *in situ* morcellation can cause excessive blood loss; hence, the operator needs good teamwork for faster and safer morcellation.

Defect Closure

We close the defect in multiple layers (muscular and serosal) by using polygalactin 1/0 sutures in a continuous manner such that there is no dead space (Figures 11.5 and 11.6). In case of a large defect, hemostatic material like "Surgicel" can be placed *in situ* and the defect can be closed in layers. If the endometrial cavity gets opened, first the endometrial cavity is repaired

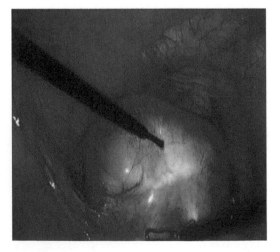

Figure 11.3 Injecting vasopressin using the standard injection needle.

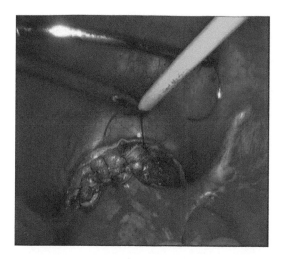

Figure 11.5 The myoma bed closed in layers using polygalactin suture 1'0.

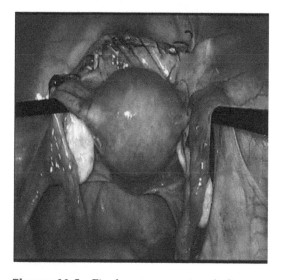

Figure 11.6 Final anatomy restored after myomectomy.

with 3'0 polygalactin sutures and then the myoma bed closure is carried out in layers. The patient is given a high dose of estrogen postoperatively.

Prevention of Adhesion Formation

In our practice, to avoid postoperative adhesion formation, we prefer the fluid barrier method of hydroflotation [23], which has had good results. We leave 2 to 3 L of fluid in the abdomen with 400 mg of hydrocortisone in it [24]. Other commonly used surface adhesion barriers are Interceed® (Gynecare, a subsidiary of Johnson & Johnson) and Seprafilm® (Baxter).

HYSTERECTOMY

In case of total laparoscopic hysterectomy (TLH), port placement remains the same as for myomectomy. In large myomas, we prefer four accessory ports. Tackling the adnexal pedicles with a vessel-sealing device is preferred, although bipolar and scissors can also be used. Before TLH, removing the myomas that are posing difficulty in tackling the uterine arteries may be a better approach. Exploring the retro-peritoneal space and performing ureteral dissection can safeguard ureteral injury or uterine artery laceration. In case of dense adhesions or associated endometriosis, the use of ICG or infrared catheters can be beneficial to prevent ureteric injuries. Rectal probes can be beneficial in case of rectum involvement and facilitate judicious dissection.

Anticipated Complications and Management

Possible complications during myomectomy include the following:

Excessive Blood Loss

Role of Vasopressin in Myomectomy

Vasopressin causes smooth muscle constriction in capillaries, small arterioles, and venules and hence minimizes blood loss during myomectomy. This technique is found to be as effective as the mechanical occlusion of uterine vessels. But extra precaution is required while using vasopressin because of reported complications like pulmonary edema [25], severe hypo-hypertension [26], bradycardia, and even cardiac arrest [27]. The most important step includes aspiration of vasopressin before every single active injection to check for vascular puncture. Avoiding intravascular injection of vasopressinn is the key in preventing above mentioned side effects.

Our standard injection needles are usually 33 cm long and opaque throughout; hence, a minor vessel puncture can be missed if aspiration cannot reach the complete column of needle since the capsule, which is the site of injection, has abundant vessels. To overcome this problem, Pisat's VVIN (visual vasopressin injection needle) has turned out to be an innovative tool for safe laparoscopic myomectomy [28, 29] (Figure 11.7). It contains a detachable, disposable, and transparent plastic hub 1 cm long at the proximal end of the instrument that can pass any 5-mm port. The idea of this 1-cm plastic segment is that it instantly shows if the needle punctured a vessel and blood is aspirated, thereby increasing the safety of vasopressin usage. Just 0.03 mL of blood (less than a single drop) is sufficient to detect a

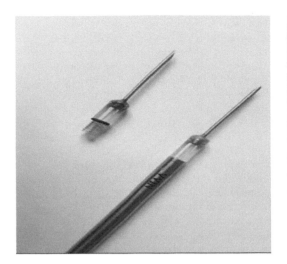

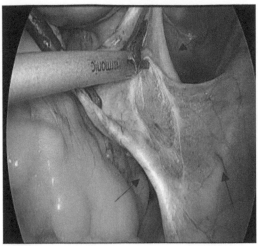

Figure 11.7 Pisat's VVIN (visual vasopressin injection needle) with a proximal transparent plastic 1-cm hub.

Figure 11.9 Approach to uterine artery ligation at origin through pelvic triangle formed by infundibulopelvic ligament, round ligament, and external iliac vessel.

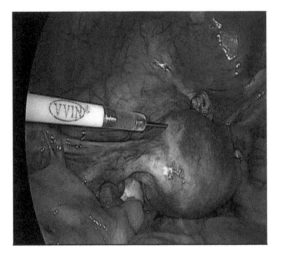

can be approached by opening the peritoneum over the pelvic triangle formed by round ligament, infundibulopelvic ligament, and external iliac vessel (Figure 11.9). Once the tissue is dissected, the ureter is seen on the medial aspect of the broad ligament. Further dissection shows the uterine artery crossing from the lateral to medial aspect in the pararectal space. It is further traced back at its origin from the hypogastric artery (Figure 11.10) and is easily identified by its pulsation, slight bulge at the point of origin, and tracing ureter under uterine artery depicting "water under the bridge."

Figure 11.8 Injecting vasopressin under correct avascular plane under capsule using VVIN (visual vasopressin injection needle).

vascular puncture and this is 27 times more sensitive than a regular injection needle [28, 29] and hence avoids major vascular complications (Figure 11.8). The dose of vasopressin is a maximum of 20 IU diluted in 400 mL saline. (For details on precaution for vasopressin, refer to Chapter 12.)

Laparoscopic Uterine Artery Ligation
In huge cervical myomas, bilateral uterine artery ligation helps to reduce blood loss [30, 31]. However, the role of this permanent method in a patient who desires future fertility is still under study [32, 33]. The uterine artery

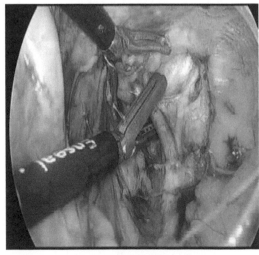

Figure 11.10 Coagulation of uterine artery at its origin using vessel sealer—Enseal.

If the myoma is large enough with distorted anatomy, "backyard theory" can be applied and may be beneficial. As per backyard theory, a transverse incision is given anteriorly on the most bulging part of myoma such that uterine arteries and ureter stay behind and safe posteriorly. (For details about backyard theory, see Chapter 12.)

Temporarily Blocking Methods

The titanium vascular clips [34, 35] can be used for temporarily blocking the vessels in the patient wanting to preserve fertility but these clips are usually not readily available. Thus, to overcome this, a temporary removable "shoelace knot" [36] (Figure 11.14) that requires little surgical expertise can serve the purpose. If it is a myomectomy, then permanent ligature of the uterine artery may compromise the blood supply of the uterus. So it is advisable to use a "shoelace" reversible technique of uterine artery occlusion. In this, we take a suture by making a small knot on the shorter free end of the suture. Then we tie the knot with the other end of the suture which is doubled up (Figures 11.11 and 11.12). So, in a way, we make the knot with three threads. After making the knot, we tighten the short limb of the free end, which can be identified by the knot put on the thread in the beginning (Figures 11.13 and 11.14). Only one knot is enough to occlude the uterine artery. It is done bilaterally. After the suturing of the myoma bed, the reversible shoelace knot is removed. The reperfusion of the uterine artery is complete within 5 to 10 min of removal of suture (1–0 polygalactin). It can even

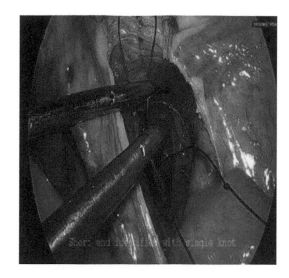

Figure 11.12 Shoelace knotting with a short knotted end while long end doubled up to form three-threaded knot.

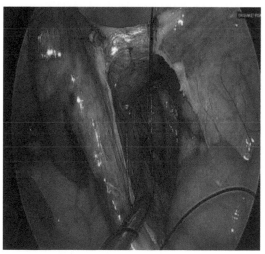

Figure 11.13 A single three-threaded knot placed over the uterine vessel.

be converted to a permanent knot if required by pulling the short end that further tightens the knot [36].

Ureteric Injury

This is a common possibility but can be prevented by judicious assessment.

1. Tracking the course of ureters.

2. Opening the retroperitoneum to explore the ureters.

3. In difficult cases of dense adhesions or coexisting endometriosis, use of illuminated

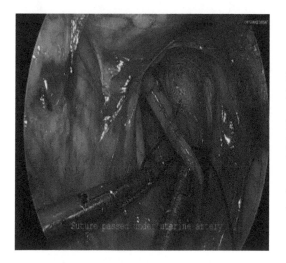

Figure 11.11 First step of "shoelace knot" (temporary knot) to pass the suture below the uterine vessel.

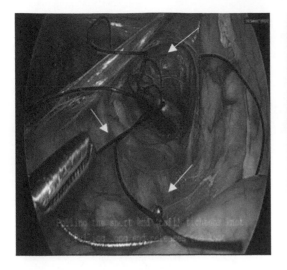

Figure 11.14 Final placed knot with three ends a short tail knotted end, doubled up end and a long pulling end.

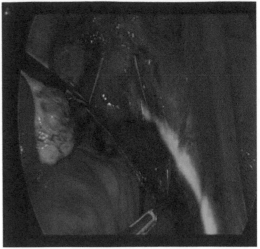

Figure 11.16 1688 Stryker advanced imaging modality (AIM) 4K platform using indocyanine green (ICG) dye. Fluorescent green appearance of ureters.

stents (infrared) [37] (Figure 11.15) or injecting ICG dyes directly into ureters during cystoscopy and visualizing the fluorescent glow can be helpful in ureteric mapping and ease of dissection [38–40]. The fluorescence from the tri-carbocyanine dye ICG shows an absorption peak at 805 nm, whereas the fluorescence emission peak is at 835 nm. ICG binds to the proteins in plasma that glows green in the near-infrared spectrum on illumination with light at 806 nm. Hence, we need a dedicated system that uses the infrared mode or contrast for fluoroscopic images like Stryker 1588 or 1688) (Figures 11.16 and 11.17). The main

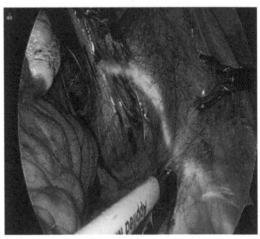

Figure 11.17 1588 Stryker advanced imaging modality (AIM) 4K platform using indocyanine green (ICG) dye. Fluorescent green appearance of ureters with black and white background.

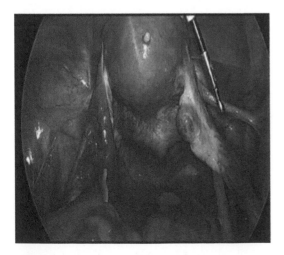

Figure 11.15 Illuminated red appearance of ureters using infra red intra ureteric stents.

contraindication and side effect of ICG dye is allergic reaction. It is therefore contraindicated in patients allergic to iodine as the dye contains a small amount of iodine. It should also be used carefully in patients with any history of allergy to penicillin or sulfa drugs [40].

4. Finally, a "check cystoscopy" at the end of surgery is a good practice to detect and assess the ureteric function. Not only ureteric peristalsis but also spurt of urine should be checked during cystoscopy.

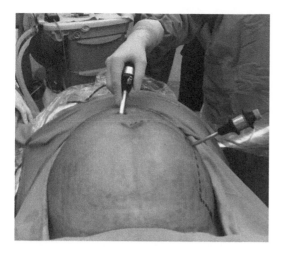

Figure 11.18 10-mm 30° telescope being inserted supraumbilically higher up under the vision of 5-mm telescope at "Jain point."

POSTOPERATIVE

The laparoscopic technique gives the benefit of early ambulation. We usually allow oral sips within 4 h of surgery, and the patient is ambulatory within 6 h and discharged the next day. Postoperative lower limb and breathing exercises are explained to the patient.

POINTS TO REMEMBER

1. Prior myomectomy before proceeding for definitive steps for hysterectomy can be helpful.

2. To reduce blood loss, take precautionary measures like the use of vasopressin, uterine artery ligation at the origin for TLH, or temporary blocking uterine arteries before myomectomy.

3. Minimize the risk for surrounding organs, giving judicious incisions depending on the location of the myoma.

4. Suture the defect in multiple layers to avoid leaving a dead space and suture the endometrial cavity as a separate layer in case the cavity opens.

5. Surgery must have good hemostasis and less blood loss and take necessary measures to prevent adhesion formation.

6. Using advanced modalities like infrared ureteric stents or ICG dye for ureteric mapping can prevent injuries to the ureter.

7. Managing cervical fibroids depends on its size, location, and surgical expertise; hence, a good clinical evaluation helps in deciding the approach to such cases.

8. Laparoscopic surgeries need innovation that can ease and facilitate the surgical procedures, especially large, complicated, and distorted anatomy.

REFERENCES

1. Tiltman AJ. Leiomyomas of the uterine cervix: a study of frequency. *Int J Gynecol Pathol.* 1998;17:231–234.

2. Jeffcoate N. Tumors of corpus uteri. In: Bhatla N (ed). *Jeffcoate's Principles of Gynaecology*, 6th Delhi, Arnold Publication; 2001:466–497.

3. Jayashree V, Mahjabeen B, Thariq IA. A case of huge cervical fibroid with characteristic "Lantern on St. Paul's Cathedral" appearance. *IJBAMR.* 2015;4,3:455–458.

4. Suneja A, Taneja A, Guleria K, Yadav P. Incarcerated procidentia due to cervical fibroid: an unusual presentation. *Aust NZJ Obstet Gynecol.* 2003;43:252–253.

5. Jones HW III, Rock JA. *Te Linda's Operative Gynecology*, 11th ed. Philadelphia, PA, Wolters Kluwer Health; 2015. Section V, Chapter 31:656–696.

6. Singh S, Chaudhary P. Central cervical fibroid mimicking as chronic uterine inversion: a case report. *Int J Reprod Contracept Obstet Gynecol.* 2013;2(4):687–688.

7. Kumar S. Huge cervical fibroid causing urinary retention. *Int J Reprod Contracept Obstet Gynecol.* 2016;5:4070–4072.

8. Verma ML, Sambharam K, Bhalerao AN. Delivery of huge impacted cervical fibroid using Wrigley's obstetrics forceps. *Pan Asian J Obs Gyn.* 2019;2(2):90–92.

9. Samal SK, Rathod S, Rajsekaran A, Rani R. An unusual presentation of central cervical fibroid: a case report. *Int J Res Med Sci.* 2014;2(3):1226–1228.

10. Kavitha B, Jyothi R, Rama Devi A, Madhuri K, Sachin Avinash K, Murthy SGK. A rare case of central cervical fibroid with characteristic "Lantern on top of ST. PAUL" appearance. *Int J Res Dev Health.* 2014;2(1):45–47.

11. Goto A, Takeuchi S, Sugimura K, Maruo T. Usefulness of Gd-DTPA contrast-enhanced dynamic MRI and serum determination of LDH andits isozymes in the differential diagnosis of leiomyosarcoma from degenerated leiomyoma of the uterus. *Int J Gynecol Cancer* 2002;12:354–361. doi:10.1046/j.1525-1438.2002.01086.x.

https://obgyn.onlinelibrary.wiley.com/doi/pdf/10.1576/toag.9.2.088.27309.

12. Reddy DN, Rao GV, Sriram PV. Efficacy and safety of oral sodium phosphate versus polyethylene glycol solution for bowel preparation for colonoscopy. *Indian J Gastroenterol.* 2002;21(6):219–221.

13. Shi R. Clinical analysis of laparoscopic myomectomy for patients with cervical myoma. *J Minim Invasive Gynecol.* 2010;17. 10.1016/j.jmig.2010.08.294.

14. Chang WC, Chen SY, Huang SC, Chang DY, Chou LY, Sheu BC. Strategy of cervical myomectomy under laparoscopy. *Fertil Steril.* 2010;94:2710–2715.

15. Mihmanli V, Cetinkaya N, Kilickaya A, Kilinc A, Köse D. Giant cervical myoma associated with urinary incontinence and hydroureteronephrosis. *Clin Exp Obstet Gynecol.* 2015;42(5):690–691.

16. Jain N. Jain point: a new safe portal for laparoscopic entry in previous surgery cases. *J Minim Invasive Gynecol.* 25(7). 1 Nov 2018. https://doi.org/10.1016/j.jmig.2018.09.723.

17. Jain N, Sareen S, Kanawa S, Jain V, Gupta S, Mann S. Jain point: a new safe portal for laparoscopic entry in previous surgery cases. *J Hum Reprod Sci.* 2016;9:9–17.

18. Jain N, Jain V, Agarwal C, Bansal P, Gupta S, Bansal B. Left lateral port: safe laparoscopic port entry in previous large upper abdomen laparotomy scar. *J Minim Invasive Gynecol.* 2019;26(5):973–976.

19. Mulayam B, Aksoy O. Direct trocar entry from left lateral port (Jain point) in a case with previous surgeries. *J Gynecol Surg.* 2020;37–39. http://doi.org/10.1089/gyn.2019.0077.

20. Patel P, Banker M, Munshi S, Bhalla A. Handling cervical myomas. *J Gynecol Endosc Surg.* 2011;2(1):30–32. doi: 10.4103/0974-1216.85277.

21. Lee EM, Delgado S, Hendessi P. Surgical approach to a large cervical fibroid. *J Minim Invasive Gynecol.* 2019;26. https://doi.org/10.1016/j.jmig.2019.09.015.

22. Sinha R, Hegde A, Warty N, Mahajan C. Laparoscopic myomectomy: Enucleation of the myoma by morcellation while it is attached to the uterus. *J Minim Invasive Gynecol.* 2005;12:284–289.

23. Ahmad G, Mackie FL, Iles DA, O'Flynn H, Dias S, Metwally M, et al. Fluid and pharmacological agents for adhesion prevention after gynaecological surgery. *Cochrane Database Syst Rev.* 2014;(7):CD001298.

24. Torres-De La Roche LA, Campo R, Devassy R, Di Spiezio Sardo A, Hooker A, Koninckx P, et al. Adhesions and anti-adhesion systems highlights. *Facts Views Vis Obgyn.* 2019;11(2):137–149.

25. Tulandi T, Béique F, Kimia M. Pulmonary edema: a complication of local injection of vasopressin at laparoscopy. *Fertil Steril.* 1996;66(3):478–480. https://doi.org/10.1016/S0015-0282(16)58523-9.

26. Nezhat F, Admon D, Nezhat CH, Dicorpo JE, Nezhat C. Life-threatening hypotension after vasopressin injection during operative laparoscopy, followed by uneventful repeat laparoscopy. *J Am Assoc Gynecol Laparosc.* 1994;2(1):83–86. doi: 10.1016/S1074-3804(05)80837-0.

27. Chudnoff S, Glazer S, Levie M. Review of vasopressin use in gynecologic surgery. *J Minim Invasive Gynecol.* 2012;19(4):422–433. doi: 10.1016/j.jmig.2012.03.022.

28. Pisat S, van Herendael B. Pisat's visual vasopressor injection needle: an innovative tool for increasing patient safety in laparoscopic myomectomy. *Surg Technol Int.* 2017;30:197–204.

29. Pisat SV. Pisat's visual vasopressor injection needle: a new device for increasing patient safety in laparoscopic myomectomy. *J Obstet Gynecol India* 2017;67(6):451–453.

30. Dubuisson J, Ramyead L, Streuli I. The role of preventive uterine artery occlusion during laparoscopic myomectomy: a review of the literature. *Arch Gynecol Obstet.* 2015;291:737–743.

31. Chang KM, Chen MJ, Lee MH, Huang YD, Chen CS. Fertility and pregnancy outcomes after uterine artery occlusion with or without myomectomy. *Taiwan J Obstet Gynecol.* 2012;51:331–335.

32. Vercellino G, Erdemoglu E, Joe A, Hopfenmueller W, Holthaus B, Köhler C, et al. Laparoscopic temporary clipping of uterine artery during laparoscopic myomectomy. *Arch Gynecol Obstet.* 2012;286:1181–1186.

33. Roman H, Sentilhes L, Cingotti M, Verspyck E, Marpeau L. Uterine devascularization and subsequent major intrauterine synechiae and ovarian failure. *Fertil Steril.* 2005;83:755–757.

34. Voss M, Koehler C, Elger F, Kruppa S, Schneider A. Temporary clipping of the uterine artery during laparoscopic myomectomy—a new technique and the results of first cases. *Gynecol Surg.* 2007;4:101–105.

35. Matsuoka S, Kikuchi I, Kitade M, Kumakiri J, Kuroda K, Tokita S, et al. Strategy for laparoscopic cervical myomectomy. *J Minim Invasive Gynecol.* 2010;17:301–305.

36. Pisat S, van Herendael BJ. Temporary ligation of the uterine artery at its origin using a removable "shoelace" knot. *J Minim Invasive Gynecol.* 2020;27(1):26. doi: 10.1016/j.jmig.2019.06.011. Epub 2019 Jun 26.

37. Kim K, Schwaitzberg S, Onel E. An infrared ureteral stent to aid in laparoscopic retroperitoneal lymph node dissection. *J Urol.* 2001;166(5):1815–1816.

38. Siddighi S, Yune JJ, Hardesty J. Indocyanine green for intraoperative localization of ureter. *Am J Obstet Gynecol.* 2014;211(4):436.e1–436.e2. doi: 10.1016/j.ajog.2014.05.017. Epub 2014 May 14.

39. Slooter MD, Janssen A, Bemelman WA, Tanis PJ, Hompes R. Currently available and experimental dyes for intraoperative near-infrared fluorescence imaging of the ureters: a systematic review. *Tech Coloproctol.* 2019;23:305–313. https://doi.org/10.1007/s10151-019-01973-4.

40. Long Y, Yao Y, Yao D-S. Indocyanine green angiography for preserving the ureteral branch of the uterine artery during radical hysterectomy. *Medicine (Baltimore).* 2018;97(40):e12692. doi: 10.1097/MD.0000000000012692.

12 Broad Ligament Fibroids

Techniques for Myomectomy and Hysterectomy

Nutan Jain and Shalini Singh

CONTENTS

INTRODUCTION

Fibroids are benign, monoclonal smooth muscle tumors of the myometrium and are aggregates of extracellular matrix containing collagen, elastin, proteoglycans, and fibronectins [1]. Forty percent are associated with chromosomal abnormalities like translocation of chromosome 12 and 14, deletion of chromosome 7, and trisomy of chromosome 12 [2, 3]. Although these are benign tumors, the incidence of sarcomas in fibroids is reported to be 0.29 to 0.05% of cases. Hence, diagnosis and proper management are necessities, especially in symptomatic and large fibroids.

Uterine fibroids are commonly intramural, submucosal, or subserosal as classified in FIGO (International Federation of Gynecology and Obstetrics) classification types 1 to 7. They can also have extrauterine origin classified as type 8 in the FIGO classification (Table 12.1). They arise from broad ligament, round ligament, ovarian ligament, and the ovaries [4]. Broad ligament is the most common extrauterine site for the occurrence of leiomyoma [5]; the incidence is less than 1% [6]. They are of great clinical and surgical importance because of their location involving ureters.

Type 8: Fibroids that do not arise from myometrium but include cervical lesions, round or broad ligaments without direct attachment to the uterus, and other "parasitic" lesions [7] (https://obgyn.onlinelibrary.wiley.com/doi/pdf/10.1002/ijgo.12666).

Broad ligament fibroids are classified as true and pseudo broad ligament fibroids (Table 12.2). True broad ligament fibroids arise from the muscle fibers in the mesometrium commonly located in round ligament, utero-ovarian ligament, and the connective tissue surrounding

TABLE 12.1: Classification of fibroids

Intrauterine	Extrauterine
0. Pedunculated intracavitary	8. Others (cervical/broad ligament/parasitic)
1. <50% intramural	
2. ≥50% intramural	
3. Contacts endometrium, 100% intramural	
4. Intramural	
5. Subserosal ≥50% intramural	
6. Subserosal <50% intramural	
7. Subserous pedunculated	

TABLE 12.2: Differentiating features of true and pseudo-broad ligament fibroids

True broad ligament fibroid	Pseudo broad ligament fibroid
It is not connected with the uterus; it arises from the muscle fibers in the mesometrium.	It arises or is connected via the pedicle to the uterus.
The ureter can lie medial, lateral, below, or within the fibroid.	It arises above uterine vessels and as it enlarges the ureter lies lateral or below it.
It has no pseudocapsule; hence, enucleation is difficult with high chances of ureteric injury.	It has a pseudocapsule; hence, dissection is easier within the capsule to avoid ureteric injury.

the ovarian and uterine vessels. Those arising from connective tissue can attain a very big size and can distort the fallopian tubes. However, they are entirely separate from the uterus and hence can displace but not distort the uterus. Pseudo (false) broad ligament fibroids actually originate from the lateral walls of the uterus or supravaginal cervix and grow toward the broad ligament. It is also considered that the false broad ligament fibroid with long and thin pedicles further elongates and loses its blood supply through the pedicle, leading to necrosis of the pedicle. It starts receiving its blood supply through connective tissue of the broad ligament and becomes a true broad ligament fibroid.

The anatomical location of broad ligament fibroids may cause local pressure effects, including ureteric obstruction, chronic pelvic pain, compression of the bladder causing urinary retention, and bowel dysfunction. It can lead to menstrual abnormalities with a coexisting intrauterine myoma. These fibroids have a tendency to attain a large size and undergo degenerative changes also. There have been case reports where broad ligament fibroid with cystic degeneration and intervening septations raised the suspicion of ovarian neoplasm on ultrasonography [8]. Even its surgery is associated with the risk of complications, particularly ureteric and uterine vessel injuries and concealed hematoma formation [9]. Broad ligament fibroids are also a diagnostic challenge on imaging because of their locations (Figure 12.1a–f). They may be confused with ovarian tumors appearing adnexal in location [8, 10] or may have an alternative histological diagnosis following myomectomy; suspected broad ligament fibroid has been reported as Schwannoma in histology [11]. True broad ligament tumors usually lie lateral to the ureter and uterine vessels, whereas a pseudotumor always lies medial to it. Hence, correct diagnosis and evaluation of location of fibroids help in better management and prevention of complications in the surgical procedure.

DIAGNOSIS

Diagnosis of broad ligament fibroid is also a challenge. Imaging techniques helpful in detecting extrauterine leiomyoma are ultrasonography, transvaginal sonography, computed tomography, and magnetic resonance imaging (MRI). MRI with its multiplanar imaging capabilities can be useful in differentiating broad ligament fibroids from ovarian tubal masses. The differential diagnosis for broad ligament fibroids includes pedunculated subserosal leiomyoma projecting into broad ligament, solid ovarian neoplasms (commonly ovarian fibroma or fibro-thecoma), and broad ligament cyst. Because it allows clear visual separation of the uterus and ovaries from the mass, transvaginal ultrasound with color Doppler helps in diagnosing broad ligament fibroid. The triad of lactate dehydrogenase (LDH), color Doppler, and MRI is helpful in the diagnosis of sarcomatous changes in huge fibroids. Goto et al. showed that, for dynamic MRI, the specificity, positive predictive value, negative predictive value, and diagnostic accuracy were 93%, 83%, 100%, and 95%, respectively [7]. Combined use of dynamic MRI and serum measurement of LDH isozymes increased all of these values to 100% [7]. On pelvic ultrasound, broad ligament fibroid is usually seen as a hypoechoic, solid, well-circumscribed adnexal mass, although that can be heterogeneous when large. In case of pseudo broad ligament fibroid, generally there is no interface between the tumor and the uterus. There are bridging vessels between the uterus and the myoma in case of pseudo broad ligament fibroids but they are absent in true broad ligament fibroid. Intravenous urography, ureteric stenting, and infraureteric catheters can be required to trace ureters for any displacement or obstruction, especially in cases of true broad ligament fibroids where ureters can even run medial to, through, or just below the fibroid. As an innovation, the use of radioactive dye (indocyanine green, or ICG) and fluorescent imaging during surgery is also a preferred method to trace the ureters during surgery to prevent ureteric complications. According to Rajanna et al. [8], broad ligament fibroid may be associated with pseudo-Meigs syndrome with elevated CA 125 levels; hence, MRI plays a vital role in the differentiation of broad ligament fibroids from ovarian tumors.

PREOPERATIVE PREPARATIONS

As for any other major surgery, the patient is investigated with a complete hemogram, blood grouping cross-matching, and all mandatory investigations. As per recent evidence, there is no need of bowel preparations before surgery, but in case of large tumors, it is desirable to have a flat bowel, so it may be recommended in this situation. The patient is kept on a liquid diet for 2 days prior to surgery.

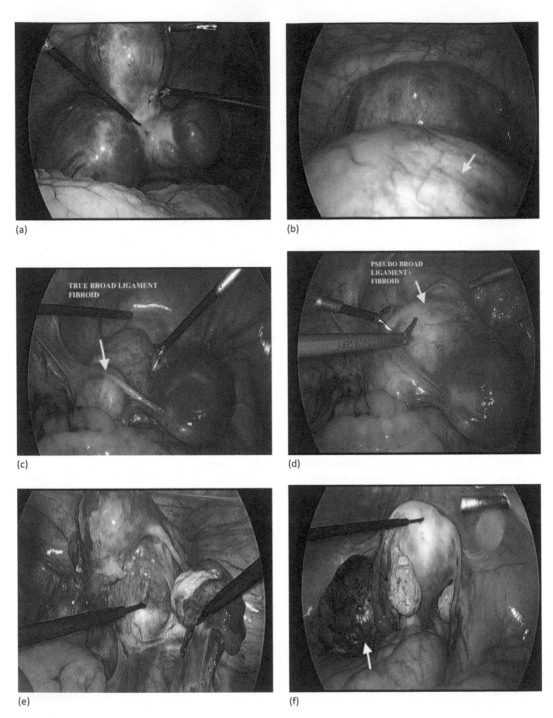

Figure 12.1 (a) Multiple uterine and extrauterine (round ligament fibroids in location) planned for total laparoscopic hysterectomy. (b) Giant posterior wall cervical fibroid giving the appearance of "Lantern on top of St. Paul's Cathedral" planned for laparoscopic myomectomy. (c) Pseudo-broad ligament fibroid arising from lateral wall of uterus and supravaginal part of cervix. (d) True broad ligament fibroid arising from round ligament. (e) A broad ligament fibroid with posterior bulge significance explained in "Backyard theory." (f) A true broad ligament fibroid with degenerative changes.

SURGICAL APPROACH

Hysterectomy is the definitive management for fibroids, but myomectomy becomes the treatment of choice in women who have symptomatic fibroids and who desire fertility or uterine preservation. Growing surgical expertise, safer techniques, and advantages of laparoscopy over laparotomy have enabled laparoscopic excision of large fibroids. Laparoscopy is considered the best route for broad ligament fibroid management. It causes a safe approach in tackling such fibroids, faster recovery, shorter hospital stay, and less morbidity. Because of the location and size of broad ligament fibroids, surgery is challenging, especially because of the risk of injury to surrounding organs such as ureters, intestines, and urinary bladder. Hence, the ureteric course must be identified during surgery.

Surgical Technique

Broad ligament fibroids become a challenge in many cases. With the appropriate techniques, such myomectomies can be accomplished safely. Myomectomy of broad ligament myoma before total laparoscopic hysterectomy (TLH) can facilitate surgery, although TLH can be carried out with myoma *in situ* as well.

Port placement is carried out in a usual preferred way. We have found that the "Jain point" can be beneficial as a first entry port in very large cases or in cases with previous surgeries (Figure 12.14b), especially where Palmer's point entry has doubtful safety [12, 13]. Jain point is a more lateral entry point located in the left paraumbilical region at the level of the umbilicus, in a straight line drawn vertically upward from a point 2.5 cm medial to the anterior superior iliac spine (Figure 12.14a). With this technique, the 10-mm 30° telescope can be inserted under the vision of a 5-mm telescope in accordance with the mandate of the case. We begin myomectomy by injecting vasopressin in large dilution (20 IU in 400 mL saline) (Figure 12.3). The incision is given on the most bulging part of the myoma on the anterior aspect considering the "Backyard theory" (described later). Usually, these myomas are just beneath the serosa and have an easy plane of cleavage. A myoma screw is applied, and once we reach a good plane, the myoma just walks out of its bed. At the base, we carefully coagulate any connections between the myoma and uterus (Figure 12.8). As the base may be large, we apply an absorbable hemostatic "Surgicel" made of oxidized regenerated cellulose in the dead space and close the serosa

loosely. This is a standard technique of laparoscopic myomectomy.

In case of TLH, port placement remains the same as for myomectomy. In large myomas, we prefer four accessory ports. Tackling the adnexal pedicles with a vessel-sealing device is preferred, although bipolar and scissors can also be used. Before proceeding to the uterine artery ligation, we usually perform a myomectomy, as it may be difficult to approach the uterine artery on the side of the myoma. To ensure the safety of the ureters and uterine arteries, broad ligament myomas are one indication where myomectomy before the uterine pedicle is a good technique. The rest of the procedure remains the same as for any other indication for TLH. A routine cystoscopy to see the ureteric spurt after completion can be good practice and is preferred by the authors.

Backyard Theory

We have devised a novel way of tackling broad ligament fibroids as they have high risk of injury to ureters. The concept of "Backyard theory" can help in these cases. We start by using a large volume of diluted vasopressin to aid in hydrodissection (Figure 12.3). This helps in reducing the blood loss and getting the correct plane, especially in cases of broad ligament fibroids that attain large sizes. According to our "Backyard theory," we always make an incision on the anterior aspect of the broad ligament myoma (Figure 12.4) irrespective of its location, even in cases where the myoma is bulging more posteriorly. In such cases, an assistant pushes the posteriorly bulged myoma anteriorly with the help of an atraumatic grasper (Figure 12.5). The myoma becomes prominent anteriorly, and an incision can be made on the anterior aspect and the myoma can be pried out (Figure 12.6) with a screw or spiral. Our technique has never failed us; thus, when this "Backyard theory" is adhered to, broad ligament myomas do not pose any challenge for us. They are taken up easily with a lot of vasopressin, and the anterior incision keeps ureters and uterine arteries secured in their location; it's just like we are operating in a living room and the rest of the stuff in the backyard doesn't bother us. In this endeavor, the myoma is brought out anteriorly and the ureter remains posteriorly and never comes across in the field of surgery (Figure 12.7). This technique can be followed for myomectomy or TLH for broad ligament myomas.

Removal of Fibroids

Methods for the removal of myomas could be morcellation, colpotomy, or minilaparotomy. The authors have been using all these modalities according to the mandate of the case, marital status, parity, size and number of the myomas, and levels of LDH, color Doppler, and MRI study. (Further details of each technique are beyond the purview of this chapter.)

Anticipated Complications

The probability of complications during myomectomy for intraligamentous fibroids is more than that of other uterine fibroids. Sizzi et al. indicated an 18.8% complication rate and reported an odds ratio of 2.43 for developing any complication [14]. Here, we mention a few common complications that can be prevented by appropriate techniques.

Concealed Hematoma Formation

Since broad ligament fibroids are larger (Figure 12.2.), enucleation leaves a large dead space (Figure 12.9) which can have oozers that can lead to collection and hematoma formation. So careful inspection of the dead space is a must, especially after releasing carbon dioxide (CO_2) pneumo-peritoneum. Cauterization can be carried out, and absorbable hemostatic material made of oxidized regenerated cellulose, commonly available as "Surgicel" (Figure 12.10), can be placed in the dead space. The serosa is closed loosely (Figure 12.11).

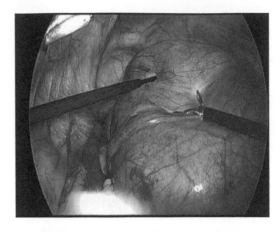

Figure 12.3 Injecting Pitressin turns the uterus pale.

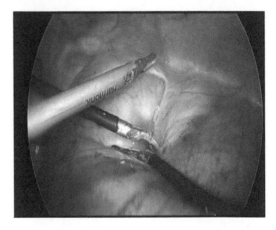

Figure 12.4 Incision must be given on the anterior side so that ureter and uterine lie safe in their position as explained by "Backyard theory."

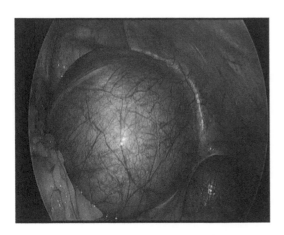

Figure 12.2 Large broad ligament fibroid in a young woman planned for myomectomy.

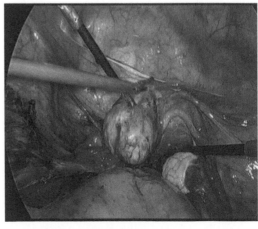

Figure 12.5 Case of posteriorly bulging broad ligament fibroid that is pushed anteriorly by a grasper to make an incision anteriorly: "Backyard theory."

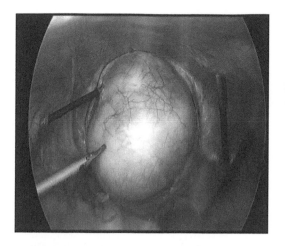

Figure 12.6 Myoma in process of enucleation.

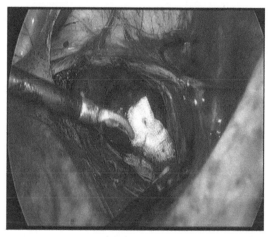

Figure 12.9 The large dead space left after myomectomy can have multiple oozers, hence the risk of hematoma formation.

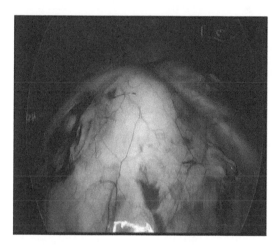

Figure 12.7 Enucleated large myoma.

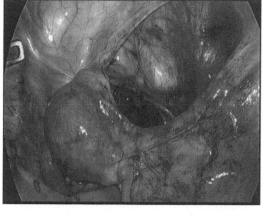

Figure 12.10 Placing "Surgicel" absorbable hemostat in the dead space is a good technique to stop generalized oozing.

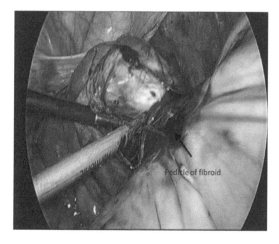

Figure 12.8 Pedicle of the large fibroid being cut by harmonic.

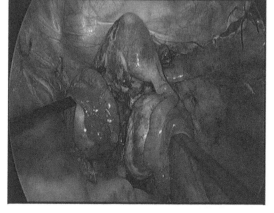

Figure 12.11 The leaflets of broad ligament should be stitched back loosely to restore anatomy.

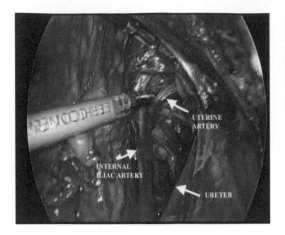

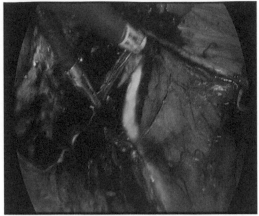

Figure 12.12 Tracking the course of ureters can help to prevent ureteric injuries.

Figure 12.13 Ureteric mapping by injecting indocyanine green (ICG) dye in ureters and florescence imaging also facilitate surgery and trace ureters in such cases.

Ureteric Injury

This is a common possibility but can be prevented by judicious assessment:

- Tracking the course of ureters (Figure 12.12).

- Opening the retroperitoneum to explore the ureters and do a uterine artery ligation at the origin in cases of TLH (laparoscopic uterine artery ligation).

- Following the "Backyard theory" and making an anterior incision and totally avoiding ureters and uterine arteries.

- In difficult cases of dense adhesions or coexisting endometriosis, the use of illuminated stents or injecting ICG dyes directly into ureters during cystoscopy and visualizing the fluorescent glow can be helpful in ureteric mapping and ease dissection (Figure 12.13). We need a dedicated system that uses infrared mode or contrast for fluoroscopic images (1588 or 1688 Stryker system).

- Finally, a "check cystoscopy" at the end of surgery can be good practice to detect and assess the ureteric status; not only ureteric peristalsis but also spurt of urine should be checked during cystoscopy.

Role of Vasopressin in Myomectomy

Vasopressin is an antidiuretic hormone that causes smooth muscle constriction in capillaries, small arterioles, and venules and hence minimizes blood loss during myomectomy. This technique is found to be as effective as the mechanical occlusion of uterine vessels. But extra precaution is required while giving vasopressin as it can have complications on the table.

- Total dose of vasopressin is a maximum of 20 IU diluted in 400 mL saline.

- The half-life of vasopressin is 20 min and so the dose can be repeated after 20 to 25 min if required.

- Always inform the anesthetist while giving the injection since strict monitoring of vitals is required.

- Complications like bradycardia, hypertension, and cardiovascular collapse have been reported. Hence, intravascular injection should be avoided and vitals should be carefully monitored.

- If there is persistent hypertension, then nitroglycerine (NTG) infusion should be started.

- Anticholinergic (glycopyrolate 0.2 mg i.v.) can be given before induction since it has a protective role against bradycardia induced by vasopressin.

- Keep diluted NTG ready at hand.

- Keep a finger on the radial pulse and watch the monitor continuously.

- A 15% rise in blood pressure (systolic and diastolic) is tolerable; above this, NTG is required.

- A 0.5 mg i.v. bolus NTG causes a fall in blood pressure within 2 min. If blood pressure is still high, further i.v. NTG 0.5 mg can be given.

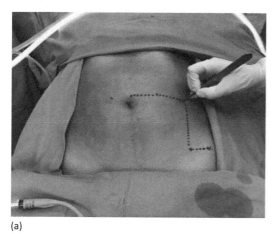
(a)

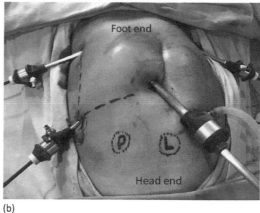
(b)

Figure 12.14 (a) Location of Jain point (explained in the text). (b) Ports position with Jain point as an entry port in case of previous surgery with large broad ligament.

POSTOPERATIVE

The laparoscopic technique gives the benefit of early ambulation. We usually allow oral sips within 4 h of surgery, and the patient is ambulatory within 6 h and discharged the next day. Postoperative lower limb and breathing exercises are explained to the patient and post operative DVT prophylaxis or compression stockings must be given especially in long surgeries.

POINTS TO REMEMBER

- Broad ligament fibroids are frequently under-reported in ultrasound. There is a need for a high level of suspicion of broad ligament in case of lateral fibroids.

- Vasopressin causes smooth muscle constriction in capillaries, small arterioles, and venules; hence, all the cautions outlined in the chapter need to be practiced in every case.

- "Backyard theory" gives us a safe approach to deal with such large broad ligament myomas and makes our surgery easy by keeping ureters and uterine behind.

- Illuminated stents or injecting ICG dyes are advanced and good techniques for ureteric mapping and make safe dissection easier.

- A routine "check cystoscopy" at the end of surgery can be a good practice.

REFERENCES

1. Leppert PC, Catherino WH, Segars JH. A new hypothesis about the origin of uterine fibroids based on gene expression profiling with micro-arrays. *Am J Obstet Gynecol.* 2006:195:415–420.

2. Hashimoto K, Azuma C, Kamiura S, Kimura T, Nobunaga T, Kanai T, et al. Clonal determination of uterine leiomyoms by analyzing differential inactivation of the X chromosome-linked phosphoglycerokinase gene. *Gynecol Obstet Invest.* 1995:40:204–208.

3. Ligon AH, Morton CC. Genetics of uterine leiomyomata. *Genes Chromosomes Cancer* 2000;28:235–245.

4. Rajesh S, Adam M. Benign metastasizing leiomyoma: "a sheep in wolf's clothing." *Community Oncol.* 2013;10:122–125.

5. Bhatta N. *Tumours of the corpus uteri. Jeffcoats Principles of Gynaecology.* 6th ed. London: Arnold Printers; 2001:470.

6. Parker WH. Uterine myomas: an overview of development, clinical features, and management. *Obstet Gynecol.* 2005;105:216–217.

7. Goto A, Takeuchi S, Sugimura K, Maruo T. Usefulness of Gd-DTPA contrast-enhanced dynamic MRI and serum determination of LDH and its isozymes in the differential diagnosis of leiomyosarcoma from degenerated leiomyoma of the uterus. *Int J Gynecol Cancer.* 2002;12:354–361. doi:10.1046/j.1525-1438.2002.01086.x. https://obgyn.onlinelibrary.wiley.com/doi/pdf/10.1576/toag.9.2.088.27309

8. Rajanna DK, Pandey V, Janardhan S, Datti SN. Broad ligament fibroid mimicking as ovarian tumor on ultrasonography and computed tomography scan. *J Clin Imaging Sci.* 2013;3:8.

9. Sinha R, Hegde A, Warty N, Patil N. Laparoscopic excision of very large myomas. *J Am Assoc Gynecol Laparosc.* 2003;10(4):461–468.

10. Yıldız P, Cengiz H, Yıldız G, Sam AD, Yavuzcan A, Çelikbaş B, et al. Two unusual clinical presentations of broad-ligament leiomyomas:

a report of two cases. *Medicina (Kaunas)*. 2012;48(3):163–165.

11. Sinha R, Sundaram M, Hegde A, Mahajan C. Pelvic schwannoma masquerading as broad ligament myoma. *J Minim Invasive Gynecol*. 2008;15(2):217–219.

12. Palmer R. Safety in laparoscopy. *J Repro Med*. 1974;13(1):1–5.e6.

13. Tulikangas PK, Nicklas A, Falcone T, Price LL. Anatomy of the left upper quadrant for cannula insertion. *J Am Assoc Gynecol Laparosc*. 2000;7(2):211–214. doi:10.1016/s1074-3804(00)80042-0.

14. Sizzi O, Rossetti A, Malzoni M, Minelli L, La Grotta F, Soranna L, et al. Italian multicenter study on complications of laparoscopic myomectomy. *J Minim Invasive Gynecol*. 2007;14(4):453–462.

13 Breach of the Endometrial Cavity during Myomectomy and Its Implications for Subsequent Fertility

Olarik Musigavong

CONTENTS

INTRODUCTION

Uterine fibroids are the most common benign gynecologic tumor; the lifetime risk is about 70–80% [1]. The clinical features can present in one of three ways:

1. Heavy and prolonged menstrual bleeding

2. Bulked-related symptoms

3. Reproductive dysfunction

Uterine fibroids affect reproductive dysfunction in two ways: infertility and obstetric complications [2]. There are many modalities to treat uterine fibroids, such as expectant management, medical therapy, surgery, and interventional radiology. The goal of treatment is to relieve the symptoms. In reproductive age, patients who need to preserve fertility function should discuss the plan and choice of treatment.

UTERINE FIBROID AND INFERTILITY

Fibroid causes infertility by several mechanisms depending on the type of fibroid.

Submucous Myoma

Increased uterine contractility, disturbances in endometrial cytokine expression, abnormal vascularization, and chronic endometrial inflammation are mechanisms that harm embryo implantation [3]. Another mechanism that has undergone evaluation is the reduction of HOXA-10 levels in the endometrium [4].

Intramural Myoma

According to recent evidence, the effect of intramural myoma on infertility is inconclusive. Several studies include a systematic review showing the adverse impact of intramural myoma on implantation rate [5–10]. However, some studies did not show the impact of intramural myoma [11–14]. Other studies show size of myoma do not affect fertility, subserosal or intramural myoma less than 4 cm does not impact on IVF-ICSI (*in vitro* fertilization–intracytoplasmic sperm injection) outcomes (abortion, implantation, and pregnancy rate), but patients with intramural myoma greater than 4 cm had lower pregnancy rate [13, 15–17].

Nonspecific Myoma

Several studies show endometrial gene expression based on myoma size and mechanical stretch of the myometrium or endometrium or both [18–20].

INDICATIONS FOR PRECONCEPTION MYOMECTOMY

The most frequent question is when to perform myomectomy. It seems that we are dealing with a disease that has a lot of heterogeneities (location, numbers, and volume). There are durable pieces of evidence that FIGO (International Federation of Gynecology and Obstetrics) L0–L2 should be removed to improve pregnancy rate [21–24]. In some cases, FIGO L3–L5 greater than 5 cm should be removed before IVF or prenatural conception in infertile patients. In some instances, FIGO L6 or L7 should be removed to prevent pregnancy complications or to improve symptoms [25].

HOW TO AVOID A BREACH IN ENDOMETRIAL CAVITY?

Breach of the endometrial cavity during myomectomy is the chaos of treatment. Prevention is better than the treatment of complications.

The technique to avoid entering the endometrial cavity can be divided into two categories: preoperative preparation and intraoperative technique.

■ Preoperative preparation

- *Uterine mapping*: The standard procedure for clinical diagnosis of uterine fibroid is pelvic ultrasonography. Advanced imaging such as 3D ultrasonography or magnetic resonance imaging can provide more accurate information on the number of fibroids, their volume, vascularization, relationship with the endometrial cavity, serosal surface, and boundary of normal myometrium [26].

- *Reducing uterine size*: Preoperative medical treatment of gonadotropin-releasing hormone agonist or selective progesterone receptor modulator can reduce the size of uterine fibroid up to 50% [27–30].

- *Decrease vascularization*: Uterine artery embolization preoperation can decrease blood loss and facilitate successful myomectomy [31].

■ Intraoperative technique

- *Identify the uterine cavity*: Intrauterine balloon during the operation can help to identify the uterine cavity. A precise and diligent hemostasis technique helps to identify capsule of the fibroid to avoid entering into the endometrial cavity.

HOW TO REPAIR AN ENDOMETRIAL CAVITY

There is no gold-standard procedure for repair once the endometrial cavity is breached. Some studies suggest a single layer by absorbable monofilament suture material to repair the endometrial cavity [32], and others suggest repair of two layers with continuous 2–0 vicryl suture. The first layer of the edges of the breach was inverted to create a smooth internal surface. The second layer increases the strength by approximating the myometrium. This pilot study shows the benefit of postoperation Foley catheter balloon for the prevention of intrauterine adhesion [33]. Some centers use hyalobarrier gel to prevent intrauterine adhesion [34].

THE COMPLICATION OF BREACH OF ENDOMETRIAL CAVITY DURING MYOMECTOMY

Intrauterine Adhesion and Infertility

The incidence of breach of the endometrial cavity during myomectomy is as high as 52.8%

[34]. The three significant factors that cause intrauterine adhesion are endometrial trauma, infection, and hypoxia [35]. Intrauterine adhesion causes infertility by several mechanisms such as cervical occlusion canal, uterine cavity, tubal ostia, and interfere with the implantation of the embryo [36]. The incidence of recurrent pregnancy loss increases in the woman who has intrauterine adhesion due to abnormalities of implantation in areas of denuded endometrium or insufficient vascularization [36].

CONCLUSION

Uterine fibroid can cause infertility per se. Moreover, the surgical treatment of uterine fibroid should not additionally add to the infertility problems. Preoperative preparation and intraoperative technique, can prevent the breach of endometrial cavity during myomectomy and prevent the untoward sequalae.

REFERENCES

1. Baird DD, Dunson DB, Hill MC, Cousins D, Schectman JM. High cumulative incidence of uterine leiomyoma in black and white women: ultrasound evidence. *Am J Obstet Gynecol.* 2003;188(1):100–107.

2. Stewart EA. Clinical practice. Uterine fibroids. *N Engl J Med.* 2015;372(17):1646–1655.

3. Munro MG. Uterine polyps, adenomyosis, leiomyomas, and endometrial receptivity. *Fertil Steril.* 2019;111(4):629–640.

4. Rackow BW, Jorgensen E, Taylor HS. Endometrial polyps affect uterine receptivity. *Fertil Steril.* 2011;95(8):2690–2692.

5. Sunkara SK, Khairy M, El-Toukhy T, Khalaf Y, Coomarasamy A. The effect of intramural fibroids without uterine cavity involvement on the outcome of IVF treatment: a systematic review and meta-analysis. *Human Reprod.* 2009;25(2):418–429.

6. Hart R, Khalaf Y, Yeong C-T, Seed P, Taylor A, Braude P. A prospective controlled study of the effect of intramural uterine fibroids on the outcome of assisted conception. *Human Reprod.* 2001;16(11):2411–2417.

7. Khalaf Y, Ross C, El-Toukhy T, Hart R, Seed P, Braude P. The effect of small intramural uterine fibroids on the cumulative outcome of assisted conception. *Human Reproduction.* 2006;21(10):2640–2644.

8. Guven S, Kart C, Unsal MA, Odaci E. Intramural leiomyoma without endometrial cavity distortion may negatively affect the ICSI – ET outcome. *Reprod Biol Endocrinol.* 2013;11(1):102.

9. Eldar-Geva T, Meagher S, Healy DL, MacLachlan V, Breheny S, Wood C. Effect of intramural, subserosal, and submucosal uterine fibroids on the outcome of assisted reproductive technology treatment. *Fertil Steril.* 1998;70(4):687–691.

10. Christopoulos G, Vlismas A, Salim R, Islam R, Trew G, Lavery S. Fibroids that do not distort the uterine cavity and IVF success rates: an observational study using extensive matching criteria. *BJOG.* 2017;124(4):615–621.

11. Farhi J, Ashkenazi J, Feldberg D, Dicker D, Orvieto R, Ben Rafael Z. Effect of uterine leiomyomata on the results of in-vitro fertilization treatment. *Human Reprod.* 1995;10(10):2576–2578.

12. Surrey ES, Lietz AK, Schoolcraft WB. Impact of intramural leiomyomata in patients with a normal endometrial cavity on in vitro fertilization–embryo transfer cycle outcome. *Fertil Steril.* 2001;75(2):405–410.

13. Oliveira FG, Abdelmassih VG, Diamond MP, Dozortsev D, Melo NR, Abdelmassih R. Impact of subserosal and intramural uterine fibroids that do not distort the endometrial cavity on the outcome of in vitro fertilization–intracytoplasmic sperm injection. *Fertil Steril.* 2004;81(3):582–587.

14. Yan L, Ding L, Li C, Wang Y, Tang R, Chen ZJ. Effect of fibroids not distorting the endometrial cavity on the outcome of in vitro fertilization treatment: a retrospective cohort study. *Fertil Steril.* 2014;101(3):716–721.

15. Klatsky PC, Tran ND, Caughey AB, Fujimoto VY. Fibroids and reproductive outcomes: a systematic literature review from conception to delivery. *Am J Obstet Gynecol.* 2008;198(4):357–366.

16. Pritts EA, Parker WH, Olive DL. Fibroids and infertility: an updated systematic review of the evidence. *Fertil Steril.* 2009;91(4):1215–1223.

17. Klatsky PC, Lane DE, Ryan IP, Fujimoto VY. The effect of fibroids without cavity involvement on ART outcomes independent of ovarian age. *Human Reprod.* 2006;22(2):521–526.

18. Rogers R, Norian J, Malik M, Christman G, Abu-Asab M, Chen F, et al. Mechanical homeostasis is altered in uterine leiomyoma. *Am J Obstet Gynecol.* 2008;198(4):474.e1–474e11.

19. Payson M, Malik M, Siti-nur Morris S, Segars JH, Chason R, Catherino WH. Activating transcription factor 3 gene expression suggests that tissue stress plays a role in leiomyoma development. *Fertil Steril.* 2009;92(2):748–755.

20. Norian JM, Owen CM, Taboas J, Korecki C, Tuan R, Malik M, et al. Characterization of tissue biomechanics and mechanical signaling in uterine leiomyoma. *Matrix Biology.* 2012;31(1):57–65.

21. Strobelt N, Ghidini A, Cavallone M, Pensabene I, Ceruti P, Vergani P. Natural history of uterine leiomyomas in pregnancy. *J Ultrasound Med.* 1994;13(5):399–401.

22. De Vivo A, Mancuso A, Giacobbe A, Savasta LM, De Dominici R, Dugo N, et al. Uterine myomas during pregnancy: a longitudinal sonographic study. *Ultrasound Obstet Gynecol.* 2011;37(3):361–365.

23. Piazze Garnica J, Gallo G, Marzano PF, Vozzi G, Mazzocco M, Anceschi MM, et al. Clinical and ultrasonographic implications of uterine leiomyomatosis in pregnancy. *Clin Exp Obstet Gynecol.* 1995;22(4):293–297.

24. Gojnic M, Pervulov M, Petkovic S, Papic M, Jeremic K, Mostic T. Indication of myomectomy during pregnancy from Doppler ultrasonography. *Clin Exp Obstet Gynecol.* 2004;31(3):197–198.

25. Milazzo GN, Catalano A, Badia V, Mallozzi M, Caserta D. Myoma and myomectomy: poor evidence concern in pregnancy. *J Obstet Gynaecol Res.* 2017;43(12):1789–1804.

26. Donnez J, Dolmans MM. Uterine fibroid management: from the present to the future. *Hum Reprod Update.* 2016;22(6):665–686.

27. Chen I, Motan T, Kiddoo D. Gonadotropin-releasing hormone agonist in laparoscopic myomectomy: systematic review and meta-analysis of randomized controlled trials. *J Minim Invasive Gynecol.* 2011;18(3):303–309.

28. Friedman AJ, Lobel SM, Rein MS, Barbieri RL. Efficacy and safety considerations in women with uterine leiomyomas treated with gonadotropin-releasing hormone agonists: The estrogen threshold hypothesis. *Am J Obstet Gynecol.* 1990;163(4, Part 1):1114–1119.

29. Donnez J, Donnez O, Matule D, Ahrendt HJ, Hudecek R, Zatik J, et al. Long-term medical management of uterine fibroids with ulipristal acetate. *Fertil Steril.* 2016;105(1):165–173.e4.

30. Donnez J, Hudecek R, Donnez O, Matule D, Arhendt HJ, Zatik J, et al. Efficacy and safety of repeated use of ulipristal acetate in uterine fibroids. *Fertil Steril.* 2015;103(2):519–527.e3.

31. Butori N, Tixier H, Filipuzzi L, Mutamba W, Guiu B, Cercueil J-P, et al. Interest of uterine artery embolization with gelatin sponge particles prior to myomectomy for large and/or multiple fibroids. *Eur J Radiol.* 2011;79(1):1–6.

32. Bean EM, Cutner A, Holland T, Vashisht A, Jurkovic D, Saridogan E. Laparoscopic myomectomy: a single-center retrospective review of 514 patients. *J Minim Invasive Gynecol.* 2017;24(3):485–493.

33. Gupta S, Talaulikar VS, Onwude J, Manyonda I. A pilot study of Foley's catheter balloon for prevention of intrauterine adhesions following breach of uterine cavity in complex myoma surgery. *Arch Gynecol Obstet.* 2013;288(4):829–832.

34. Conforti A, Krishnamurthy GB, Dragamestianos C, Kouvelas S, Micallef Fava A, Tsimpanakos I, et al. Intrauterine adhesions after open myomectomy: an audit. *Eur J Obstets Gynecol Reprod Biology.* 2014;179:42–45.

35. Papoutsis D, Georgantzis D, Dacco MD, Halmos G, Moustafa M, Mesquita Pinto AR, et al. A rare case of Asherman's syndrome after open myomectomy: sonographic investigations and possible underlying mechanisms. *Gynecol Obstet Invest.* 2014;77(3):194–200.

36. Yu D, Li TC, Xia E, Huang X, Liu Y, Peng X. Factors affecting reproductive outcome of hysteroscopic adhesiolysis for Asherman's syndrome. *Fertil Steril.* 2008;89(3):715–722.

14 Predictors of Uterine Rupture and Recurrence after Myomectomy

Manou Manpreet Kaur

CONTENTS

INTRODUCTION

Uterine fibroids are the most common benign tumors of the female reproductive tract. Despite several medical and other non-medical management options for symptomatic fibroids, myomectomy remains the most common approach in women desiring fertility or preservation of their uterus or both. Uterine rupture (UR), defined as a complete disruption of the uterine wall, is rare but is one of the fearful complications associated with a myomectomy during a subsequent pregnancy and represents an obstetric emergency as it can be catastrophic, causing serious morbidity and mortality for the mother and unborn child. If UR occurs, the risk of a hysterectomy can be as high as 12%. In developed countries, UR is almost exclusively observed in the setting of a previous surgery on the uterus.

The overall risk of UR with a history of myomectomy has been estimated to be between 0.5% and 1% [1–5]. Specifically, it is 0.47% when stratified to the subgroup of women who undergo a trial of labor (TOL); however, it can be much higher (around 1.5%) in the category of women in whom it occurs before the onset of labor [2]. About one third of the URs tend to occur within 36 weeks of gestation [2]. Transabdominal myomectomy (TAM) is associated with a UR incidence of 0.67 to 1.7%, whereas this incidence is 0.49 to 0.99% after a laparoscopic myomectomy (LM) [5].

Several risk factors have been investigated in the literature to predict the potential event of UR and recurrence of fibroids after myomectomy. An outline of these risk factors is presented by critically appraising the current literature available on this subject.

UTERINE RUPTURE

Obstetrical Aspects

The interval between myomectomy and an attempt to conceive has not been clearly established, and the suggested time frame is 6 to 12 months. Obstetricians have been assessing the risk for UR on the basis of their clinical judgment to crystallize the mode and timing of delivery. At present, it is unclear whether an elective cesarean section can prevent UR during labor after previous myomectomy. Despite the lack of evidence about the role of entering the uterine cavity at the time of myomectomy and the subsequent risk of UR, this has been a commonly held tenet, which has resulted in a routine management of scheduling a cesarean delivery between 36 and 39 weeks in these patients [1, 4, 6, 7]. It is reasonable to recommend that steps be taken to recognize an inadvertent entry into the uterine cavity. History of a cesarean section with a "classical vertical incision" produces a substantially higher risk factor for UR in a subsequent pregnancy than having a history of myomectomy [6, 8]. Risk of UR is also higher after a conventional cesarean section with a low transverse incision when compared with previous myomectomy. Landon et al. reported 1.9% URs in a population of 105 women with a prior classical, inverted T, or J incision [3].

The systematic review and meta-analysis by Claeys et al. revealed a trend for increased occurrence of UR after LM (24 events per 2017 or 1.2%) versus following an open myomectomy (OM) by laparotomy (3 events per 705 or 0.4%) [5]. However, this difference was not statistically significant (*P* = 0.119). Nevertheless, the likelihood of a "primary" cesarean section was significantly increased after an LM compared with a TAM. However, there was no significant difference for the risk of "secondary" cesarean section between the two groups (*P* = 0.090), whereas none of the secondary cesarean sections was reportedly carried out for an impending UR. Their observation of a higher primary cesarean section rate after LM compared with following an OM can partially result from confounding and performance bias as there has been an overall increase in the cesarean section rates over the last two or three decades, which is also the "era of laparoscopy," making laparoscopy the preferred approach to perform a myomectomy. However, the latter may induce altered recommendations on delivery mode because of surgeon anxiety during their learning curve for laparoscopic suturing and presuming that laparoscopic uterine wall closure may entail a higher risk of UR compared with the open approach. The available evidence in the literature does not contraindicate a childbirth per viam naturalem with a previous myomectomy, regardless of the surgical technique [5]. However, this requires caution as there is a paucity of data to support this belief and therefore the evidence is graded as low.

Furthermore, the relationship between the mechanical stress during labor and event of UR remains unclear as most of the reported cases of UR following a myomectomy occurred before the onset of labor as opposed to following a previous cesarean section where it happens mainly during labor [2, 4, 5, 9]. As the majority of the myomectomies are performed in the corporeal part of the uterus versus a lower uterine segment incision during a cesarean section, this could partly explain the aforementioned difference. There is a lack of research on how to monitor women with a history of myomectomy in their third trimester, when most of the URs occur. Planning a cesarean section at early term may not be effective to avoid the risk for UR, whereas it is still unclear how to identify those who are at risk [1].

Pistofidis et al. reported an early UR at 24 weeks' gestation which involved a twin pregnancy and suggested that even though a single case would not allow firm recommendations to be made, it is reasonable to advise against a multiple pregnancy after having undergone an LM [10]. Awareness to avoid a multiple pregnancy with a history of myomectomy especially should require more attention when assisted reproductive treatments are offered to this patient population, thereby preferring a single embryo transfer in in vitro fertilization and avoiding ovarian stimulation in intrauterine insemination [10].

The literature is scarce around the correct myometrial thickness post-myomectomy for vaginal delivery attempts, but recommendations on thickness of the lower uterine segment in gravid women who have a history of cesarean section have suggested a threshold of 2.8 mm [11]. Some authors have prospectively evaluated the outcome of TOL after a previous LM achieving a vaginal delivery and have reported success rates of 79 to 80% [12, 13]. TOL

may be considered a feasible and relatively safe option as compared with vaginal birth after cesarean section, but it should be executed only at a center with emergency operating facilities as the risk of UR is very unpredictable.

Surgical Aspects

Nowadays, most cases of intramural and subserosal fibroids are removed by a minimally invasive approach, although sometimes open TAM is the most optimal route (for example, when dealing with very large fibroids) [1]. In addition to the surgical approach, the extent of uterine incision, characteristics of myomas removed, hemostasis, and suturing technique(s) at the time of myomectomy have been proposed to be considered in determining the risk factors of UR [1, 7, 14].

A recent literature review by Nahum and Pham [15] suggests that there is heterogeneity on reporting the true UR rate after a TAM as often factors deemed important for assessing the risk of UR are not delineated whereas most studies are focused on LMs only [2]. Another retrospective analysis, of 92 post-TAM pregnancies beyond 20 weeks' gestation over a 16-year period, reported that whilst 54 of these women were allowed to labor, 45 achieved a vaginal delivery with no cases of UR whereas the most common indication for intrapartum cesarean section was poor labor progress [16]. Similarly, there is scarcity of clear data on UR rate after laparoscopic/robotic-assisted myomectomy, but as UR has been reported to occur as late as 8 years after an LM, there is a need for further investigations with long-term follow-up [15, 17]. Several authors have reported on UR rates after LM, ranging from 0 to 1% [18–20]. One spontaneous UR at 33 weeks' gestation following an LM was reported in a multicenter study from Italy from a cohort of 386 patients, which involved an 8-cm adenomyoma [14].

Interestingly, one of the largest series of LM from nearly 20 years of data in a single institution could not identify any correlation between their UR cases (3/523 deliveries, 0.6%) and the characteristics of the myomas removed (size, location, and number) [20]. However, the retrospective nature of study does imply that complete data were missing on specific surgical techniques, including the learning curve – both during the uptake of laparoscopy and the individual variation in skill set alongside this learning curve among the 20 surgeons involved U.S.—and the associated complications which may have affected the analyzed outcome. Nonetheless, the published data in the literature suggest that the suturing technique, or whether the surgery was performed in a teaching hospital or a non-teaching hospital, is not associated with an increased risk [5]. From a clinically logical point of view, a large intramural location is more likely to implicate a risk factor for UR as this would involve full myometrial thickness. Given the difficulty to achieve evidence from a randomized trial in assessing the outcomes after myomectomy because of obstetrical issues, the retrospective cohorts on a large scale can help tailor the clinical practice when used within the limits of the clinical characteristics of the individual patient.

The residual strength of the myometrium after a myomectomy procedure is determined by a combination of factors consisting of the number of fibroids excised, their size and location, identification of a correct cleavage plane, entry into the uterine cavity, and completeness of the excision. In regard to adenomyomas, the depth and extent of the lesion, the time to local inflammation exposure, and the amount of extirpation play pivotal roles in weakening of the uterine muscle. As adenomyosis infiltrates the normal myometrium, its excision subtracts myometrial mass from the total uterine volume, therefore producing scars with reduced tensile strength [10, 14]. In addition to this, excessive cauterization, suboptimal uterine wall approximation, postoperative hematoma formation, and wound infection can compromise the uterine musculature strength and form a risk factor for UR during pregnancy following a myomectomy [2, 4, 10, 18].

High-frequency electrosurgery is a commonly used surgical tool in the form of monopolar and bipolar devices and has the advantage of reduced blood loss when compared with cold knife/cold scissors. However, as cauterization heat leads to denaturation of proteins and clots, it causes high fibrin deposition and highly cohesive agglomerates affecting angiogenesis, adhesion formation, and tissue healing, whereas the discoloration makes the margins of the dissection planes of resection less clear, which also can lead to wound dehiscence. Studies have demonstrated delayed wound healing in tissues handled with electrocautery compared with the cold-knife surgery as high collagen concentrations with fewer smooth muscle fibers have been found near the UR areas when histological examination is carried out in cases of previous myomectomies [9]. Although there is a trend in encountering more URs when electrocautery is used, no statistically significant difference has been seen when comparison is made between bipolar versus monopolar or between electrocautery versus none [2]. Alternative energy sources such as ultrasonic energy can be considered.

The presence of neuropeptide substance P and vasoactive intestinal peptide in the pseudocapsule of uterine myomas may affect wound healing and myometrial function in subsequent pregnancy. These can be preserved by avoiding excessive coagulation to protect the pseudocapsule neurovascular bundle and by using the intracapsular myomectomy technique proposed by Tinelli et al., in which a subserous or intramural myoma is enucleated through an opening in the fibrovascular capsule whilst using a selective, low-energy hemostasis on the pseudocapsule vessels; this allows the myometrial bed to collapse after the enucleation without excessive bleeding [21, 22].

A good hemostasis after fibroid enucleation is important to facilitate optimal healing. Severe postoperative pain following a myomectomy can indicate a hematoma of a hysterotomy wound, which can be diagnosed by ultrasound scan [4]. Diluted vasopressin can be used around the fibroid wall (extracapsular) to minimize the bleeding during dissection, whereas a selective diathermy of larger vessels only with a bipolar is preferable to monopolar. Excessive coagulation and carbonization, especially of the micro bleeders, should be avoided [9, 10, 18].

Furthermore, correct suturing technique is paramount to achieve good wound healing. Excessive tension sutures or incomplete approximation of edge-to-edge seromuscular planes can be a risk factor for tissue necrosis, increased scarring, and collagen deposition which can contribute to a weak myometrium exposed to the risk of rupture during pregnancy and labor. Figure-of-eight sutures or separated single sutures are preferred in the deep myometrial layers, whereas continuous sutures can be used in the superficial layers. The literature reports that, depending on the depth of fibroid into the myometrium, single- or double-layer sutures can be used [19]. Intramural fibroid enucleation often requires a double-layer suture, especially when more than 50% of the myometrial thickness is involved [4, 10, 18]. The potential value of multiple-layer stitching was reflected by the multicenter, case-control study by Bujold et al., who suggested that a single-layer closure of the lower uterine segment is associated with a twofold risk of UR during labor when compared with a double-layer closure [23]. Parker et al. reported on 19 UR cases following LM, the mean diameter of myoma was 4.5 cm (range of 1 to 11 cm), and only three cases were sutured in multiple-layer; moreover, in all but two cases, electrosurgery was used for hemostasis [9]. However, others have found no association between single-layer closure and UR [2, 24, 25].

In cases where there is an inevitable gap between the edges of the myometrial incision, such as after excision of a large intramural fibroid with concomitant focal adenomyosis, postoperative follow-up becomes paramount and it is good practice to make a comment about this in the patient's discharge notes [26]. In the follow-up process, Tepper et al. highlighted the importance of ultrasonographic features of solid hyperplastic myometrial tissue which has the potential to be misinterpreted as a remaining fibroid or focal hematoma [27].

Absorbable poligleacaprone monofilament, polydioxanone suture (PDS), and polyglicolic vicryl 0, 1, or 2–0 are often used. Nowadays, barbed sutures, such as Stratfix®, are used by some for continuous suturing of the myometrial layers which not only can reduce operative time but also can increase the tensile strength of the defect. The suture pedicles should be inside the wound, and the serosal layer can be closed by performing mattress suturing, which can minimize the rough area left and thereby reduce the risk of adhesions [4]. Utilization of hemostatic oxidized regenerated cellulose or other physical anti-adhesive barriers has been documented by some but there is no conclusive evidence about their effectiveness at present.

RECURRENCE

There is no clear evidence in the literature regarding risk factors for recurrence of uterine leiomyomas (ULs) following their surgical removal. The overall recurrence rates reported vary from 14.5 to 31.6%, and the cumulative risk of UL recurrence at 60 months ranges from 16.7 to 52.8%, reflecting heterogeneous methodological approaches in defining a UL recurrence as not all recurrences are symptomatic and therefore have a debatable clinical significance [28–30]. The cumulative probability of reoperation for recurrent UL has been suggested by some to define a clinically significant recurrence [29]. Others have suggested an imaging-based diagnosis of a UL of at least 2 cm in diameter in combination with reappearance of fibroid-related symptoms [30].

Commonly Proposed Potential Risk Factors

The *total number of removed ULs* has been suggested to be inversely correlated with the risk of recurrence giving an increased risk when a higher number is removed. Therefore, patients with more than two or three ULs should be informed about the potential risk of recurrence. A recent meta-analysis from a multicenter cohort ($N = 2566$) found similar UL recurrence

rates after laparoscopic and transabdominal OM in women ages 18 to 44 years when not more than five ULs were removed, but the UL recurrence was higher in the laparoscopic group when myomectomy involved more than five ULs, including a higher rate of reoperation for ULs in the latter group when more than three myomas were removed at index surgery [31]. The relationship between a higher number of ULs removed and increased recurrence rate has been echoed by other authors [30, 32, 33]. This relationship could be explained by the difficulty faced in the removal of multiple ULs, which can include tiny ULs with multifocal small UL nuclei resulting in continuous development of new symptomatic lesions. Furthermore, another causal relationship is a higher potential of the myometrium to produce leiomyomas as myometrial cells can undergo spontaneous chromosomal rearrangements to initiate proliferation of myoma cells in unicellular growth [30].

Emanuel evaluated the probability of avoiding recurrent surgery after a hysteroscopic removal of submucosal ULs and found that it drops from 90.3% in a normal-size uterine with not more than two ULs to 64.8% when the uterus is enlarged and three or more ULs are involved [34]. About 50% of the patients with incomplete resections required surgery within 2 years. The latter is often associated with a greater than 50% intramural penetration of ULs, representing FIGO type 3 ULs. Aksoy et al. showed similar results in their cohort of LM and OM with a follow-up ranging from 2 to 8 years that 17.7% recurred and a higher number of ULs were involved in the recurring group [28].

Pregnancy after myomectomy was shown by the same authors to increase the risk of recurrence by 2.8 fold [28]. This risk factor was suggested by Yoo et al. as well [29]. Sex steroids and growth factors influence myometrial proliferation. The literature includes evidence that estrogen increases cell responsiveness to progesterone but that the number of progesterone receptors is elevated around ULs. A combined effect of increased growth factors and estrogen and progesterone during pregnancy is potentially the attributing factor [35]. However, some authors have also reported a reduced risk for reoperation among patients who achieved subsequent parity [32, 33, 36]. The mechanism for the latter relationship remains unclear, but postpartum uterine remodeling has been suggested to lead to selective apoptosis of the residual small lesions [37].

Size or location of the ULs as a risk factor for recurrence has not been consistently reported [28, 38].

Surgical approach in relation to recurrence rate is also not consistent in the literature. Some authors have reported a higher recurrence rate following an LM [30]. At 8 years of follow-up, Kotani et al. reported a cumulative recurrence rate of 76.2% in LM versus 63.4% in the group of OM, suggesting that fewer residual (smaller) myoma masses were the contributing factor for the lower recurrence rates in OM [36]. Their Cox hazard testing also revealed that an absence of postoperative gestation significantly contributed to the recurrence rate of UL, as discussed above [36]. On the other hand, a retrospective analysis of 122 LMs and 38 cases requiring a minilaparotomic myomectomy with a minimum follow-up of 2 years showed no significant difference in the recurrence rates [39]. Relative contraindications for a minimally invasive approach for myomectomy, including the presence of an intramural myoma of more than 10 to 12 cm in size or more than four ULs in different sites of the uterus (or both), have been reported [37].

Preoperative gonadotropin-releasing hormone (GnRH) agonist therapy was found by the same authors to be the only significant recurrence factor after myomectomy [39]. Analyzing the recurrence risk after GnRH agonist pretreatment in robotically assisted myomectomy patients, Sangha et al. reported an overall symptomatic recurrence rate of 14.4% in a cohort of 118 patients with at least 2 years' follow-up with a significantly higher recurrence rate in the GnRH agonist group; 65% of the recurrences had received GnRH agonist, whereas 90% without recurrence were not given GnRH agonists [38]. Consistently, GnRH agonist use was significantly higher in the reoperation group (56% vs. 9%) [38]. Although GnRH agonists have been associated with a reduction in volume of a fibroid uterus and with increased hemoglobin and hematocrit levels, their role in shrinking the ULs may not be beneficial when the risk of recurrence is measured against their presumed advantages. Another factor that potentially leads to an indirectly increased risk of recurrence is that GnRH agonists given for more than 6 to 8 weeks can obscure the tissue planes between ULs and myometrium, resulting in a more challenging complete enucleation of the ULs [40]. A similar correlation with regard to preoperative use of the selective progesterone receptor modulator, ulipristal acetate, was proposed recently [41]. However, there remains a paucity of data on this potential correlation with mixed results, which does not allow us to ascertain these risks [42].

Long-term efficacy of adenomyomectomy is rarely reported. A recent report published a significantly lower recurrence rate when post-surgically a combined treatment with GnRH agonist and a levonorgestrel-releasing intrauterine system (LNG-IUS) or oral contraceptive is given compared with GnRH agonists only [43]. In addition, a significantly higher recurrence rate was found in this subgroup of patients who had coexistent endometriosis. Their results also suggested a superiority of an open adeno-myomectomy as surgical approach when more than 5 cm adenomyoma is involved to facilitate a complete excision [43]. These results need to be interpreted with caution as further studies with a larger subset of patients are required to confirm these findings.

Vascular occlusion. With regard to optimal hemostatic technique in LM, the role of temporary bilateral uterine artery occlusion alone or in combination with utero-ovarian vessel occlusion compared with no vascular occlusion was assessed in 200 patients undergoing an LM. No difference in recurrence rates was found at 30-month follow-up. Furthermore, no statistical difference was noted in anti-Müllerian hormone between the groups preoperatively or at 3, 6, and 12 months postoperatively [44]. A better hemostasis during the myomectomy may allow a more efficient eradication of smaller residual ULs. However, there is currently no convincing biological rationale for reduction in recurrence rate associated with uterine artery occlusion at the index surgery. Sanders et al. analyzed 25 studies involving 2871 patients on uterine artery occlusion at the time of myomectomy and reported to have found a significantly reduced fibroid recurrence rate [45]. However, these results should be interpreted with caution as fibroid recurrence was evaluated as a secondary outcome whereas only a small number of the included studies reported data on recurrence rates and the follow-up time was relatively short. It is noteworthy that there are no data on long-term reproductive implications.

Other Factors to Be Considered

Age. The relationship between age at index surgery and UL recurrence is not well established. Whereas some report a lower recurrence rate when index surgery was performed at an age of less than 35 years, others have reported a decreased recurrence rate in patients operated after the age of 35 years and some have found no relationship [29, 30, 32].

Early menarche is a known risk factor for fibroid development. However, its role in UL recurrence following myomectomy has not been well investigated [37].

Race constitutes an important risk factor for UL development; African-American and African women have a high incidence of UL by the age of 35 years. Akin to these observational findings, an increased risk for UL recurrence after myomectomy was found in this subgroup of women [37].

Genetics. Although some specific genetic alterations were shown to be linked to UL growth, the possible role of inheritance pattern in UL recurrence needs to be elucidated [28, 37].

Certain histopathological characteristics have been suggested to be linked to a higher risk of recurrence. ULs with higher mitotic activity, epithelioid differentiation, or cellular leiomyomas can present as a relative challenge to the clinicians when fertility is desired. ULs with myxoid changes, characterized by accumulation of glycosaminoglycans rich in hyaluronic acid, present as a focal finding in about 12% of all benign ULs [32]. Very few authors have reported the outcomes following myomectomy for these non-ordinary ULs [32, 46, 47]. The clinical behavior of these ULs is still unknown and contradictory. Therefore, a long duration of follow-up is important because of their potential of recurrence, although a hysterectomy should be performed as first-line treatment if fertility preservation is not an issue.

Obesity has been suggested by some to increase the risk of UL recurrence. The hormonal imbalance caused by increased peripheral aromatase activity is potentially an attributing factor.

CONCLUSION

Rising myomectomy rates worldwide represent an increase in uterine scarring leading to an increased risk of UR during a subsequent pregnancy, which generally occurs in the third trimester or during labor and delivery. The reported incidence of UR after myomectomy is low and this likely reflects the cautionary practice patterns which include measures to prevent UR. Although there is a lack of evidence regarding entry into the cavity, many obstetricians seem to be influenced by this when deciding for mode of delivery. Enucleation of intramural fibroid(s) has been found to be more commonly associated with the UR cases after myomectomy. No statistically significant difference has been reported in surgical approach for TAM and LM. Prudence dictates that preventive measures for UR can consist of using correct and preferably double-layer suturing, limiting the use of electrosurgery and

minimizing the risk for hematoma formation and postoperative infections. Current evidence suggests that TOL is at least as safe as it is after cesarean section and can be considered a feasible and possible safe option under optimal obstetrical care facilities.

The choice of management of UL recurrence with distinctive symptoms and age groups can be tailored to the individual patient. The number of ULs removed at index surgery has been consistently shown to be an independent risk factor for UL recurrence. Women undergoing a myomectomy and having more than two to five ULs should be adequately counselled about this risk. Several authors have suggested a superior role of OM when four or more ULs are involved to reduce the recurrence risk. In addition, a complete excision, identification of a correct cleavage plane, and avoidance of excessive cauterization with high-frequency electrosurgery are the other main factors to prevent the undermining of residual myometrium during a myomectomy.

The literature classically demonstrates a publication bias due to systematic under-reporting of iatrogenic complications, which calls for more solid scientific evidence by means of randomized controlled trials. In addition to this, this chapter contains information appearing in English publications only and mostly consisting of observational studies, which therefore can represent a selection bias.

REFERENCES

1. Gambacorti-Passerini ZM, Penati C, Carli A, Accordino F, Ferrari L, Berghella V, et al. Vaginal birth after prior myomectomy. *Eur J Obstet Gynecol Reprod Biol.* 2018;231:198–203.

2. Gambacorti-Passerini Z, Gimovsky AC, Locatelli A, Berghella V. Trial of labor after myomectomy and uterine rupture: a systematic review. *Acta Obstet Gynecol Scand.* 2016;95(7):724–734.

3. Landon MB, Hauth JC, Leveno KJ, Spong CY, Leindecker S, Varner MW, et al. Maternal and perinatal outcomes associated with a trial of labor after prior cesarean delivery. *N Engl J Med.* 2004;351(25):2581–2589.

4. Tanos V, Toney ZA. Uterine scar rupture – Prediction, prevention, diagnosis, and management. *Best Pract Res Clin Obstet Gynaecol.* 2019;59:115–131.

5. Claeys J, Hellendoorn I, Hamerlynck T, Bosteels J, Weyers S. The risk of uterine rupture after myomectomy: a systematic review of the literature and meta-analysis. *Gynecol Surg.* 2014;11:197–206.

6. Landon MB, Lynch CD. Optimal timing and mode of delivery after cesarean with previous classical incision or myomectomy: a review of the data. *Semin Perinatol.* 2011;35(5):257–261.

7. Gyamfi-Bannerman C, Gilbert S, Landon MB, Spong CY, Rouse DJ, Varner MW, et al. Risk of uterine rupture and placenta accreta with prior uterine surgery outside of the lower segment. *Obstet Gynecol.* 2012;120(6):1332–1337.

8. Rosen MG, Dickinson JC, Westhoff CL. Vaginal birth after cesarean: a meta-analysis of morbidity and mortality. *Obstet Gynecol.* 1991;77(3):465–470.

9. Parker WH, Einarsson J, Istre O, Dubuisson JB. Risk factors for uterine rupture after laparoscopic myomectomy. *J Minim Invasive Gynecol.* 2010;17(5):551–554.

10. Pistofidis G, Makrakis E, Balinakos P, Dimitriou E, Bardis N, Anaf V. Report of 7 uterine rupture cases after laparoscopic myomectomy: update of the literature. *J Minim Invasive Gynecol.* 2012;19(6):762–767.

11. Bujold E, Jastrow N, Simoneau J, Brunet S, Gauthier RJ. Prediction of complete uterine rupture by sonographic evaluation of the lower uterine segment. *Am J Obstet Gynecol.* 2009;201(3):320.e321–326.

12. Makino S, Tanaka T, Itoh S, Kumakiri J, Takeuchi H, Takeda S. Prospective comparison of delivery outcomes of vaginal vagina births after cesarean section versus laparoscopic myomectomy. *J Obstet Gynaecol Res.* 2008;34(6):952–956.

13. Kumakiri J, Takeuchi H, Itoh S, Kitade M, Kikuchi I, Shimanuki H, et al. Prospective evaluation for the feasibility and safety of vaginal birth after laparoscopic myomectomy. *J Minim Invasive Gynecol.* 2008;15(4):420–424.

14. Sizzi O, Rossetti A, Malzoni M, Minelli L, La Grotta F, Soranna L, et al. Italian multicenter study on complications of laparoscopic myomectomy. *J Minim Invasive Gynecol.* 2007;14(4):453–462.

15. Nahum GG, Pham KQ. *Uterine rupture in pregnancy 2018*; http://emedicine.medscape.com/refarticle-srch/275854-overview, 2010.

16. Kelly BA, Bright P, Mackenzie IZ. Does the surgical approach used for myomectomy influence the morbidity in subsequent pregnancy? *J Obstet Gynaecol.* 2008;28(1):77–81.

17. Zaami S, Montanari Vergallo G, Malvasi A, Marinelli E. Uterine rupture during induced labor after myomectomy and risk of lawsuits. *Eur Rev Med Pharmacol Sci.* 2019;23(4):1379–1381.

18. Landi S, Fiaccavento A, Zaccoletti R, Barbieri F, Syed R, Minelli L. Pregnancy outcomes and deliveries after laparoscopic myomectomy. *J Am Assoc Gynecol Laparosc.* 2003;10(2):177–181.

19. Malzoni M, Sizzi O, Rossetti A, Imperato F. Laparoscopic myomectomy: a report of 982 procedures. *Surg Technol Int.* 2006;15:123–129.

20. Koo YJ, Lee JK, Lee YK, Kwak DW, Lee IH, Lim KT, et al. Pregnancy outcomes and risk factors for uterine rupture after laparoscopic myomectomy: A single-center experience and literature review. *J Minim Invasive Gynecol.* 2015;22(6):1022–1028.

21. Malvasi A, Tinelli A, Cavallotti C, Morroni M, Tsin DA, Nezhat C, et al. Distribution of substance P (SP) and vasoactive intestinal peptide (VIP) in pseudocapsules of uterine fibroids. *Peptides.* 2011;32(2):327–332.

22. Tinelli A, Hurst BS, Hudelist G, Tsin DA, Stark M, Mettler L, et al. Laparoscopic myomectomy focusing on the myoma pseudocapsule: technical and outcome reports. *Hum Reprod.* 2012;27(2):427–435.

23. Bujold E, Goyet M, Marcoux S, Brassard N, Cormier B, Hamilton E, et al. The role of uterine closure in the risk of uterine rupture. *Obstet Gynecol.* 2010;116(1):43–50.

24. Durnwald C, Mercer B. Uterine rupture, perioperative and perinatal morbidity after single-layer and double-layer closure at cesarean delivery. *Am J Obstet Gynecol.* 2003;189(4):925–929.

25. Paul PG, Koshy AK, Thomas T. Pregnancy outcomes following laparoscopic myomectomy and single-layer myometrial closure. *Hum Reprod.* 2006;21(12):3278–3281.

26. Tanos V, Berry KE. Benign and malignant pathology of the uterus. *Best Pract Res Clin Obstet Gynaecol.* 2018;46:12–30.

27. Tepper R, Beyth Y, Klein Z, Aviram R. Postmyomectomy sonographic imaging: uterus remodeling and scar repair. *Arch Gynecol Obstet.* 2009;280(3):509–511.

28. Aksoy RT, Tokmak A, Guzel AI, Yildirim G, Kokanali MK, Doganay M. Effect of pregnancy on recurrence of symptomatic uterine myomas in women who underwent myomectomy. *Hippokratia.* 2018;22(3):122–126.

29. Yoo EH, Lee PI, Huh CY, Kim DH, Lee BS, Lee JK, et al. Predictors of leiomyoma recurrence after laparoscopic myomectomy. *J Minim Invasive Gynecol.* 2007;14(6):690–697.

30. Radosa MP, Owsianowski Z, Mothes A, Weisheit A, Vorwergk J, Hudelist G, Tsin DA, Stark M, Mettler L, et al. Long-term risk of fibroid recurrence after laparoscopic myomectomy. *Eur J Obstet Gynecol Reprod Biol.* 2014;180:35–39.

31. Ming X, Ran XT, Li N, Nie D, Li ZY. Risk of recurrence of uterine leiomyomas following laparoscopic myomectomy compared with open myomectomy. *Arch Gynecol Obstet.* 2020;301:235–242.

32. Sukur YE, Kankaya D, Ates C, Sertcelik A, Cengiz SD, Aytac R. Clinical and histopathologic predictors of reoperation due to recurrence of leiomyoma after laparotomic myomectomy. *Int J Gynaecol Obstet.* 2015;129(1):75–78.

33. Hanafi M. Predictors of leiomyoma recurrence after myomectomy. *Obstet Gynecol.* 2005;105(4):877–881.

34. Emanuel MH. Hysteroscopy and the treatment of uterine fibroids. *Best Pract Res Clin Obstet Gynaecol.* 2015;29(7):920–929.

35. Pavone D, Clemenza S, Sorbi F, Fambrini M, Petraglia F. Epidemiology and risk factors of uterine fibroids. *Best Pract Res Clin Obstet Gynaecol.* 2018;46:3–11.

36. Kotani Y, Tobiume T, Fujishima R, Shigeta M, Takaya H, Nakai, et al. Recurrence of uterine myoma after myomectomy: Open myomectomy versus laparoscopic myomectomy. *J Obstet Gynaecol Res.* 2018;44(2):298–302.

37. Donnez J, Dolmans MM. Uterine fibroid management: from the present to the future. *Hum Reprod.* 2016;22(6):665–686.

38. Sangha R, Katukuri V, Palmer M, Khangura RK. Recurrence after robotic myomectomy: is it associated with use of GnRH agonist? *J Robot Surgery.* 2016;10(3):245–249.

39. Shin DG, Yoo HJ, Lee YA, Kwon IS, Lee KH. Recurrence factors and reproductive outcomes of laparoscopic myomectomy and minilaparotomic myomectomy for uterine leiomyomas. *Obstet Gynecol Sci.* 2017;60(2):193–199.

40. Saridogan E. Surgical treatment of fibroids in heavy menstrual bleeding. *Womens Health (Lond).* 2016;12(1):53–62.

41. Mallick R, Oxley S, Odejinmi F. The use of ulipristal acetate (Esmya) prior to laparoscopic myomectomy: help or hindrance? *Gynecol Minim Invasive Ther.* 2019;8(2):62–66.

42. Lethaby A, Puscasiu L, Vollenhoven B. Preoperative medical therapy before surgery for uterine fibroids. *Cochrane Database Syst Rev.* 2017;11:CD000547.

43. Zhu L, Chen S, Che X, Xu P, Huang X, Zhang X. Comparisons of the efficacy and recurrence of adenomyomectomy for severe uterine diffuse adenomyosis via laparotomy versus laparoscopy: a long-term result in a single institution. *J Pain Res.* 2019;12:1917–1924.

44. Jin L, Ji L, Shao M, Hu M. Laparoscopic myomectomy with temporary bilateral uterine artery and utero-ovarian vessels occlusion compared with traditional surgery for uterine fibroids: blood loss and recurrence. *Gynecol Obstetric Invest.* 2019;84(6):548–554.

45. Sanders AP, Chan WV, Tang J, Murji A. Surgical outcomes after uterine artery occlusion at the time of myomectomy: systematic review and meta-analysis. *Fertil Steril.* 2019;111(4):816–827.e814.

46. Sahin H, Karatas F, Coban G, Özen Ö, Erdem Ö, Onan MA, et al. Uterine smooth muscle tumor of uncertain malignant potential: fertility and clinical outcomes. *J Gynecol Oncol.* 2019;30(4):e54.

47. Guntupalli SR, Ramirez PT, Anderson ML, Milam MR, Bodurka DC, Malpica A. Uterine smooth muscle tumor of uncertain malignant potential: a retrospective analysis. *Gynecol Oncol.* 2009;113(3):324–326.

15 Secondary Hemorrhage after Myomectomy

Latika Chawla

CONTENTS

Myomectomy is a surgical procedure well known for its morbidity due to the potential for serious intraoperative and postoperative complications. Immediate complications include intraoperative hemorrhage, requirement for blood transfusion [1], risk of hysterectomy due to uncontrollable bleeding, and conversion from a minimally invasive route to laparotomy. Short-term complications include febrile morbidity, bleeding, infection, and thromboembolism [2]. Long-term complications include pelvic adhesions [3], post-myomectomy intrauterine adhesions, recurrent fibroids [4], and associated risk of uterine rupture in subsequent pregnancies [5, 6]. Intraoperative blood loss is deemed one of the most significant of the lot; thus, principles of myomectomy and measures (both preoperative and intraoperative) to decrease intraoperative blood loss [7] have been extensively described in the literature.

SECONDARY HEMORRHAGE FOLLOWING MYOMECTOMY

Secondary hemorrhage after myomectomy, though rare, is conceivably a life-threatening complication of the procedure. It happens usually when it is least expected. Evidence regarding secondary hemorrhage after myomectomy and its etiology and management is sparse; the evidence is limited to a few case reports and case series and its incidence has yet not been documented in the literature. Secondary hemorrhage after any surgical procedure usually happens after 7–10 days of surgery and is most often linked to local infection. It may be of varying intensity from minimal spotting to life-threatening exsanguination. However, most evidence related to secondary hemorrhage following myomectomy is related to the development of pseudoaneurysms of the uterine artery. These have been reported as early as 7 days [8] to as late as 97 days [9] after surgery.

Pseudoaneurysm is a complication of vascular injury secondary to trauma or inflammation. It is a blood-filled cavity that communicates with lumen of the artery because of a focal deficiency in all three layers of the arterial wall [10, 11]. Pseudoaneurysms have been reported after uterine curettage, abortion, normal vaginal delivery, and cesarean section [10, 12–14]. A uterine artery pseudoaneurysm is a rare complication of myomectomy. Removal of the myoma or postmyomectomy local site infection can very rarely lead to disruption of a small part of the three-layered wall of the uterine artery with extravasation of blood and formation of a pseudosac in the myometrium. As more blood dissects into the myometrium, the pseudosac enlarges and can communicate with the uterine cavity and its rupture can lead to torrential bleeding per vaginum [15]. The exact incidence of uterine artery aneurysm after myomectomy is unknown [15] and these may be largely underreported as their presence may be realized only when they lead to hemorrhage.

MANAGEMENT OF SECONDARY HEMORRHAGE

As a dictum, when a patient presents with severe bleeding, management includes hemodynamic resuscitation, stabilization, and control of the source of bleeding. Tranexamic acid can be tried initially for control of bleeding. If bleeding does not respond to conservative approaches, conventional surgery and pelvic angioembolization must be kept in mind. As evidence suggests, for any patient with secondary hemorrhage after myomectomy (hysteroscopic, laparotomy, or laparoscopic), a high index of suspicion for a pseudoaneurysm must be kept in mind. On ultrasonography, a pseudoaneurysm appears like a well-defined hypoechoic/anechoic cystic structure which may be associated with a hematoma at the previous myomectomy site [16] with turbulent blood flow on color Doppler. However, 3D computed tomography (CT) angiography is the preferred modality for a more accurate diagnosis of a pseudoaneurysm [17]. Once the diagnosis of a pseudoaneurysm has been established, management by transarterial embolization of the pseudoaneurysm should be discussed in detail with the patient [15–20]. Even in the absence of a pseudoaneurysm, if there is an obvious bleeder on angiography, embolization of the uterine artery has been shown to be a safe and effective method in stopping hemorrhage from its pseudoaneurysm/bleeding branch, as shown in various past studies. At the time of embolization, it is important that along with all the major feeding vessels, collateral supply from the opposite uterine artery is also taken care of to prevent a recurrence and rebleed.

The first report of transarterial embolization for secondary hemorrhage after myomectomy was made by Zorlu et al. [18], where the patient was embolized on postoperative day 7. On angiography, the authors found bilaterally dilated uterine arteries with complex dispersion of distal parts of the artery on the side of removal of myoma. However, no obvious pseudoaneurysm was described. Bilateral uterine arteries were successfully embolized. Pseudoaneurysm after myomectomy was first reported by Higón et al. [19] in a patient who had secondary hemorrhage 40 days after laparoscopic myomectomy. It was embolized successfully by using gelatin sponge pledgets. The patient resumed normal menstrual cycle after embolization.

A retrospective review from Korea [20] described the efficacy and safety of uterine artery embolization in eight patients who had hemorrhage after myomectomy. The time interval between myomectomy and the embolization was from 0 to 47 days with a median interval of 1.5 days. Two patients who underwent transcervical and hysteroscopic myomectomy had to be embolized on the very same day as surgery because of persistent vaginal bleeding and low hemoglobin levels. Two patients who underwent open myomectomy were embolized on day 1, and another patient had to undergo embolization on day 2 after surgery. Three patients had secondary hemorrhage after open myomectomy on days 22, 28, and 47. Two of them were hemodynamically unstable. Pelvic angiography of the eight patients revealed hypervascular staining without obvious bleeding focus in five patients, active extravasation of contrast from the uterine artery in two patients, and a pseudoaneurysm in one patient. Peritoneal hematoma was noted on CT in one patient. Uterine artery embolization was technically and clinically successful in all eight patients. Gelatin sponge particles were used in all eight patients. All patients resumed normal menstrual cycles after the procedure.

In another retrospective review, Takeda et al. [15] described outcomes of 854 patients who underwent laparoscopic-assisted myomectomy. Nine of the 854 patients who underwent laparoscopic-assisted myomectomy developed a pseudoaneurysm. Patients were routinely subjected to postoperative ultrasounds. Pseudoaneurysms were diagnosed without any symptoms on a median postoperative day 8 in eight of the patients. One patient, who remained undiagnosed, presented with torrential secondary hemorrhage on day 79 of myomectomy. Eight patients underwent successful embolization. Spontaneous resolution of the pseudoaneurysm was noted in one of the patients. A decision to not intervene was taken only after discussion with the patient and her family.

Fertility issues following uterine artery embolization are always a concern. Since patients may want fertility after myomectomy, they should be adequately counselled prior to the procedure. Takeda et al. [16] reported successful embolization of a uterine artery pseudoaneurysm in a patient who developed hemorrhage 79 days after laparoscopic myomectomy. The patient could conceive naturally following the embolization and had one spontaneous abortion followed by a successful delivery by cesarean section. Another report of successful pregnancy following embolization was made by Ito et al. [21]. The patient underwent embolization for secondary hemorrhage after hysteroscopic myomectomy 22 days following the surgery. She had two successful deliveries following the embolization. Of the eight patients who underwent embolization as reported by Takeda et al. [15], five were desirous of fertility; four of the five conceived, resulting in three live births and two spontaneous abortions. However, larger long-term follow-up studies would be required before we can consider angioembolization as a useful fertility-sparing method, and patients need to be counseled in detail about the limited evidence regarding fertility issues related to uterine artery embolization.

Pelvic angioembolization (uterine/internal iliac artery) has been accepted as a standard method of treatment of postpartum hemorrhage and for management of fibroids [21]. According to the limited evidence available to date, transarterial embolization has proven to be a safe, effective, and reliable modality for management of secondary hemorrhage following myomectomy as well. Nonetheless, in clinical setups where facility for intervention radiology is not available or if the patient is hemodynamically unstable or not expected to maintain intravascular volume/vitals for the time duration required for the procedure, laparotomy may be required for hemorrhage control. However, securing control of the source of bleeding may be challenging as it might require opening up the myomectomy site, evacuating myomectomy site hematoma, and digging in deep in the myometrium to secure the bleeder and may eventually end up in a hysterectomy. Bilateral uterine artery ligation or internal iliac artery ligation may also be considered as viable options. Embolization of the uterine artery has definite advantages as it avoids morbidity associated with laparotomy, does not require anesthesia, entails less pain and decreased hospital stay, and preserves the uterus [15].

However, pelvic angioembolization has a unique set of complications. Non-ischemic complications include allergic reaction to contrast media, femoral hematoma at the puncture site, pelvic hematoma, dissection of the internal iliac or uterine artery, pulmonary embolism, and post-embolization syndrome. Post-embolization syndrome is a common side effect of embolization that includes nausea, vomiting, pelvic pain, and fever. It is a self-limiting condition and usually resolves within 3–4 days of the procedure. Ischemic complications occur as a result of non-target embolization because of migration of the embolizing material to other arteries via the anastomotic channels [22]. This includes buttock claudication, acute lower limb ischemia [23, 24], transient sciatic nerve ischemic neuropathy [25], and rarely labial, vaginal, cervical, buttock, or bladder necrosis [26–28].

A case of secondary hemorrhage after hysteroscopic myomectomy is being described here. A 34-year-old woman underwent resection of submucous myoma of 4×5 cm^2 and then presented with intractable bleeding per vaginum 3 days after hysteroscopic resection. Magnetic resonance imaging showed a large hematoma in the cavity (Figure 15.1). Since the bleeding was not being controlled by medical management, she underwent uterine artery embolization and recovered well. Figures 15.2 and 15.3 show pre- and post-embolization pictures. (Case and image are courtesy of Dr. Rooma Sinha.)

CONCLUSION

Delayed hemorrhage after myomectomy, though rare, can be a life-threatening complication. Time-trusted laparotomy for control of secondary hemorrhage following myomectomy is always an option; however, it should be reserved as the last alternative. If available, pelvic angioembolization should always be thought of as a viable strategy to avoid a laparotomy.

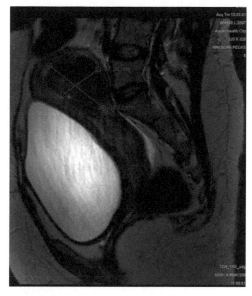

Figure 15.1 Magnetic resonance imaging picture showing large hematoma in the endometrial cavity.

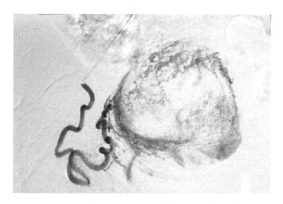

Figure 15.2 Installation of dye before the embolization outlines the hemorrhage in the uterine cavity.

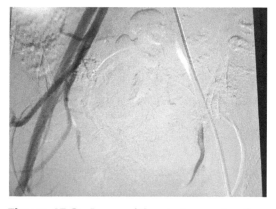

Figure 15.3 Image of the uterine cavity after the embolization.

REFERENCES

1. LaMote AI, Lalwani S, Diamond MP. Morbidity associated with abdominal myomectomy. *Obstet Gynecol.* 1993;82:897–900.

2. Iverson RE Jr, Chelmow D, Strohbehn K. Myomectomy fever: testing the dogma. *Fertil Steril.* 1999;72:104–108.

3. Frederick J, Hardie M, Reid M, Fletcher H, Wynter S, Frederick C. Operative morbidity and reproductive outcomes in secondary myomectomy: a prospective cohort. *Hum Reprod.* 2002;17:2967–2971.

4. Nishiyama S, Saito M, Sato K, Kurishito M, Itasaka T, Shioda K. High recurrence rate of uterine fibroids on transvaginal ultrasound after abdominal myomectomy in Japanese women. *Gynecol Obstet Invest.* 2006;61:155–159.

5. Dubuisson JB, Chapron C, Fauconnier A, Kreiker G. Laparoscopic myomectomy and myolysis. *Curr Opin Obstet Gynecol.* 1997;9:233–238.

6. Somigliana E, Vercellini P, Benaglia L, Abbiati A, Barbara G, Fedele L. The role of myomectomy in fertility enhancement. *Curr Opin Obstet Gynecol.* 2008;20(4):379–385.

7. Kongnyuy EJ, Wiysonge CS. Interventions to reduce haemorrhage during myomectomy for fibroids. *Cochrane Database Syst Rev.* 2014;(8):CD005355. doi: 10.1002/14651858.CD005355.pub5.

8. Sauerbrun-Cutler M, Kanos J, Friedman A, Bernstein S. Pseudoaneurysm after abdominal myomectomy: a rare but catastrophic complication. *Open J Obstet Gynecol* 2013;3:123–125.

9. Asai S, Asada H, Furuya M, Ishimoto H, Tanaka M, Yoshimura Y. Pseudoaneurysm of the uterine artery after laparoscopic myomectomy. *Fertil Steril.* 2009;91:929.e1–929.e3.

10. Zimon AE, Hwang JK, Principe DL, Bahado-Singh RO. Pseudoaneurysm of the uterine artery. *Obstet Gynecol.* 1999;94:827–830.

11. Saad NE, Saad WE, Davies MG, Waldman DL, Fultz PJ, Rubens DJ. Pseudoaneurysms and the role of minimally invasive techniques in their management. *Radiographics* 2005;25:S173–S189.

12. Henrich W, Fuchs I, Luttkus A, Hauptmann S, Dudenhausen JW. Pseudoaneurysm of the uterine artery after cesarean delivery: sonographic diagnosis and treatment. *J Ultrasound Med.* 2002;21:1431–1434.

13. Kovo M, Behar DJ, Friedman V, Malinger G. Pelvic arterial pseudoaneurysm—a rare complication of cesarean section: diagnosis and novel treatment. *Ultrasound Obstet Gynecol.* 2007;30:783–785.

14. McGonegle SJ, Dziedzic TS, Thomas J, Hertzberg BS. Pseudoaneurysm of the uterine artery after an uncomplicated spontaneous vaginal delivery. *J Ultrasound Med.* 2006;25:1593–1597.

15. Takeda A, Koike W, Imoto S, Nakamura H. Conservative management of uterine artery pseudoaneurysm after laparoscopic-assisted myomectomy and subsequent pregnancy outcome: case series and review of the literature. *Eur J Obstet Gynecol Reprod Biol.* 2014;182:146–153.

16. Takeda, A., Kato K., Mori M., Sakai K., Mitsui, T., Nakamura, H. Late massive uterine hemorrhage caused by ruptured uterine artery pseudoaneurysm after laparoscopic assisted myomectomy. *J Minim Invasive Gynecol.* 2008;15:212–216.

17. Takeda A, Koyama K, Mori M, Sakai K, Mitsui T, Nakamura H. Diagnostic computed tomographic angiography and therapeutic emergency transcatheter arterial embolization for management of postoperative hemorrhage after gynecologic laparoscopic surgery. *J Minim Invasive Gynecol.* 2008;15:332–341.

18. Zorlu CG, Akar ME, Seker-Ari E, Yilmaz S, Sindel T. Uterine artery embolization to control bleeding after myomectomy. *Acta Obstet Gynecol Scand.* 2005;84:606–607.

19. Higón MA, Domingo S, Bauset C, Martínez J, Pellicer A. Hemorrhage after myomectomy resulting from pseudoaneurysm of the uterine artery. *Fertil Steril.* 2007;87:417.e5–417.e8.

20. Wan A-YH, Shin JH, Yoon H-K, Ko G-Y, Park S, Seong N-J, et al. Postoperative hemorrhage after myomectomy: safety and efficacy of transcatheter uterine artery embolization. *Korean J Radiol.* 2014;15:356–363.

21. Ito N, Natimatsu Y, Tsukada J, Sato A, Hasegawa I, Lin BL. Two cases of postmyomectomy pseudoaneurysm treated by transarterial embolization. *Cardiovasc Intervent Radiol.* 2013;36:1681–1685.

22. Palacios Jaraquemada JM, García Mónaco R, Barbosa NE, Ferle L, Iriarte H, Conesa HA. Lower uterine blood supply: extrauterine anastomotic system and its application in surgical devascularization techniques. *Acta Obstet Gynecol Scand.* 2007;86:228–234.

23. Bishop S, Butler K, Monagham S, Chan K, Murphy G, Edozien L. Multiple complications following the use of prophylactic internal iliac artery balloon catheterization in a patient with placenta percreta. *Int J Obstet Anesth.* 2011;20:70–73.

24. Greenberg JI, Suliman A, Inranpour P, Angle N. Prophylactic balloon occlusion of the internal iliac arteries to treat abnormal placentation:

a cautionary case. *Am J Obstet Gynecol.* 2007; 197:470.e1–470.e4.

25. Lingman K, Hood V, Carty MJ. Angiographic embolization in the management of pelvic hemorrhage. *BJOG.* 2000;107: 1176–1178.

26. Cottier JP, Fignon A, Tranquart F. Herbreteau D. Uterine necrosis after arterial embolization for postpartum hemorrhage. *Obstet Gynecol.* 2002;100:1074–1077.

27. Pirard C, Squifflet J, Gilles A, Donne ZJ. Uterine necrosis and sepsis after vascular embolization and surgical ligation in a patient with postpartum hemorrhage. *Fertil Steril.* 2002;78: 412–413.

28. Zanati J, Resch B, Roman H, Brabant G, Sentilhes L, Verspyck E, et al. Buttock necrosis after subtotal hysterectomy, bilateral internal iliac arteries ligature and pelvic embolization for control of severe post-partum haemorrhage. *J Gynecol Obstet Biol Reprod.* 2010;39:57–60.

16 Laparoscopic Surgery for Fibroid Uterus

When to Convert to Laparotomy

Rooma Sinha

CONTENTS

INTRODUCTION

There is an inherent risk of conversion to conventional laparotomy during any laparoscopic surgery and the conversion should not be regarded as an adverse event [1]. Conversion to laparotomy has been reported in 0–19% of patients [2]. This risk depends on a number of factors like indication, severity of disease, patient characteristics, and the surgeon's skill. In their study, Sandberg et al. found that the risk of conversion at the time of laparoscopic myomectomy was low (1.09%) [3]. These converted cases were associated with more intraoperative blood loss and a longer hospital stay compared with cases that underwent either a laparoscopic myomectomy or a planned abdominal myomectomy. It is important to assess the risk factors for conversion during preoperative evaluation and make a planned decision regarding the approach to surgery.

So How Do We Define Conversion from Laparoscopic Approach to Laparotomy?

It is important to define this term for meaningful use and for understanding. Shawki et al. tried to obtain a consensus on the definition of conversion [4]; 68% of respondents agreed with the definition "Any incision made earlier than initially planned to complete the procedure" [4] during laparoscopic surgery. This survey, however, was limited to colorectal surgeons.

Blikkendaal et al. conducted a web-based Delphi consensus study among general surgeons, gynecologists, and urologists: the survey included 268 respondents in the first Delphi round (response rate of 45.6%) and included 43% general surgeons, 49% gynecologists, and 8% urologists [5]. Based on this survey, a consensus definition was compiled. Conversion was defined as "an intraoperative switch from a laparoscopy to an open abdominal approach." There are two types of conversions: strategic and reactive [5]. When a standard laparotomy is carried out immediately after the initial assessment of the feasibility of the procedure by laparoscopic surgery, it is called strategic conversion. Such a strategic conversion is made by the surgical team when they feel their lack of competence to complete the procedure by laparoscopic surgery or due to logistic considerations of available equipment.

An enlarged uterus that is difficult to mobilize has the potential perception of hemorrhage as the vascular pedicles are inaccessible. The presence of severe adhesions obscuring the vision can further prompt the surgical team to make a decision to do strategic conversion. It can be interpreted as a reactive conversion when a laparotomy is performed because of an intraoperative complication or when there is an operative difficulty due to poor visualization of the operating field after a considerable amount of dissection (i.e., 15 min of operative time). Conversions done in cases with uncontrollable hemorrhage or organ damage is termed as reactive conversion. Anesthesia-related issues leading to conversion, like ventilation problems or inability to attain sufficient Trendelenburg (or both), should be regarded as reactive conversion [5]. Technical failure of the equipment leading to a decision for conversion should be regarded as a complication and interpreted as a reactive conversion [6]. A laparotomy after a diagnostic laparoscopy (i.e., to assess the surgical curability of the disease) or an incision made for specimen retrieval should not be considered a conversion at all [5].

WHY WORRY ABOUT CONVERSION AND WHEN IS THAT DECISION MADE?

It is difficult to preoperatively identify some of the factors (e.g., pelvic adhesion or associated pathologies) that may become a reason for conversion. An intraoperative reactive conversion is usually associated with worse outcomes; these patients have longer hospital stay and more postoperative complications. In short, such conversions have higher morbidity compared with a procedure completed by laparoscopic surgery [7, 8]. Patients with conversion had a higher chance of surgical site infection, severe sepsis, or need for blood transfusion or reoperation even if no intraoperative complication had occurred. Magnetic resonance imaging (MRI) can be an important investigation for the evaluation of fibroids, their location, associated endometriosis, or pelvic adhesions in the preoperative evaluation with high accuracy [9]. These MRI evaluations can preoperatively estimate the difficulty of laparoscopic surgery with either myomectomy or hysterectomy and a decision can be made appropriately.

An evidence-based cutoff would be 15 min of dissection, either starting after establishment of the pneumoperitoneum or at any point during the progress of the surgery. If there is no meaningful progress of the intended surgery in 15 min, it may be wise to make it into a strategic conversion rather than to face a complication and make it into a reactive conversion [10]. It may be a good idea to inform the nurse or anesthetist to watch the time and inform the surgeon of the lapse of 15 min so that he or she is aware of the time lapse and can take a call. Reactive conversion due to lack of progress after a considerable amount of laparoscopic operating time indirectly implies an inadequate judgment in the preoperative or an intraoperative assessment. Such a conversion should be carried out as early as possible as any further delay in this decision adds to the postoperative morbidity. Reactive conversion is usually a result of suboptimal preoperative patient evaluation. During their learning curve, a surgical team ends up with more reactive conversions which over the years should be brought down. Strategic conversions can be achieved by good preoperative evaluation and timely and sound surgical judgement. An understanding of one's own surgical skills can help the timely decisions by the surgical team. A balance between strategic (70%) and reactive (30%) conversion should be maintained by a good surgical team [2].

REASONS FOR CONVERSION

The most important factor in preventing conversion during laparoscopic surgery is the surgeon's experience and appropriate patient selection for complex procedures. There is no doubt that surgeon volume determines the conversion rate. But a successful surgery is a combination of the surgeon's skill and their surgical volume and experience. The ability to make timely decisions and, of course, the assistance of a reliable team can make most conversions strategic. In general, the presence of large masses in terms of either their weight or volume makes vision during laparoscopy difficult and is one of the most common reasons for conversion. Specimen weight of more than 500 g, which corresponds to a uterus of about 16 weeks' gestation, was associated with a greater risk of conversion in either laparoscopic hysterectomy or myomectomy. Poor visibility or difficulty to move the uterus freely or both are the primary reasons for this type of conversion [11, 12]. We need to understand that the volume of the uterus poses more problems in laparoscopy than the absolute weight of the uterus. This clinical assessment during preoperative evaluation can help in decision making. A larger transverse diameter of the uterus is a risk factor for difficult surgery. This wide uterus with fibroids prevents access to the uterine pedicles, leading to difficulty in controlling the bleeding and thus compromising the safety of the surgical procedure.

Obstruction of a clear view of the anatomy is common in the presence of severe adhesions. These can be due to previous surgery or associated conditions like endometriosis or advanced malignancy. Encountering unexpected endometriosis is an important factor that increases the risk of conversion in cases with fibroid uterus as the two are seen together in many patients. Obesity in women can make laparoscopy complicated right from the placement of primary port to manipulation of instruments, thus compromising the safety of a successful surgery. Obese women also have increased visceral fat and that can make vision and dissection challenging. Uncontrollable bleeding was the most important primary adverse event leading to a reactive conversion. Adequate repair of unexpected damage to bowel, bladder, ureter, or a large vessel may necessitate reactive conversion as not all gynecological surgeons may be proficient in repairing these defects laparoscopically. It is better to timely recognize the organ damage and do the best possible repair during the surgery even if conversion is needed. At times, the gynecological surgeon may ask for help from the concerned specialty colleague, and the surgeon responding in the emergency may not be proficient in laparoscopy; hence, conversion for repair of a damaged organ may be warranted.

Strategic or pre-emptive conversion can be carried out for various reasons. In a prospective cohort study, Twijnstra et al. reported that 69% of conversions were strategic in nature [2]. Decision of strategic conversion may be made if additional disease (more advanced stage of cancer or severe endometriosis) is encountered unexpectedly. Body mass index (BMI) and higher uterus weight were independent risk factors for conversion. In the same paper, they reported that the risk increases with BMI greater than 35 (about 6.5-fold), age greater than 65 years (about 7-fold), uterus weight 200–500 g (about 4-fold), and uterus weight greater than 500 g (about 30-fold). Higher conversion in age of more than 65 years could be due to a higher probability of finding malignancy within this subgroup [2].

We reported a conversion rate of 10.9% in our series of laparoscopic hysterectomy for fibroid uterus. This study had all selected patients with a uterus greater than 16 weeks. The conversion was significantly correlated with excessive hemorrhage and bladder injury but not with difficult bladder dissection or the presence of adhesions per se. When the data were analyzed year-wise, the need for conversion gradually decreased over the years. In fact, there were no conversions after the first 3 years (completion of 53 cases). Considering this analysis, we proposed that about 50 cases are needed as a learning curve to be able to complete laparoscopic hysterectomy for a large uterus with fibroids [13]. Proficiency of learning curve of laparoscopic hysterectomy irrespective of the size of uterus is about 30 cases, according to studies reported in the literature. After this experience, the surgeon acquires a steady rate of successful surgical outcomes, reducing the need for conversion [14]. We further reported conversion rates in a comparative study between laparoscopic and robot-assisted hysterectomy for fibroid uterus (all cases >16 weeks). The conversion rates were 4.3% in the robotic group and 10.9% in the laparoscopic hysterectomy group but this difference was not statistically significant [15]. Other authors have also reported the advantage of robotic assistance in reducing the conversion rate. Robotic assistance and surgeon volume are strongly associated with decreased odds of conversion in robotic hysterectomy [16]. With the use of robotic surgical system, a lower conversion rate has also been seen in other surgeries like radical prostatectomy and surgery for colorectal cancer [17].

CONCLUSION

By understanding that the risk of conversion is inherent in laparoscopic surgery, gynecological surgeons can accurately select the best mode of surgical access and counsel patients with fibroid uterus during preoperative assessment. Conversion should not be taken as a failure or complication but should be considered as a strategy to complete the surgery safely and efficiently for good postoperative outcome. The chance of conversion increases during laparoscopy for fibroid uterus while performing either myomectomy or hysterectomy due to the large size of specimen. The risk of conversion further increases if there is a history of open abdominal myomectomy, presence of cervical or oddly located fibroids especially in the lower segment of uterus, dense bowel adhesions, and presence of associated endometriosis. Knowledge of these risk factors during the preoperative evaluation can help the surgeon to decide the best approach. The women can be counselled for realistic expectations about their surgical outcome. Proper consent can be taken after carefully explaining all of the possible surgical scenarios. Awareness of these factors should help surgeons decide for strategic conversion where appropriate while doing laparoscopic surgery for fibroid uterus.

REFERENCES

1. Atkinson SW. Results of eVALuate study of hysterectomy techniques: Conversion to open surgery should not be regarded as major complication. *BMJ (Clinical Research Ed.).* 2004;328(7440):642–643. doi:10.1136/bmj.328.7440.642-a.

2. Twijnstra ARH, Blikkendaal MD, van Zwet EW, Jansen FW. Clinical relevance of conversion rate and its evaluation in laparoscopic hysterectomy. *J Minim Invasive Gynecol.* 2013;20(1):64–72.

3. Sandberg EM, Cohen SL, Jansen FW, Einarsson JI. Analysis of risk factors for intraoperative conversion of laparoscopic myomectomy. *J Minim Invasive Gynecol.* 2016;23(3):352–357.

4. Shawki S, Bashankaev B, Denoya P, Seo C, Weiss EG, Wexner SD. What is the definition of "conversion" in laparoscopic colorectal surgery? *Surg Endosc.* 2009;23(10):2321–2326.

5. Blikkendaal MD, Twijnstra ARH, Stiggelbout AM, Beerlage HP, Bemelman WA, Jansen FW. Achieving consensus on the definition of conversion to laparotomy: A Delphi study among general surgeons, gynecologists, and urologists. *Surg Endosc.* 2013;27(12):4631–4639.

6. Twijnstra ARH, Zeeman GG, Jansen FW. A novel approach to registration of adverse outcomes in obstetrics and gynaecology: A feasibility study. *Qual Saf Heal Care.* 2010;19(2):132–137.

7. Chew MH, Ng KH, Fook-Chong MCS, Eu KW. Redefining conversion in laparoscopic colectomy and its influence on outcomes: Analysis of 418 cases from a single institution. *World J Surg.* 2011;35(1):178–185.

8. Yang C, Wexner SD, Safar B, Jobanputra S, Jin H, Li VKM, et al. Conversion in

laparoscopic surgery: Does intraoperative complication influence outcome? *Surg Endosc.* 2009;23(11):2454–2458.

9. Byrne H, Ball E, Davis C. The role of magnetic resonance imaging in minimal access surgery. *Curr Opin Obstet Gynecol.* 2006;369–373.

10. Slim K, Pezet D, Riff Y, Clark E, Chipponi J. High morbidity rate after converted laparoscopic colorectal surgery. *Br J Surg.* 1995;82(10): 1406–1408.

11. Stoelinga B, Huirne J, Heymans MW, Reekers JA, Ankum WM, Hehenkamp WJK. The estimated volume of the fibroid uterus: A comparison of ultrasound and bimanual examination versus volume at MRI or hysterectomy. *Eur J Obstet Gynecol Reprod Biol.* 2015;184:89–96.

12. Twijnstra AR, Blikkendaal MD, Van Zwet EW, Van Kesteren PJM, De Kroon CD, Jansen FW. Predictors of successful surgical outcome in laparoscopic hysterectomy. *Obstet Gynecol.* 2012;119(4):700–708.

13. Sinha R, Swarnasree G, Rupa B, Madhumathi S. Laparoscopic hysterectomy for large uteri: Outcomes and techniques. *J Minim Access Surg.* 2019;15(1):8–13.

14. Tunitsky E, Citil A, Ayaz R, Esin S, Knee A, Harmanli O. Does surgical volume influence short-term outcomes of laparoscopic hysterectomy? *Am J Obstet Gynecol.* 2010;203(1):24.e1–24. e6.

15. Sinha R, Bana R, Sanjay M. Comparison of robotic and laparoscopic hysterectomy for the large uterus. *J Soc Laparoendosc Surg.* 2019;23(1):e2018.00068. doi:10.4293/JSLS.2018.00068.

16. Lim CS, Mowers EL, Mahnert N, Skinner BD, Kamdar N, Morgan DM, et al. Risk factors and outcomes for conversion to laparotomy of laparoscopic hysterectomy in benign gynecology. *Obstet Gynecol.* 2016;1295–1305.

17. Tanis PJ, Buskens CJ, Bemelman WA. Laparoscopy for colorectal cancer. *Best Pract Res Clin Gastroenterol.* 2014;28(1):29–39.

17 Cesarean Section in the Setting of Fibroid Uterus and Cesarean Myomectomy

Andrea Tinelli, Marina Vinciguerra, Antonio Malvasi, and Michael Stark

CONTENTS

INTRODUCTION

Conditions that require surgical intervention in women become prevalent with advanced age. Although pregnancy occurs more often in the young population, in recent decades the age of pregnancies advanced with higher risk of uterine (Figure 17.1) and adnexal (Figure 17.2) tumors. Therefore, some operations are indicated during pregnancy.

The most common indications are cholecystectomy (45%), ovary operations due to cysts or tumors (mostly benign) (34%), appendectomies (15%), and others (6%) [1]. One publication reported three cholecystectomies: an adnexal procedure and two operations for abdominal pain [2]; 33% of the surgeries during pregnancy were performed in the first trimester, 56% in the second, and 11% in the third trimester. Until

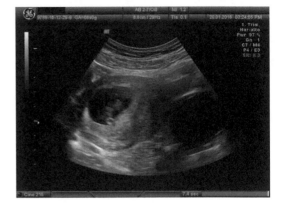

Figure 17.2 Image of transvaginal ultrasound in pregnancy at 8 weeks, with ovarian cyst adherent to the uterus.

recently, myomectomy during cesarean section (CS) was considered a controversial operation because of intrasurgical and post-surgical risk, but since the beginning of the last decade, removal of fibroids during delivery has been frequently reported [3]. For example, Bhatla et al. performed successful myomectomy in the second trimester for a huge subserous fibroid (weighing 3900 g) and the pregnancy continued until term [4].

EPIDEMIOLOGY AND SYMPTOMS OF FIBROIDS

Fibroids are the most common tumors in women and are the most common indication for hysterectomy. In India, in the Kasturba Hospital in Manipal, 39.8% of all hysterectomies were due to fibroids [5]. By the age of 50, fibroids are found in 70% of white women

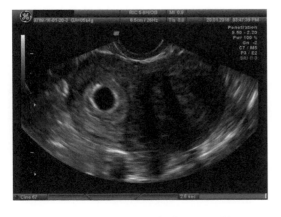

Figure 17.1 Transvaginal ultrasound image in early pregnancy at 5 weeks, with uterine fibroma occupying most of the uterine volume.

in the United States and in more than 80% of black women. Similar data come from Italy; however, in Sweden, the prevalence of fibroids is lower. The incidence of fibroids in pregnancy increases with age, and the prevalence rates of fibroids is 10% in pregnant Hispanic women in the United States [6] but only 3.9% in Greece [7]. The prevalence of uterine fibroids ranged from 4.5% (the UK) to 9.8% (Italy), reaching 9.4% (the UK) to 17.8% (Italy) in the age group of 40 to 49 years [8]. Often, fibroids are asymptomatic and found only by a routine gynecological examination.

Fibroids are found in any part of the uterus, not necessarily obstructing the birth canal (Figure 17.3). However, they might cause a variety of symptoms, including uncontrolled bleeding, dysmenorrhea, pelvic pain, reproductive failure, and symptoms which are the result of compression on adjacent viscera or even obstruct the lower segment of the uterus (Figure 17.4). But during pregnancy, the major complications are pain, bleeding, unexplained fever, tenderness of the abdomen, and

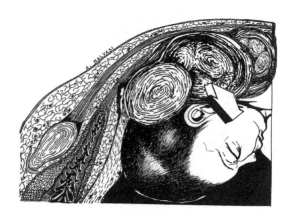

Figure 17.4 Sagittal anatomical section of the Lower Uterine Segment (LUS) in pregnant at term uterus with anterior fibroid that obstructed the LUS and cause flexion of fetal head (arrow). (Modified by: Ecografia intraparto e il parto. Antonio Malvasi e Gian Carlo Di Renzo. Edit. Laterza, Bari, Italy, 2012).

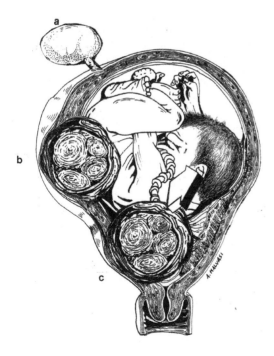

Figure 17.3 Longitudinal anatomical section of pregnant uterus at 38 gestational weeks with fibroids. Fibroids localization: (a) subserosal fundal fibroid, (b) intramural lateral right fibroid in the body of the uterus, anterior right intramural fibroid located in the lower uterine segment (LUS). (Modified by Semeiotica Ostetrica. Antonio Malvasi e Gian Carlo Di Renzo. C.I.C. Edit. Intern. Rome, Italy, 2012).

occasionally malpresentations and premature rupture of the membranes [9]. About 39.95% of women with fibroids during pregnancy have CS deliveries [10]. These days, when more women in advanced age become pregnant, mainly in Western countries, due to social reasons as well as for the development of *in vitro* fertilization as egg donation enables even menopausal women to become pregnant, it is only natural that more fibroids will be found in pregnant women (Figure 17.5). The rate of CS increases gradually all over the world and certainly in women who receive treatment for

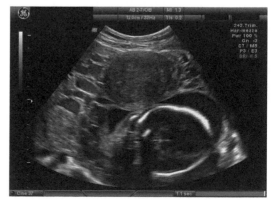

Figure 17.5 Transabdominal ultrasound scan during pregnancy at 17 weeks, with fetal skull topped by transmural fibroma.

infertility or those who deliver at advanced age; therefore, more fibroids are present during the CS.

TREATMENT OF FIBROIDS

In recent years, a big shift happened concerning indications for hysterectomy because of the development of alternative methods to reduce the size of the fibroid or abolish its symptoms. The use of magnetic resonance–guided focused ultrasound, performed without general anesthesia, causes local heat inside the fibroid and produces its shrinkage [11, 12].

An innovative diagnostic procedure, currently still under development, is laparoscopic intra-abdominal ultrasound-guided radiofrequency ablation. A recent case series showed the great outcomes obtained with this technique, but more evidence is needed before it can be used clinically on a widespread basis [13]. Other methods are hysteroscopic resection of fibroids that protrude into the uterine cavity [14], which should be done while avoiding extensive, high-wattage diatherml coagulation or excessive tissue manipulation or muscular trauma in order to preserve the myoma's pseudocapsule as new scientific evidenced suggest method [15].

Although no single medical treatment can be officially labeled as an effective and, at the same time, a permanent cure of uterine myoma, many randomized controlled trials (RCTs) and meta-analyses recently tried to define the role of several classes of compounds with the aim of giving a reasonable alternative to surgery or at least making myomectomy or hysterectomy easier and safer for the patient [16–18].

In this regard, the most investigated drugs are the so-called SPRMs (selective progesterone receptor modulators), also mistakenly called "anti-progestins," which have a chemical structure similar to that of progesterone. Owing to this structure, they can interact with co-repressors and co-activators of progesterone receptor (PR), obtaining at the same time agonistic and antagonistic effects according to tissue type, cell type, or physiological context [18–20].

Mifepristone, also named RU486, was the first of the SPRMs to have been synthesized and successfully used for treatment of myomas [16], reducing both epidermal growth factor (EGF) expression progesterone related [21] and PR [22] and also negatively modulating glutathione pathway [23]. Even if the first studies considered effective in reducing uterine volume, anemia and dysmenorrhea with doses of 50 or 25 mg daily of mifepristone [24, 25]. Subsequent

RCTs showed that good results can be obtained with doses between 2.5 and 25 mg daily for 3 to 6 months [26, 27]; according to recent studies, mifepristone can be a valid choice for long-term fibroid treatment in symptomatic perimenopausal or premenopausal women who are not eligible for surgery using a very low dosage like 50 mg weekly for 6 months [28] or declining the initial dosage of 25 mg every 3 months for a total period of 9 months in 1 year [29]. Even a vaginal administration of 10 mg daily of mifepristone showed good results [30].

In the last decade, the most promising results among SPRMs have been achieved by ulipristal acetate (UPA), also known as CDB-2914 or VA-2914, whose effectiveness in significantly reducing uterine fibroids volume is attributed to its triple action on myoma cells: it inhibits their proliferation, promotes their apoptosis, both modulates PR myoma isoform and downregulates factors involved in the myoma growth and survival (i.e., PCNA, Bcl-2, VEGF, and adrenomedullin) [31–33], and increases the expression of metalloproteinase-2 (MMP-2) [34]. These effects seem to be incremented by the combination with vitamin D_3, which could become a favorable clinical option in the future [35]. Moreover, UPA controls signs and symptoms which are myoma-related, like dis/hypermenorrhea or bleeding resulting with anemia [36], exerting its action on the following:

■ Pituitary gland, through inhibition of P activity, reduction of follicle-stimulating hormone (FSH) release, continuance of estradiol levels within mid-follicular range (60–150 pg/mL) and hence inhibition or retardation of ovulation [36, 37].

■ Endometrium, promoting unique and class-specific endometrial changes, labelled as PEAC (Progesterone Receptor Modulator Associated Endometrial Changes), which is represented by a thickening easily detectable during treatment by ultrasound or MRI in 41 to 78.8% of patients, whose benign and completely reversible nature was widely reported in a recent Cochrane review [38].

VENUS I and II, two phase 3 RCTs of North America, examined more than 400 premenopausal women (18–50 years) with uterine leiomyomas and abnormal uterine bleeding. The RCTs divided them into a once-daily 5 mg ulipristal group, a 10 mg ulipristal group, and a placebo group in two 12-week treatment courses separated by a drug-free interval of two periods. The 5 mg and 10 mg ulipristal groups were superior to the placebo group in achieving amenorrhea (42% and 54.8% vs. 0.0%) with a significant improvement of health-related quality of life and a low rate of adverse effects like hot flushes (7.5% and 11.6% vs. 1.7%) [39–41]. Good evidences regarding effectiveness of UPA were obtained by the four PEARLs (PGL4001 Efficacy Assessment in Reduction of symptoms due to uterine Leiomyomata) phase 3 trials [42]. Unfortunately, the spread of UPA caused discussion due to several cases of liver damage which were reported by the EMA (European Medicines Agency), four of which resulted with hepatic transplantations. Therefore, although there are uncertainties around causality, EMA's PRAC (Pharmacovigilance Risk Assessment Committee) review officially warned about the use of UPA; in 2018, EMA's CHMP (Committee for Medicinal Products for Human) defined the new conditions for its use:

■ Contraindicated in patients affected by liver disorders

■ Indicated for only one course of treatment in patients eligible for surgery

■ Intermittent treatment is indicated only for moderate to severe symptoms in adult women of reproductive age not eligible for surgery.

■ Every patient should be informed about signs or symptoms of liver injury, and treatment should be stopped.

■ Liver function tests must be performed before starting each treatment course, monthly during the first two treatment courses, thereafter as clinically indicated and 2 to 4 weeks after stopping treatment.

■ UPA should not to be started if AST (aspartate aminotransferase) and ALT (aspartate alanine-transferase) are more than two times ULN (the upper normal limits).

■ UPA should be stopped if AST and ALT are more than three times ULN [43].

On the other hand, conditioned by post-marketing reports, US Food and Drug Administration did not approved UPA for the treatment of abnormal uterine bleeding in women with uterine fibroids, requiring additional information for the future [44].

Also gonadotropin-releasing hormone-agonist became a valid method to significantly reduce the size of fibroids as a 3 or 6 months pre-treatment before any type of surgery procedure (laparotomy, laparoscopic or hysteroscopic myomectomy, etc.) [45], although this class of drug, inducing a sort of "medical menopause"

or "medical oophorectomy" and being its effects on myoma reversible, is not fit for a long-term treatment in patients not eligible for surgery [16]. Some scientists proposed the possibility of an "add-back therapy" in order to reduce signs and symptoms related to the persistent hypo-estrogenism [46], but they do not have a great feedback from medical community in this set of patients.

In the last years, gynecologists became associated with interventional radiologists who perform uterine artery embolization (UAE) [47], which seems to give good results for symptomatic leiomyoma with a high technical success rate [48] and a low re-intervention rate [49], the latter often due to an incomplete infarction or to the presence of more than one submucous myoma [50]. A retrospective cohort pilot study in 2014 claimed that UAE could cause reduction of the ovarian reserve over time (>12 months), but more evidence about it is needed [51]. All these methods can be used in women during childbearing age prior to their pregnancies or after pregnancies as a valid alternative for myomectomy or hysterectomy.

MYOMECTOMY DURING CESAREAN SECTION: A HISTORICAL OVERVIEW

Despite lack of evidence, myomectomy during CS was not recommended until recently and even discouraged unless these fibroids were pedunculated (Figure 17.6). The main reason was the fear of massive bleeding during the

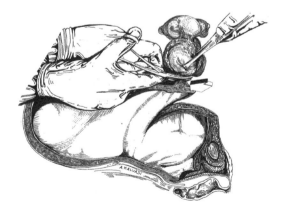

Figure 17.6 Myomectomy of pedunculated fibroids of the LUS (arrow), during Cesarean Section (CS), after fetal extraction and removal of the placenta. (Modified by: *Cesarean Delivery. A Comprehensive Illustrated Practical Guide.* Gian Carlo Di Renzo e Antonio Malvasi. CRC Press/ Taylor & Francis Group 2017).

procedure due to the well-developed vascularization of the uterus in pregnancy which increases toward the end of the pregnancy. Therefore, many obstetricians used to perform hysterectomies following the delivery as a definitive treatment whenever the family planning was completed. Others used to leave the fibroids *in situ* and perform a planned myomectomy after involution of the uterus which usually takes up to six weeks.

Fibroids found during CS shrink often during the involution of uterus, and sometimes, no indication for myomectomy is given during the follow-up examination. One of the reasons that removal of fibroids during CS was considered as a contraindication and was discouraged was the expressed judgment of opinion leaders, such as "Te Linde." His opinions are unquestionable, citations from his book are often used in courts in matters of malpractice. He stated in his book: "Myomectomy delivery in conjunction with Cesarean section, is contraindicated. If there is a pedunculated sub-serous fibroid attached to the uterus with a small pedicle, suturing and excision of the pedicle may be done easily. However, the removal of intramural myoma from the pregnant uterus is inadvisable due to recognized difficulty in controlling blood loss" [52].

Another opinion leader was Danforth. In his book he states that the reason for not performing myomectomy during CS is bleeding which may be profuse and therefore hysterectomy may be required. He believes as well that because fibroids often undergo remarkable involution after delivery, they may become pedunculated postpartum, which makes myomectomy safer as a postpartum operation than at the time of the CS [53]. Some obstetricians who tried to perform myomectomies during CS received non-favorable outcomes. For example, Exacoustos et al. reported nine myomectomies performed during CS delivery. Of these, three resulted with severe hemorrhage necessitating hysterectomy. They emphasized the myoma size, position, location, relationship to the placenta, and echogenic structure, as factors which must be considered when identifying women at risk for myoma-related complications [54]. It is certainly important to respect time-honored knowledge, but at the same time we always have to be open to new ideas, re-examine our routines using new knowledge and research, and constantly challenge old traditions. Therefore, we must find out whether in the twenty-first century conservative attitude to fibroids found in CS should prevail, and if not, what are the measures we must take in order to make myomectomy during CS safe without the involved risks (Figure 17.7).

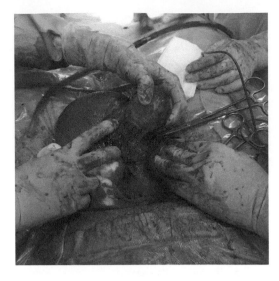

Figure 17.7 Intraoperative image of myomectomy during cesarean section with removal of large anterior myoma of the body, after hysterorraphy.

CESAREAN MYOMECTOMY

In the last years, more reports are published concerning successful removal of fibroids during CS. In the literature search, which included PubMed, MEDLINE, EMBASE, and Cochrane Library, relevant studies were identified. Nine studies, including 1082 women with leiomyomas, met the inclusion criteria; 443 (41.0%) patients had CS followed by removal of fibroids and 639 (59.1%) had only CS. Also, the blood loss was higher in the myomectomy group, but the difference was not significant. The operative time was 4.94 min longer, and there was not difference in febrile morbidity. No conversion to hysterectomies occurred in either group. The authors concluded that fibroid removal during CS is a valid option which should be considered [55].

In 1989, four years before Exacoustos, Burton and colleagues reported on 13 successful cesarean myomectomies with the sole complication of intraoperative hemorrhage. They concluded that surgical management of leiomyomata during pregnancy and CS is safe in carefully selected patients [56].

Hsieh et al. reviewed 47 incidental cesarean myomectomies. The procedure added 11 min to the operation time, 112 mL to the blood loss and extended hospital stay of one and a half day in comparison to the control group. There were no wound infections or serious morbidity involved [57].

In 1997, Michalas et al. reported eight fibroids obstructing the lower part of one uterus which were removed during CS at 39th week of pregnancy. There was no maternal or fetal complication [58].

Ehigiegba et al. have assessed the intra- and postoperative complications of cesarean myomectomy (CM) in 25 pregnancies. Five patients required blood transfusion, and no one necessitated hysterectomy. They concluded, that "With adequate experience and the use of high dose of oxytocin infusion (intra- and postoperatively), myomectomy at cesarean section is not as hazardous as many now believe" [59].

A recent case report described a 1500-g fibroid successfully removed during a CS [55].

In a report from India, three fibroids were found during CS, two of them were removed without any complications and the third one was left in situ due to extended vascularity found around the fibroid [60]. This accentuates the necessity to individualize each case and make decisions according to the findings and to be flexible enough to recalculate the indication when necessary.

O'Sullivan and Abder reported two cases of myomectomy during CS: 10 cm diameter sub-serosal and another one was found in the fundus. Both were removed without any complications. The authors also concluded that myomectomy at the time of cesarean delivery is safe and reasonable procedure [61].

Ramya et al. in a retrospective review reported their last 10 years' experience in a tertiary care-level teaching institution. In this review 20 women underwent CM, of which 6 multiparous with previous lower segment CS and 3 previously subjected to myomectomy. There were no exclusion criteria about patient characteristics and the procedure was executed regardless location, type, size or number of myomas. The biggest myoma was 8 cm in size and they were three myomas in the same patient. The risk of intraoperative bleeding was avoided as far as possible by tranexamic acid infusion, vasopressin instillation, uterine artery ligation, electrocautery (Figure 17.8)

and high-dose oxytocin during 24 hours infusion, so that the blood loss was 876 ± 386.9 mL and only two patients needed intraoperative blood transfusion. The conclusion was that the security of the procedure is linked more than any other factor to the experience of the gynecologist [62].

In mainland China, where myomectomy during CS is becoming a common medical practice, Zhao et al. collected data in 39 hospitals for a recent retrospective cohort study, in which the comparison of postpartum hemorrhage, neonatal weight, fetal distress, and neonatal asphyxia showed no statistical significance between the CM group and the cesarean group. The only suggestion they give to a surgeon evaluating the possibility of a myomectomy during CS is to consider a birth weight of at least 4000 g (odds ratio [OR] 3.1, 95% confidence interval [CI] 1.6–6.0) and presence of a fibroid with diameter of more than 5 cm (OR 2.2, 95% CI 1.3–4.0) as high-risk factors for peripartum hemorrhage, meant as blood loss of at least 1000 mL [63].

In another study by Sparic et al. 36 cases of CM were compared with 17 CS without the removal of fibroids. In this study as well, no significant differences were found in the sociodemographic and clinical findings between the groups. The average size of the fibroids in the study and control group ($P = 0.873$) was 55.44 and 47.25 mm, respectively. The average duration of the operation was 62.5 min in the study group and 53.82 in the control group ($P = 0.058$). Intraoperative hemorrhage was more frequent in the study group ($P = 0.045$). Neither the number nor the volume of intraoperative transfusions was significantly different. No complications were recorded, and the duration of hospitalization was similar in both groups. The authors concluded that CM in patients with single anterior wall (Figure 17.9)

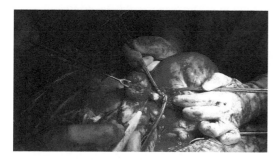

Figure 17.8 Removal of fibroma during cesarean section using an electric scalpel.

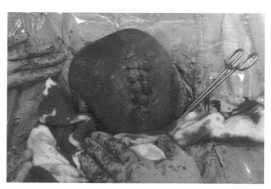

Figure 17.9 Suture of the anterior uterine wall after cesarean myomectomy.

and low uterine segment fibroids does not cause increased perioperative morbidity and is considered as a safe procedure [64].

Kwon et al. compared 96 cases of women who had CS without myomectomy, and 65 women who underwent CM. They compared the maternal characteristics, neonatal weight, fibroid types, and operative outcomes between two groups and analyzed CM group according to fibroid size. The large fibroids were defined as more than 5 cm in size. The maternal characteristics, neonatal weight, and fibroid types were compared between two groups. They also compared the operative outcomes such as pre-operative and postoperative blood loss, operative time, and hospitalization days between two groups. There were no significant differences in the maternal characteristics, fibroid types, neonatal weight and operative outcomes between the two groups. The subgroup analysis according to fibroid size (>5 cm or not) in CM group revealed that there were no significant differences in the mean hemoglobin drop (1.2 vs. 1.3 mg/dL, $P = 0.6$), operative time (90.5 vs. 93.1 mins, $P = 0.46$), and the length of hospital stay (4.7 vs. 5.2 days, $P = 0.15$) between the two groups. They concluded that CM in patients with large fibroids is a safe and effective procedure [65].

In a recent retrospective study, Sparic et al. compared women who had a single myomectomy during CS not only against women who had a CS alone, but also compared with non-pregnant women who had a laparotomic myomectomy; unlike the previous studies cited all the women with multiple fibroids were excluded. There were no significant differences in minor or major complications (like intraoperative hemorrhage) in the three groups, they also remark that the only variables predictive of complications in the CM group are the fibroid size, with a diameter cutoff of 75.00 mm, and the duration of surgery, which was 87.5 min. Moreover, they conclude that CM is a safe procedure not only for the women but also for the baby, not affecting in any way the Apgar score [66]. The conclusions of this study are particularly interesting because they raise the question of when and how to treat women in childbearing age affected by myoma, whether it is correct to propose a myomectomy before becoming pregnant or, instead, ascertained that there are not myoma-related fertility problems, it is more appropriate to delay myomectomy at the time of delivery by cesarean section (Figure 17.10).

It is important to keep in mind that having a pregnancy after a myomectomy could expose a woman to one of the most feared risks in

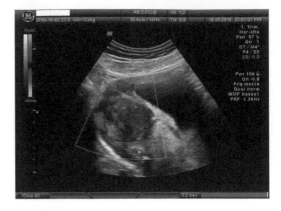

Figure 17.10 Image of transmural fibroma in pregnancy at 12 weeks, with important peripheral fibroma vasculature using echo-color Doppler.

obstetrics: the *uterine rupture*. As a matter of fact, although to date the uterine rupture is a very uncommon event (its incidence ranging from 1/40000 and 1/50000) [67], it is often associated with the worst possible complications for the women (i.e., massive blood loss, severe anemia, hysterectomy, death) and, when it happens during pregnancy, also for the baby (i.e., severe prematurity, cerebral palsy and death) [68–70].

Even if RCOG (Royal College of Gynecology) in its Green Top Guideline No. 45 "Birth after previous cesarean birth" it says that there is insufficient and conflicting information on whether the risk of uterine rupture is increased in women with previous myomectomy [71], many authors have described up to nowadays several cases of uterine ruptures during pregnancy and they are often scarred ones, that means related to previous surgery procedures on uterus, whom the most relevant is just myomectomy (Figures 17.11 and 17.12) [67–69, 72–75]. Different data are reported in several studies about it, however from a recent review the scarred uterine rupture following myomectomy seems to have an incidence ranging from 1 to 3.7% [76] and it can occur not only after the 30 weeks and during the peripartum period, contrary to past opinions, but also during each trimester of pregnancy, regardless the presence of uterine contractions [67, 69, 73, 74, 77, 78].

Furthermore, although according to some authors, an interval ranging from 3 to 6 up to 12 months should be enough for an adequate uterine wound healing [79], according to a recent review the longer is the time between pregnancies leads to a reduction of uterine rupture rate, which becomes significantly

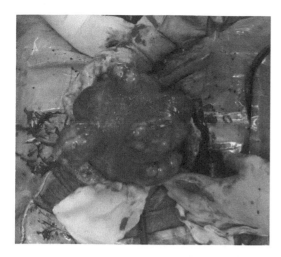

Figure 17.11 Uterus rich in fibroids during cesarean section in a patient over 40 years of age after assisted reproductive techniques. On the right of the image, there is the posterior uterine wall rich in fibroids, which will be removed during the cesarean section.

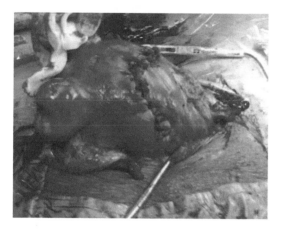

Figure 17.12 The same uterus of Figure 17.11, after multiple cesarean myomectomy, with evident scar of the posterior wall after removal of some myomas.

lower after a period at least of 19 months [80]; however there is no agreement between experts about the optimal interval between myomectomy and conception in order to completely avoid uterine rupture [67]. By surgeon point of view not even the type of approach used for myomectomy seems to definitively avoid this complication, in fact, besides the cases after laparotomic or laparoscopic myomectomy [67, 69, 73, 75, 77, 78, 80–83], nowadays scientific literature reports uterine ruptures following robotic-assisted myoma removal [74]. Even

hysteroscopic myomectomy could represents a risk factor for uterine rupture, in fact this is the type of hysteroscopic procedure is more associated with this complication, which often occurs when the myoma has an intramural component, a G2 type according to FIGO (International Federation of Gynecology and Obstetrics) classification [84]. On the other hand, several experts suggest techniques of hysterorraphy to prevent weakness of uterine wall, hematoma formation and therefore uterine rupture: multilayer closure, preservation of endometrial cavity when possible, and avoidance of electrosurgical energy [67, 74, 81, 85].

From the neonatologist point of view, despite scarred uterine rupture in compared with unscarred uterine rupture usually tends to occur earlier during pregnancy [86], both these types are equally associated to infant morbidity and death [79]. Over the decades, intrapartum/neonatal death after complete uterine rupture decreased significantly thanks to new medical strategies planned to reduce time to fetal extrusion and placenta separation as much as possible less than 20 min and to give good neonatal support in intensive care units [79]. According to the available scientific articles is difficult to correctly estimate the incidence of scarred uterine rupture after myomectomy, but it seems to be approximately 1% when hysterorraphy is well done [86]. However, a recent Japanese report of the last 5 years showed that among the cases of scarred uterine rupture, neonatal prognosis is poorer in cases of pregnancy after myomectomy in comparison with women with a prior CS [69].

Despite of the indication of the ACOG (American College of Obstetrics and Gynecologists) to prefer a cesarean delivery for women who underwent a prior myomectomy in order to avoid scarred uterine rupture [87], a retrospective cohort study conducted by Gimovsky et al. using the Maternal Fetal Medicine Units Cesarean Registry highlight that a prior myomectomy significantly exposes women who are having a CS to several complications beyond uterine rupture: 180% increased risk of intraoperative transfusion, 57% more likely to need uterotonics, 713% more likely to have a bowel injury due to postoperative adhesions, 243% more likely to undergo a cesarean hysterectomy [70].

So, in view of all this, why do not promote CM in order to reduce all these risks during pregnancy and delivery? Certainly, the available literature is inconsistent about it and we also need the correct indications and the best surgical technique of CM to be officially define and needless.

TECHNIQUES OF CESAREAN SECTION WITH MYOMECTOMY

There are many studies describing myomectomy during cesarean section. The location of fibroid during CS can be in the lower uterine segment (LUS) (Figure 17.13), in the body of the uterus or in the fundus. Pedunculated fibroids can easily be removed by suturing the pedicle before removal of the fibroid. Usually, this procedure does not cause bleeding and does not influence the outcome of the operation. However, cutting the uterine wall following CS usually causes bleeding. The surgeon performing myomectomy during CS should be in the position and have the knowledge to identify the Internal Iliac Artery and, if necessary, to identify the ureter, as fibroid due to its size might cause the distortion of the anatomy; therefore, the ureter might take an unusual pathway and be damaged when the suturing of the Internal Iliac Artery becomes necessary. It is needless to explain the importance of the knowledge needed when performing the operation and

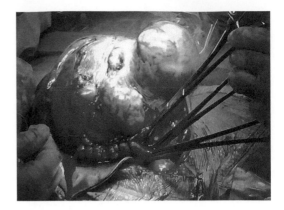

Figure 17.14 Suture of the hysterotomic incision on the lower uterine segment (LUS), before performing cesarean myomectomy.

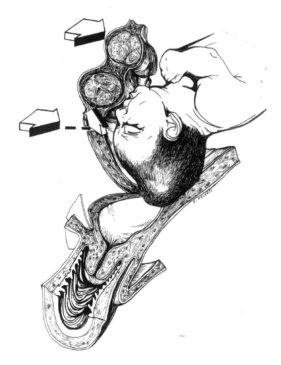

Figure 17.13 Sagittal section of the LUS during CS in occiput posterior position of the fetal head. Transverse uterine incision under two intramural fibroids in the LUS (arrow near discontinuous line). (Modified by: *Cesarean Delivery. A Comprensive Illustrate Practical Guide.* Gian Carlo Di Renzo e Antonio Malvasi. CRC Press/Taylor & Francis Group 2017).

certainly a planned Cesarean Myomectomy should be done only if an experienced surgeon does the operation.

Ideally, one should not remove a fibroid before delivering the baby even if the fibroid blocks the lower segment of uterus. In such a case, it is advisable to perform the classical CS opening the uterus longitudinally and suturing it before the removal of the fibroid (Figure 17.14). It is always recommended in any myomectomy when possible to make the incision in the midline rather than transversely. The vascularization of the uterus goes latero-medial therefore the more lateral you are, the more vascular the tissue becomes. Also in a non-pregnant uterus where many fibroids should be removed, it is advisable to make a longitudinal midline incision and to remove as many fibroids as possible through this incision (Figure 17.15). This can be difficult to do in a pregnant uterus (Figure 17.16). The wall is softer, very vascular, and therefore uncontrolled bleeding might occur. In order to prevent it, it is advisable to occasionally use tourniquet in order to temporarily block the arteries or to clamp them with a soft-ended instrument.

Ben Rafael et al. started to perform planned myomectomy during CS in cases where the fibroid was either known to be large enough to require surgery in the future, or when the fibroid caused malpresentation. In light of the inconclusive data in the literature, the following retrospective analysis was conducted. The aim was to assess the intra- and postoperative complications of CM of 32 consecutive patients who underwent CM performed between 1997 and 2001. The files were reviewed for demographics, indication for CS, and characteristics of the fibroids. Outcome measures were mode of anesthesia, type of incision, intraoperative blood

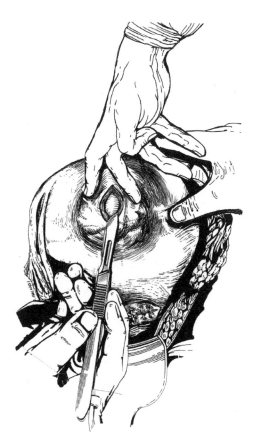

Figure 17.15 Surgical approach for cesarean myomectomy using longitudinal midline incision, in order to remove as many fibroids as possible through this incision.

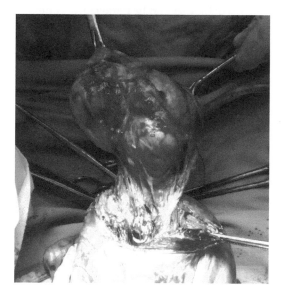

Figure 17.16 Cesarean fundal myomectomy, with myoma removal by enucleation of the same from its pseudocapsule, after uterine serosa incision.

loss, the need for blood transfusion, intra- or postoperative complications, and the length of hospital stay. In their report, all the procedures of myoma removal during cesarean section were executed only by gynecological surgeons experienced in performing myomectomies in non-gravid uteri. They performed the myomectomies even if the CS was done by another surgeon. In cases of intramural fibroids, after completion of the CS, an interlocked suture was temporarily placed on the edge of the CS uterine incision without closing it. This allows the surgeon work from the external and inner parts of the uterus with good control from the inside to prevent endometrial opening, allowing controlling bleeding by applying compression when necessary. Myomectomy was performed preferably from the edge of the incision made for the CS in the case of lower segment fibroid, or by an additional incision if the fibroid was located away from the CS incision. They used sharp dissection with scissors without using tourniquet. Oxytocin drip was given during and after the procedures. Suturing of the fibroid bed was performed by one or two layers of interrupted vicryl suture, and a baseball type suture for the serosa as third layer [88]. Thirty-nine fibroids were removed from 32 patients in 15 elective and 17 emergency procedures. The indications for CS were obstetrical (breech presentation, repeated CS, etc.) in all cases except in 6: 3 cases of fibroids blocking the pelvis, 1 of degenerative fibroid and 2 of previous myomectomy with uterine cavity penetration. Ninety percent of the fibroids were subserous or intramural and 10% submucous. The average size of fibroids was 6 cm (1.5–20), with 26 myomas >3 cm and 11 >6 cm. Four CSs (12.5%) were done with longitudinal incision and the remaining were done using the transverse low-segment incision. Three operations were done with spinal anesthesia (9.3%) and the remainder with epidural anesthesia. The difference in hemoglobin and hematocrit levels before and 12 h after the operation was statistically significant compared with the control group where CSs were done without myomectomy ($p < 0.05$), yet only 4 patients required blood transfusion. Reoperation was done in one patient after removal of 2 large fibroids due to secondary bleeding and the other due to development of a big hematoma in the scar. No patient required hysterectomy. Six developed febrile morbidity (18.7%). Average duration of hospitalization was 5.7 days, with 5 requiring more than 6 days at the hospital. There was no correlation between complications or duration of hospital stay by patient age, gravidity, parity, or the indication for CS (Table 17.1).

TABLE 17.1: Comparison of hemoglobin and Hct levels before and after CS myomectomy and without associated myomectomy [27–88]

	% Hb before	% Hb after	Hct before	Hct after
C-sections followed by myomectomy	12.4 + 1.2	10 + 1.5	66.5 + 3	30.1 + 4.4
C-sections without myomectomy	12.6 + 1.1	10.8 + 1.3	37.3 + 3	32 + 3.7
P value	NS	0.05	NS	>0.05

The authors of this study concluded that myomectomy during CS is feasible; however meticulous attention to hemostasis, enucleation using sharp dissection with Metzenbaum scissors, adequate approximation of the myometrium and abolishing dead spaces to prevention of hematoma formation are mandatory. The opinion of the authors is that myomectomy during CS is a safe procedure when done by experienced surgeon. They believe that the tradition that discouraged CM should be reassessed [88].

It seems that CM is feasible procedure which in case of experienced surgeon has favorable outcomes. However, in most of the quoted studies, the exact detailed surgical steps are not described, except general advice concerning the use of oxytocin, or meticulously abolishing the dead space. There is no standardized way to cut the uterine wall, sometimes transverse incision is used, and sometimes longitudinal one (Figure 17.4); the reason for it might be different locations of the fibroids as well as differences in training of the surgeons, depending on the institution they come from. These days, there is not yet a single evidence-based CS technique for universal use despite the existence of the one from our group, the Misgav Ladach method which is already in use in many countries. [89, 90]. It seems that also myomectomy is done by different surgeons in different ways, therefore it is important to suggest the most optimal surgical technique which could be adjustable to any situation and the location of fibroid.

We propose as the first step after removal of the fibroid to obliterate its bed and this can be done in different way according the technique chosen by surgeon. As example, Cobellis et al. sutured the hysterotomy of 322 cesarean myomectomies by placing horizontally separate "U" stitches, with a distance of 2–3 mm between each one, followed by oxytocin infusion for up to 24 h. This technique reached good results in term of hemostasis and good healing [91]. Lee JH et al. instead, introduced an unusual CM technique for sub-serosal and intramural myomas, which forms myoma-uterine reflection. They used a purse-string suture (MUPS), which allows to prevent bleeding by gradually tightening it around the myoma, thus collapsing the blood vessels. After closing the CS incision, the suture is placed intra-myometrally approximately 1–2 cm apart from the serosal reflection of the protruding myoma. The suture is tightened gradually while dissecting the fibroid, thus obliterating the dead space. Alternately, the second suture can be placed to reinforce the first suture [92].

Optimally, according to the collected experience and in agreement with the authors of this chapter, CM should be done by repeated stitching starting at the very bottom in order to secure the closure of the fibroid bed. The size of the needle in use should be individualized according to the size of the bed. After completion, the muscular wall should be closed, this time, with a big needle with big bites. It should be done continuously with locking. Thereafter, the cut edge should be meticulously examined for bleeding and if complete hemostasis has not been achieved, X stitches should be placed, and if necessary, a second layer, and again with a big needle. If a tourniquet or hemostatic clamp were used, they should be removed, and the incision should be inspected again for at least for 5 min before closing the abdomen. If the fibroid bed was not thoroughly closed, blood might collect there and will appear some minutes afterward. After the surgery, the patient should be regularly monitored for blood pressure, urine output, and repeated blood tests at least for 48 h. Each removed fibroid should be examined by the pathologist in order to ensure that no pathological elements are found; leiomyosarcoma, though rare, should always be kept in mind [93].

In 2017, Hatırnaz Ş. et al. officially introduced a novel surgical technique for CM, which has been labelled as "endometrial myomectomy" (EM), in a retrospective single institution study, and the first in the literature. This report demonstrated that this less invasive approach optimizes myomectomy outcomes and minimize adhesion formation, compared with classic cesarean serosal myomectomy (SM). Forty-six patients were enrolled, 22 women underwent to EM and the remaining to SM, including only symptomatic anterior wall fibroids and excluding all the posterior or pedunculated serosal fibroids and asymptomatic women [94]. Myomectomies in both groups were operated by a group of skilled surgeons, after baby and placenta extraction and before uterine lower segment incision closure. The EM technique involves:

- A quick evaluation of uterine surface and cavity in order to determine the number, anatomical location and size of myomas.

- Palpation of each myoma and individualization of its endometrial site.

- Endometrial and trans-myometrial incision to reach the leiomyoma, if necessary, resorting to bivalves to open even more the uterine cavity.

- Blunt and sharp dissection for fibroid removal with its entire capsule, clamping and suturing any vascular structure at the root of myoma; using a tenaculum forceps, myoma is carefully taken out from a small incision made on the endometrium or, if it is located at the lower uterine segment, between endometrium and myometrium.

- Suture of myoma bed and death spaces with # 1 vicryl, instead endometrium is sutured with absorbable suture only when the defect site is bigger than 3 cm [94].

This study reported that time of myomectomy in the SM group was 40.42 min vs. 32.36 min in the EM group ($P = 0.001$) and the amount of the intraoperative bleeding was 375 mL in the SM group vs. 209 mL in the EM ($P = 0.001$) [94]. It seems that the main benefit of the endometrial myomectomy is not to involve the uterine serosa, as there are no sutures or scars on the uterine surface, so that it drastically diminishes the risk of abdominal adhesions. Additionally, SIS (Saline Infusion Sonography) evaluation, which was done after 40 days from the cesarean endometrial myomectomy to each patient, showed no single case of endometrial damage, intracavitary adhesion formation or Ashermann syndrome. According to Hatırnaz Ş. et al., the "uterus is the major supporter of this surgery," and due its rapid involution it leads to a spontaneous dead spaces and suture sites reduction, minimizing all the related complications.

This innovative method was questioned by Tinelli et al., claiming that a fibroid's capsule removal cannot be consider a good choice for an optimal wound healing, taking into account decade of research concerning the key role of the fibrous pseudocapsule, which is rich in neurofibers and neurotransmitters important for an adequate myometrium repair process, and therefore it is the rational of the intracapsular approach for myomectomy [95]. Moreover, they did not understand the advantage of affecting the endometrium for the removal of an intramural myoma, and so intentionally damaging in fertile and young women a more delicate and complex tissue rather than the peritoneal serosa. The cutoff of 3 cm for endometrium defect suture does not seem to be mentioned anywhere in the literature [95]. According to Spariç et al, the Trans Endometrial approach for CM could be connected to a higher probability of future abnormal placentation, in terms of placental localization or myometrium infiltration as well as other possible complications [96]. It is not clear how it is possible to avoid excessive blood loss or to make endometrial myomectomy easy and feasible for the surgeon and safe for the patient, if, according to Hatırnaz Ş. et al, it should be executed before the lower uterine segment suture, immediately after fetus and placental extraction, when the uterus largely bleeds and myometrium contractions start [95]!

On the other hand, Huang S.Y. et al., in a longitudinal panel study published in 2017, demonstrated that the new and discussed transendometrial approach for CM may improve the obstetric outcomes of a subsequent pregnancy, without immediate or long-term surgical outcomes, like blood loss/transfusion, postoperative fever, hospitalization and formation of adhesions [97]. Sixty-three women after CM and who planned an elective repeat cesarean delivery, were enrolled and followed up, The authors reported that: the mean gestational age at birth and the new-born weight at the subsequent CS were higher than in the prior one ($P < 0.001$); spontaneous preterm birth ($P = 0.002$), SGA (small for gestational age) infants ($P = 0.027$) and pPROM (preterm premature rupture of membranes) ($P = 0.131$) occurred less frequently during the subsequent pregnancy [97].

Pandey S. in a farsighted and at the same time critical point of view focuses on the importance in reproductive aspects that these results could have, but remarks on the limitations of this study, in particular the short sample size and the lack of subgroup stratification by adjusting for covariates (i.e., ethnicities, socio-economic status, anamnestic findings, blood type, genetic background, clinical parameters, etc.). He also suggests the possibility to enhanced the study's overall quality by adding variables like robotic surgical outcomes, color Doppler diagnostic imaging data, mycobacterium tubercular/chlamydia/ HPV genotyping assays for further risk assessments, keeping in consideration the complexity of an overall and complete evaluation of the obstetric/surgical outcomes [98]. In the author's reply, despite the missing data detections, it emerges that color Doppler imaging data and postoperative hysteroscopic imaging, which were not mentioned in the study, have been done but revealed no anatomical changes from the EM during pregnancy. Moreover, Huang SY et al., like Hatırnaz Ş. et al, claim that an unpublished cross-sectional study derived from this report concludes the EM is significantly less related to uterine deformity, adhesion formation or perioperative complications in comparison with the classic serosal CM [99].

Unlike Hatırnaz Ş. et al., the transendometrial CM technique, described by Huang SY et al., principally differs in extraction of the myoma without its pseudocapsule, which is therefore preserved according to the reasons mentioned above. In addition the use of an infusion of 30 IU of oxytocin in 500 ml of dextrose at a rate of 60 mL/h in combination with uterine compression is mentioned and bi-manual massage after placental expulsion is done in order to promote uterine contraction and hemostasis, while the lower uterine segment incision is sutured only after the EM [97].

When myomectomy is discussed it is important not to forget that this procedure, especially when associated with CS [3], is a hemorrhagic operation, sometimes associated with life-threatening bleeding and the need for emergency blood transfusion. The last incidence of intraoperative hemorrhage reported in the literature in CM ranging from zero to 35.3% [96]. Studies in the last decades tried to asses effectiveness, safety, tolerability, and costs of interventions to reduce blood loss for any method known for myoma removal. In regard to the ability to reduce intraoperative bleeding during myomectomy according to a 2014 Cochrane review, a series of RCTs reports moderate-quality evidence for misoprostol and intramyometrial vasopressin, low-quality evidence for intramyometrial bupivacaine plus epinephrine, intravenous tranexamic acid, gelatin-thrombin matrix, a peri-cervical tourniquet, intravenous ascorbic acid, vaginal dinoprostone, loop ligation of the myoma's pseudocapsule and a fibrin sealant patch, on the other hand there are no evidences for oxytocin and enucleation of myoma by morcellation [100].

Some obstetricians advocate technique for blood loss sparing, as the use of vasopressin (use of vasoconstrictive drugs) or tourniquet, although few studies investigated the several possible methods to evaluate this risk in patients who undergo CM.

Vasopressin is a synthetic antidiuretic hormone, widely used in gynecological surgery as a vasoconstrictor agent, mostly during high risk for bleeding procedures like myomectomy. Already in 1996, Fletcher et al. showed in two cases of myomectomy that vasopressin was associated with less blood loss and lower risk for transfusion or blood loss of more than one liter [101]. Vasopressin can be administrated in different ways, but a local administration has to be preferred, because it allows the induction of local vasoconstriction lasting approximately for 30 min, avoiding as much as possible the systemic effects typical to this kind of compounds, like cardiac rhythm disorders, blood pressure alterations or other cardiovascular adverse effects [102]. Therefore, even if cases of safe myomectomies after paracervical injection of vasopressin are described [103], the technique is often done by an intramyometrial infiltration around the myoma by diluted vasopressin [100]. A recent retrospective case-control study on laparoscopic myomectomy showed that the use of intraoperative intramyometrial injection of dilute vasopressin (20 IU/100 mL normal saline), did not reduce the operation time for a skilled surgeon, but significantly reduced the blood loss in laparoscopic myomectomy without serious cardiovascular adverse events. In addition, the occurrence of hypercapnia was higher in untreated cases and contributed to conversion to laparotomy [102].

This method to prevent bleeding is described also for CM, in which the dosage is around the 20 units of vasopressin diluted in 50 mL of saline, but there are no standard indication for it. Good evidence were obtained concerning reduced intraoperative blood loss [104]. An interesting case report of a robotic-assisted myomectomy showed a new technique for maximizing vascular control, combining subserosal injection of a dilute solution of vasopressin with temporary uterine artery occlusion with soft vascular clips or after a complete skeletonization of the uterine vessels. In this way, it is possible to reduce the intraoperative blood loss effectively, mostly for patient who refuse blood transfusion, because even an innovative approach to myomectomy like the robotic one could not be completely bloodless [105]. No single study on this innovative method is available in the literature for CM.

The use of tourniquet is another widely used investigated method in laparotomic myomectomy, and many recent studies are trying to prove its effectiveness in reducing intraoperative bleeding and consequent anemia. Most of the publications are case reports or retrospective study with limitations in showing statistical validity [106]. Interesting is a RT (randomized trial), showing that there is no clinically significant difference between triple and single uterine tourniquets on blood loss during open myomectomy. Additionally, neither significant difference in AMH (anti-Müllerian hormone) postoperative levels were noted between single and triple uterine tourniquet, although the latter has been for long time considered responsible to negative effect on the reproductive function because of its presumed ischemic effect on the ovarian circulation [107].

Concerning the use of tourniquet during CM, one of the first studies was a randomized prospective one conducted in Turkey by Sapmaz et al. on 70 women which compared the use of tourniquet with the bilateral ligation of the ascending uterine artery. There were no significant differences in terms of perioperative blood loss between the two groups but it showed that just uterine artery ligation can guarantee bleeding control even in the postoperative period, so that it should be preferred in CM [108].

Incebyik et al. proposed instead the combination of tourniquet, electrosurgery and oxytocin infusion as blood loss reducing method for CM. Tourniquet was applied through a opened window in the broad ligaments at the cervical-isthmic level, and it was removed after suturing the fibroid bed and the uterine wall. Electrocautery was used for removal of the myoma and intravenous oxytocin was administered postoperatively in order to achieve adequate uterine contraction. Two out of 16 patients required blood transfusion [109]. Kwawukume reported the use of tourniquet tied around the uterine arteries and the ovarian vessels during CM, concluding that no significant difference was shown concerning blood loss in comparison with cesarean section done alone when CM is associated with the use of tourniquet [110].

Lin et al., in their case-control study, selected 72 patients with a major myoma bigger than 50 mm and investigated uterine artery occlusion (UAO) and myomectomy in women undergoing CS. During this procedure intravenous oxytocin infusion and intramyometrial injection of diluted vasopressin around the myoma were administrated. There were no statistical differences in intraoperative blood loss, postoperative recovery, complications, or wound pain between the UAO + CM group and cesarean alone group, despite of the prolonged time of surgery for the control group [111].

Desai et al. did selective uterine devascularization before the myomectomy, depending on the site of myomas. Also, in this case, a prolonged time of surgery was associated with good surgical outcome, confirming that CM is safe and favorable procedure [112].

In the most studies the employment of targeted methods to prevent bleeding during CM, like vasoconstrictors, uterine artery ligation or tourniquet, is not a routine, maybe because of the moderate-low evidence available [100]. Moreover, the use of this methods often is not a variable which is reported and investigated, because it seems not to influence blood loss better than others, considering that nowadays more and more CM trained surgeons operate in comparison with the past, when this procedure was often rejected [113]. Despite this it is generally accepted that CM is associated with an increased risk of hemorrhage [114], but is it statistically significant and should become clinically considerable?

A report by Roman and Tabsh compared retrospectively the results of cesarean myomectomies to CSs without myomectomy [115]. They evaluated 111 women who underwent a CM and 257 women with documented fibroids who underwent CS alone. The two groups were similar in age, parity, gestational age and size of the fibroids. Most patients in both groups underwent low transverse incision CS. In 86% of the patients, the fibroids were incidental findings, while in the others symptoms such as pain, dystocia and unusual appearance or consistency of the fibroids were indications for their removal. The incidence of hemorrhage in the study group was 12.6%, compared with 12.8% in the control group ($P = 0.95$). There was no significant increase in the incidence of febrile morbidity, operating time, and the length of hospital stay. The size of the fibroid did not appear to affect the incidence of hemorrhage. After categorizing the procedures by type of fibroid removed, intramural myomectomy was found to be associated with a 21.2% incidence of hemorrhage, compared with 12.8% in the control group, but this difference was not statistically significant ($P = 0.08$). No patient in either group required hysterectomy following the operation [115].

Spariç tried to define better the controversial question about risk of intraoperative bleeding and CS in a retrospective study. Included were women subjected to CM, divided into group of 36 patients in whom intraoperative hemorrhage was registered, and a control group of 66 patients in whom it was absent. Among the several parameters analyzed, the only differences found in the two group were type and size of the myoma ($P = 0.007$ and $P = 0.000$, respectively) and duration of the surgery ($P = 0.000$). As a matter of fact, in the same experience level of the surgeons, in the group with hemorrhage the myomas were 39 mm bigger and the operation time was 14.53 longer compared with the other group. So it was concluded that, considered CM as risk to bleeding procedure, factors like the size of the space in the uterus resulting from the enucleation of the fibroid and speed of the suturing could be considered as predictive to intraoperative hemorrhage, so that a correct evaluation of patient should be done in order to prepare the surgeon, in order to avoid as much as possible bleeding complication during surgery [114].

RISKS OF CESAREAN MYOMECTOMY

The calculated risk should be considered for any operation. Despite positive reports in the literature concerning the outcome of CM, the indication should consider the benefits of the procedure in comparison to possible complications. One should take into account that the size of the fibroid will anyhow diminish during the physiological involution of the uterus after the delivery, the experience and the ability of the surgeon should be considered, prior to the operation the patient should be informed about the risks and benefits and only upon her consent the myomectomy should be performed.

The literature should be evaluated critically; we know that not every complication or non-favorable outcome is reported, and we do not know how many series were not reported due the unfavorable outcome. Usually, publications report successes, mostly about short-term maternal morbidity [116]. As Sparic suggests it could be possible that the rate of complications is underestimated [96]. However, the literature did not provide so far data on long-term outcome of CM [96], but long-term morbidity seems not be higher than those expected about fertility and complications during pregnancy in agreement with Levast et al. [116]. The authors of this chapter experienced favorable outcome in their practice but strongly suggest considering seriously the ability of each surgeon confronted with this question and to calculate the benefits versus the risks of each individual case. It is advisable to work in a team and to call in an experienced colleague in case of unforeseen situation. As a matter of fact, Vitale et al. in their review claims that it is possible to make CM safe procedure when considering the experience of the surgeon and the presence of a tertiary center, because of the need of special technical care for the location of

the, recognition and preparation of the cleavage plain, hemostasis, and sutures [3].

No operation should be regarded as a minor or easy one. Even operations considered minor might end with major complications. This is the reason why these days many surgical procedures are not done by young doctors before training on simulators. Although simulators exist already for various obstetrical procedures such as for performing forceps, or even CS, there are still no simulator programs for performing CM. Simulators for endoscopic myomectomy are available but the conditions concerning the removal of fibroid from a non-pregnant uterus are completely different. Therefore, it is important that the surgeon who performs CM gathered enough experience by performing myomectomies on non-gravid uterus.

In the study by Ben-Rafael, it was shown that some of the myomectomies during CSs were not done by the same surgeon who delivered the baby. It seems to be the correct approach and it is always advisable to call in a surgeon with experience of removing fibroids in case when myomectomy is considered [88]. Such surgeons have more optimal conditions for a successful procedure. The average size of a non-gravid uterus is 7.6 cm × 4.5 cm × 3 cm weighting 100–150 g but toward the end of the pregnancy it fills the whole abdomen with increased blood supply from the uterine and the ovarian arteries. Compared with the non-pregnant state, the uterine artery diameter doubles by the week 21 from 1.4 ± 0.1 to 2.8 ± 0.2 mm, stays constant between weeks 21 and 30, and increases between weeks 30 and 36 to 3.4 ± 0.2 mm. Uterine artery mean flow velocity rises progressively from non-pregnant values to attain at week 36 a velocity nearly eight times faster (8.4 ± 2.2 versus 61.4 ± 3.0 cm/second). Unilateral uterine artery blood flow at week 36 was 312 ± 22 mL/min [117]. During CS the lower segment is opened transversely in the area where fibrous tissue prevails in contrary to the fundus where there is higher percentage of muscle tissue [118].

One should remember that also the ovarian arteries contribute to the blood flow of the uterus in a non-pregnant and pregnant state and are anastomosed with the uterine arteries [119]. This should be considered when hemorrhage occurs. A normal CS is done by opening the bladder plica, pushing down the bladder, opening the lower segment with a small transverse incision which is extended bi-digitally lateral as much as necessary. Doing so, the bleeding is minimal and usually the lower segment can be sutured with one layer and only rarely a second layer or single stitches are necessary for hemostasis [120].

Despite all possible surgical complications related to myomectomy it is important to keep in mind that one of the main advantages of the removal of myoma during cesarean delivery is to have the benefits of two operations in one, avoiding a separate myomectomy [3] and thus also the risks and costs of an additional operation [96]. Moreover, based on actual evidence, the uterine scar integrity following CM should be superior to that done in non-pregnant uterus, concerning the possibility of a future vaginal delivery [3] after a CM is not excluded [96]. Insufficient and controversial data are available about the risk of abnormal placentation after CM, and more studies concerning this risk are needed [121, 122].

SURGICAL TECHNIQUE OF INTRACAPSULAR MYOMECTOMY DURING CESAREAN SECTION

Our group headed by Tinelli was the first to describe the anatomical entity surrounding fibroids, the myoma pseudocapsule. The pseudocapsule is a neurovascular bundle or fibro-vascular network attached to the fibroids, which separates the fibroids from the myometrium (Figure 17.17). In ultrasound it appears as a white ring around the fibroid, and at echo check, it appears as a ring of fire. Pseudocapsule contains different neurofibers and neuropeptides. Consequently, damaging the pseudocapsule during myomectomy will certainly have negative impact on the healing process, although also other factors are involved. Therefore, the excision of a fibroid should be done inside the pseudocapsule even during myoma previa removal during cesarean delivery [96, 123–125] (Figure 17.18).

This technique, the intracapsular myomectomy, was used successfully in laparoscopy in non-pregnant women with single or multiple fibroids [126], the authors studied their method of fibroid removal during CS (Figure 17.19). Moreover, myomectomy should be technically easier in a pregnant uterus because of the accentuated appearance of the pseudocapsule [127]. An international research group [128] prospectively evaluated the surgical outcome of intracapsular myomectomy during CS, in university-affiliated hospitals, by a prospective case-control study on 68 patients who underwent intracapsular CM which was compared with a control group of 72 women with fibroids who underwent CS without myomectomy. All operations were performed by gynecologists experienced in intracapsular myomectomies on non-gravid uteri, and in performing CS by the

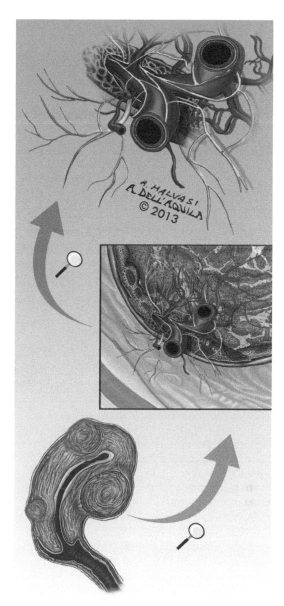

Figure 17.17 The drawing represents, from the bottom upward, the uterus with fibroids, the pseudocapsule of the myoma, the neurofibrovascular bundle inside the pseudocapsule.

Stark's method [90], under regional anesthesia. The intracapsular CM approved to be reliable, feasible and safe procedure and is associated with good intra- and post-surgical results, as also reported in the last review of Sparič et al. [96]. In this method, it is important to perform a sharp and exact pseudocapsule localization (Figure 17.20) and dissection (Figure 17.21), to approximate the edges of the myometrium and carefully close all the dead spaces.

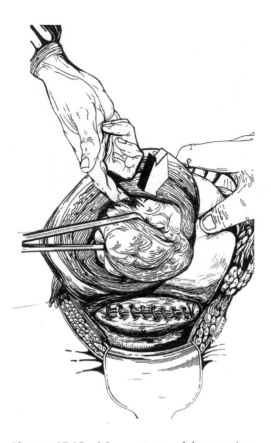

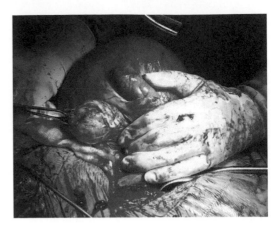

Figure 17.20 During cesarean myomectomy, the assistant highlights the pseudocapsule after incising the uterine serosa and pulling the fibroma outward.

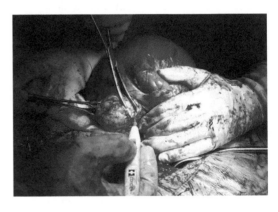

Figure 17.18 Myomectomy of the anterior intramural fibroid during CS: after the pseudocapsule incision, the surgeon performed the traction of the fibroid with Collins forceps using gentle digital enucleation of the fibroid from its pseudocapsule. (Modified by: *Cesarean Delivery. A Comprensive Illustrated Practical Guide*. Gian Carlo Di Renzo e Antonio Malvasi. CRC Press/Taylor & Francis Group 2017).

Figure 17.21 During cesarean myomectomy, a surgeon highlights the pseudocapsule with a forceps and the other surgeon cuts it with an electric scalpel.

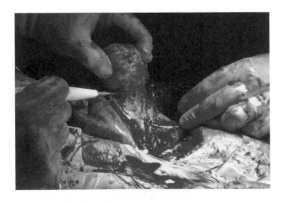

Figure 17.19 Cesarean myomectomy with removal, after hysterorraphy, of anterior wall myoma with pseudocapsule preservation.

This will prevent formation of hematomas. Obstetricians should familiarize themselves with this technique which seems to be safe and feasible. Moreover, Tinelli et al. discussed fertility-sparing myoma surgery in one of their last reviews, which focused on the correlation between pseudocapsule preservation during myomectomy and the fertility outcome, an important point especially when considering the current increasing age of the first pregnancy [125].

We conclude by stating that all available studies [3, 96, 127, 129] refer to myomectomy during pregnancy as a valid surgical option, although many authors consider this procedure

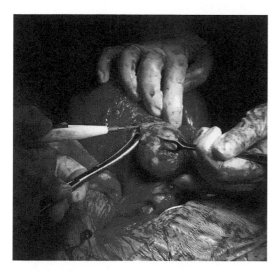

Figure 17.22 Cesarean myomectomy with removal of anterior myoma by intracapsular technique.

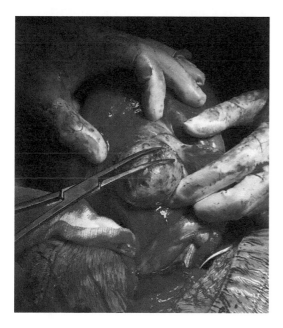

Figure 17.23 Cesarean myomectomy of right posterolateral subserosal myoma, below the area of reflection of the annex in the pelvis.

feasible only for selected patients. These are cases when myoma removal facilitates a safe delivery of the baby [3] or in cases of anterior wall myomas (Figure 17.22), subserous (Figure 17.23) and pedunculated ones, trying to avoid additional hysterotomy [127]. On the other hand, many reports suggest that a tailored surgical technique makes CM a generally

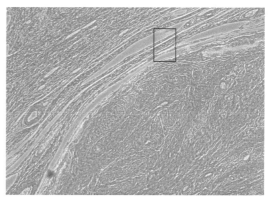

Figure 17.24 Histological examination that highlights the pseudocapsule in the black box.

safe procedure [96], as in case of preservation of the myoma pseudocapsule (Figure 17.24), even in cases associated with higher risk of surgical complications, such as multiple myomas, deep intramural, fundal and cornual myomas, and posterior uterine wall fibroids [127], although indications and contraindications for CM are still to be defined [96].

Currently, the literature provides only data concerning case-control and descriptive retrospective studies, which are low in quality due to large biases and scant conclusions, so that it would be desirable to plan a large multicenter prospective randomized trials in order to achieve strong evidence for scientific conclusion concerning CM [127]. Surely, myoma removal during CS, which was done for the first time at the beginning of the past century [96, 127], to date is about to become one of the leading novelties in obstetrics in the years to come.

CONCLUSION

- Myomectomy during CS was not recommended in the past and was contraindicated by opinion leaders.

- In recent years, this contraindication was challenged by various surgeons who performed myomectomies during CSs with favorable outcomes.

- CM should be done only when absolutely indicated and should be performed by a skilled and experienced surgeon, even if she or he is not the one who performs the CS.

- The optimal technique is midline incision and intracapsular removal. Thereafter, obliteration of the dead space with continuous suturing and closure of the uterine wall using big bites.

REFERENCES

1. Lachman E, Schienfeld A, Boldes R, Levin S, Burstein M, Stark M. Operative laparoscopy in pregnancy. *Harefuah* 1999;136(5):343–346, 420.

2. Lachman E, Schienfeld A, Voss E Gino G, Boldes R, Levine S, Borstien M, Stark M. Pregnancy and laparoscopic surgery. *J Am Assoc Gynecol Laparosc.* 1999;6(3):347–351.

3. Vitale SG, Padula F, Gulino FA. Management of uterine fibroids in pregnancy: Recent trends. *Curr Opin Obstet Gynecol.* 2015;27(6):432–437.

4. Bhatla N, Dash BB, Kriplani A, Aqarval N. Myomectomy during pregnancy: A feasible option. *J Obstet Gynaecol Res.* 2009;35:173–175.

5. Pandey D, Sehgal K, Saxena A Hebbar S, Nambiar J, Bhat RG. Research article an audit of indications, complications, and justification of hysterectomies at a teaching hospital in India. *Int J Reproduct Med..*2014;2014: 279273.

6. Laughlin SK, Schroeder JC, Baird DD. New directions in the epidemiology of uterine fibroids. *Semin Reprod Med.* 2010;28(3):204–217.

7. Lolis DE, Kalantaridou SN, Makrydimas G., Sotiriadis A, Navrozoglou I, Zikopoulos K, Paraskevaidis EA. Successful myomectomy during pregnancy. *Hum Reprod.* 2003;18(8):1699–1702.

8. Zimmermann A, Bernuit D, Gerlinger C. Prevalence, symptoms and management of uterine fibroids: an international internet-based survey of 21,746 women. *BMC Womens Health.* 2012;12:6.

9. Katz VL, Dotters DJ, Droegemueller W. Complications of uterine leiomyomas in pregnancy. *Obstet Gynecol.* 1989;73:593–596.

10. Coronado GD, Marshall LM, Schwartz SM. Complications in pregnancy, labor, and delivery with uterine leiomyomas: A Population-Based Study. *Obstet Gynecol.* 2000;95:764–769.

11. Huang X, Yu D, Zou M, Wang L, Xing HR, Wang Z. The effect of exercise on high-intensity focused ultrasound treatment efficacy in uterine fibroids and adenomyosis: a retrospective study. *BJOG.* 2017;124(Suppl 3):46–52.

12. Marret H, Bleuzen A, Guérin A, Lauvin-Gaillard MA, Herbreteau D, Patat F, Tranquart F. French first results using magnetic resonance-guided focused ultrasound for myoma treatment. *Gynecol Obstet Fertil.* 2011;39(1):12–20.

13. Iversen H, Dueholm M. Radiofrequency thermal ablation for uterine myomas: Long-term clinical outcomes and reinterventions. *J Minim Invasive Gynecol.* 2017;24(6):1020–1028.

14. Capmas P, Voulgaropoulos A, Legendre G, Pourcelot AG, Fernandez H. Hysteroscopic resection of type 3 myoma: A new challenge? *Eur J Obstet Gynecol Reprod Biol.* 2016;205:165–169.

15. Tinelli A, Favilli A, Lasmar RB, Mazzon I, Gerli S, Xue X, Malvasi A. The importance of pseudocapsule preservation during hysteroscopic myomectomy. *Eur J Obstet Gynecol Reprod Biol.* 2019;pii: S0301-2115(19)30419-1.

16. Farris M, Basyianelli C, Rosato E, Brosens I, Benagiano G. Uterine fibroids: An update on current and emerging medical treatment options. *Ther Clin Risk Manag.* 2019; 15:157–178.

17. Donnez J, Courtoy GE, Dolmans MM. Fibroid management in premenopausal women. *Climateric.* 2019;22(1):27–33.

18. Rabe T, Saenger N, Ebert AD, Roemer T, Tinneberg HR, De Wilde RL, Wallwiener M, Selective progesterone receptor modulators for the medical treatment of uterine fibroids with a focus on ulipristal acetate. *Biomed Res Int.* 2018;2018:6124628.

19. Wagenfeld A, Saunders PTK, Whitaker L, Critchley HOD. Selective progesterone receptor modulators (SPRMs): progesterone receptor action, mode of action on the endometrium and treatment options in gynecological therapies. *Expert Opin Ther Targets.* 2016;20(9):1045–1054.

20. Bouchard P, Chabbert-Buffet N, Fauser BCJM. Selective progesterone receptor modulators in reproductive medicine: Pharmacology, clinical efficacy and safety. *Fertility Sterility.* 2011;96(5):1175–1189.

21. Yang Y, Zheng S, Zhang Z. Effects of mifepristone on gene expression of epidermal growth factor in human uterine leiomyoma. *Zhonghua Fu Chan Ke Za Zhi.* 1998;33(1):38–39.

22. Sun M, Zhu G, Zhou L. Effect of mifepristone on the expression of progesterone receptor messenger RNA and protein in uterine leiomyomata. *Zhonghua Fu Chan Ke Za Zhi.* 1998;33(4):227–231.

23. Engman M, Varghese S, Lagerstedt Robinson K, Malgrem H, Hammarsjo A, Bystrom B, Lalitkumar PGR, Gemzell-Danielsson K. GSTM1 gene expression correlates to leiomyoma volume regression in response to mifepristone treatment. *PLoS One.* 2013;8(12):e80114.

24. Murphy AA, Kettel LM, Morales AJ, Roberts VJ, Yen SS. Regression of uterine leiomyomata in response to the antiprogesterone RU 486. *J Clin Endocrinol Metab.* 1993;76(2):513–517.

25. Yen SSC. Clinical use of RU 486 in the treatment of uterine fibroids. In: Donaldson MS, Dorflinger L, Brown SS, Benet LS, editors. *Clinical Applications of Mifepristone (RU 486) and Other Antiprogestins.* Washington, DC: National Academy Press. 1993;189–209.

26. Tristan M, Orozco LJ, Steed A Ramírez-Morera A, Stone P. Mifepristone for uterine fibroids. *Cochrane Database Syst Rev.* 2012;8:CD007687.

27. Shen Q, Hua Y, Jiang W, Zhang W, Chen M, Zhu X. Effects of mifepristone on uterine leiomyoma in premenopausal women: a meta-analysis. *Fertil Steril.* 2013;1006(6):1722–1726. e1–1722–1726.e10.

28. Kapur A, Angomchanu R, Dey M. Efficacy of use of long-term, low-dose Mifepristone for the treatment of fibroids. *J Obstet Gynaecol India.* 2016;66(Suppl 1):494–498.

29. Jain D. Mifepristone therapy in symptomatic leiomyomata using a variable dose pattern with a favourable outcome. *J Midlife Health.* 2018;9(2):65–71.

30. Yerushalmi GM, Gilboa Y, Jakobson-Setton A, Tadir Y, Goldchmit C, Katz D, Seidman DS. Vaginal mifepristone for the treatment of symptomatic uterine leiomyomata: an open-label study. *Fertil Steril.* 2014;101(2):496–500.

31. Xu Q, Takekida S, Ohara N Chen W, Sitruk-Ware R, Johansson ED, Maruo T. Progesterone receptor modulator CDB-2914 down-regulates proliferative cell nuclear antigen and Bcl-2 protein expression and up-regulates caspase-3 and poly(adenosine 5′-diphosphate-ribose) polymerase expression in cultured human uterine leiomyoma cells. *J Clin Endocrinol Metab.* 2005;90(2):953–961.

32. Xu Q, Ohara N, Chen W, Liu J, Sasaki H, Morikawa A, Sitruk-Ware R, Johansson ED, Maruo T. Progesterone receptor modulator CDB-2914 down-regulates vascular endothelial growth factor, adrenomedullin and their receptors and modulates progesterone receptor content in cultured human uterine leiomyoma cells. *Hum Reprod.* 2006;21(9):2408–2416.

33. Maruo T, Ohara N, Matsuo H Xu Q, Chen W, Sitruk-Ware R, Johansson ED. Effects of levonorgestrel-releasing IUS and progesterone receptor modulator PRM CDB-2914 on uterine leiomyomas. *Contraception.* 2007;75(6 Suppl):S99–S103.

34. Courtoy GE, Donnez J, Marbaix E, Dolmans MM. In vivo mechanisms of uterine myoma volume reduction with ulipristal acetate treatment. *Fertil Steril.* 2015;104(2):426–434.

35. Ali M, Shahin SM, Sabri NA, Al-Hendy A, Yang Q. 1,25 dihydroxyvitamin D3 enhances the antifibroid effects of ulipristal acetate in human uterine fibroids. *Reprod. Sci.* 2019;26(6):812–828.

36. Donnez J, Dolmans MM. Uterine fibroid management: From the present to the future. *Human Reprod. Update.* 2016;22(6):665–686.

37. Bourdet AT, Luton D, Koskas M. Clinical utility of ulipristal acetate for the treatment of uterine fibroids: Current evidence. *Int J Women's Health.* 2015;7:321–330.

38. De Milliano I, Van Hattum D, Ket JCF, Huirne JAF, Hehenkamp WJK. Endometrial changes during ulipristal acetate use: a systematic review. *Eur J Obstet Gynecol Reprod Biol.* 2017;214:56–64.

39. Liu JH, Soper D, Lukes A, Gee P, Kimble T, Kroll R, Mallik M, Chan A, Harrington A, Sniukiene V, Shulman LP. Ulipristal acetate for treatment of uterine leiomyomas: A Randomized Controlled Trial. *Obstet Gynecol.* 2018;132(5):1241–1251.

40. Lukes AS, Soper D, Harrinngton A, Sniukiene V, Mo Y, Gillard P, Schulman L. Health-related quality of life with ulipristal acetate for treatment of uterine leiomyomas: A Randomized Controlled Trial. *Obstet Gynecol.* 2019 May 133(5):869–878.

41. Coyne KS, Harrington A, Currie BM, Chen J, Gillard P, Spies JB. Psychometric validation of the 1 month recall Uterine Fibroid Symptom and Health-Related Quality of Life questionnaire (UFS-QOL). *J Patient Rep Outcomes.* 2019;3(1):57.

42. Powell M, Dutta D. Esmya® and the PEARL studies: A review. *Womens Health (Lond).* 2016;12(6):544–548.

43. EMA (European Medicine Agency). Esmya: New measures to minimise risk of rare but serious liver injury. EMA/482522/2018.

44. U.S. FDA, Allergan Complete Response Letter (CRL) from the U.S. Food and Drug Administration in response to the New Drug Application for ulipristal acetate for the treatment of abnormal uterine bleeding in women with uterine fibroids. Dublin, Aug. 21, 2018.

45. Park H, Yoon SW. Efficacy of single-dose gonadotropin-releasing hormone agonist administration prior to magnetic resonance-guided focused ultrasound surgery for symptomatic uterine fibroids. *Radiol Med.* 2017;122(8):611-616.

46. McLaren JS, Morris E, Rymer J. Gonadotrophin receptor hormone analogues in combination with add-back therapy: an update. *Menopause Int.* 2012;18(2):68–72.

47. Cao M, Qian L, Zhang X, Suo X, Lu Q, Zhao H, Liu J, Qu J, Zhou Y, Suo S. Monitoring leiomyoma response to uterine artery embolization using diffusion and perfusion indices from diffusion-weighted imaging. *Biomed Res Int.* 2017;2017:3805073.

48. Soeda S, Hiraiwa T, Takata M, Kamo N, Sekino H, Nomura S, Kojima M, Kyozuka H, Ozeki T, Ishii S, Tameda T, Asano K, Miyazaki M, Takahashi T, Watanabe T, Taki Fujimori K. Unique learning system for uterine artery embolization for symptomatic myoma and adenomyosis for obstetrician-gynecologists in cooperation with interventional radiologists: Evaluation of UAE from the point of view of gynecologists who perform UAE. *J Minim Invasive Gynecol.* 2018;25(1):84–92.

49. Yoon JK, Han K, Kim MD, Kim GM, Kwon JH, Won JY, Lee DY. Five year clinical outcomes of

uterine artery embolization for symptomatic leiomyomas: An analysis of risk factors for reintervention. *Eur J Radiol*. 2018;109:83–87.

50. Dueholm M, Langfeldt S, Mafi HM, Eriksen G, Marinovskij E. Re-intervention after uterine leiomyoma embolisation is related to incomplete infarction and presence of submucous leiomyomas. *Eur J Obstet Gynecol Reprod Biol*. 2014;178:100–106.

51. Arthur R, Kachura J, Liu G, Chan C, Shapiro H. Laparoscopic myomectomy versus uterine artery embolization: Long-term impact on markers of ovarian reserve. *J Obstet Gynaecol Can*. 2014;36(3):240-247.

52. Mattingly RF. *Te Linde's Operative Gynecology*, 5th edition, Philadelphia, PA, JB Lippincott Co, 1977, 219.

53. Scott JR, Disaia PJ, Hammond CB, Spellacy WN. *Danforth's Obstetrics and Gynecology*. Philadelphia, PA, JB Lippincott Co, 1994, 936.

54. Exacoustos C, Rosati P, Ultrasound diagnosis of uterine myomas and complications in pregnancy. *Obstet Gynecol*. 1993;82:97–101

55. Ghaemmaghami F, Karimi-Zarchi M, Gharebaghian M Kermani T. Successful myomectomy during cesarean section: Case report and literature review. *Int J Biomed Sci*. 2017;13(2):119–121.

56. Burton CA, Grimes DA, March CM. Surgical management of leiomyomata during pregnancy. *Obstet Gynecol*. 1989;74:707–709

57. Hsieh TT, Cheng BJ, Liou JD, Chiu TH. Incidental myomectomy in cesarean section. *Changgeng Yi Xue Za Zhi*. 1989 20;12:13–20

58. Michalas SP, Oreopoulou FV, Papageorgiou JS. Myomectomy during pregnancy and caesarean section. *Hum Reprod*. 1995;10:1869–1870

59. Ehigiegba AE, Ande AB, Ojobo SI. Myomectomy during cesarean section. *Int J Gynaecol Obstet*. 2001;75:21–25

60. Kathpalia SK, Arora D, Vasudeva S, Singh S. Myomectomy at cesarean section: A safe option. *Med J Armed Forces India*. 2016;72(Suppl 1):S161–S163.

61. O'Sullivan R, Abder R. Myomectomy at the time of cesarean delivery. *Ir J Med Sci*. 2016;185(4):973–975.

62. Ramya T, Sabnis S, Schitra TV, Panicker S. Cesarean myomectomy: An experience from a tertiary care teaching hospital. *J Obstet Gynaecol India*. 2019 69(5):426–430.

63. Zhao R, Wang X, Zou L, Zhang W. Outcomes of myomectomy at the time of cesarean section among pregnant women with uterine fibroids: A Retrospective Cohort Study. *Biomed Res Int*. 2019:7576934.

64. Sparic R, Malvasi A, Kadija S, Stefanović A, Radjenović SS, Popović J, Pavić A, Tinelli A. Safety of cesarean myomectomy in women with single anterior wall and lower uterine segment myomas. *J Matern Fetal Neonatal Med*. 2017:1–4.

65. Kwon DH, Song JE, Yoon KR Young Lee K. The safety of cesarean myomectomy in women with large myomas. *Obstet Gynecol Sci*. 2014;57(5):367–372.

66. Sparić R, Papoutsis D, Bukumirić Z, Kadija S, Spremović Radjenović S, Malvasi A, Lackovic M, Tinelli A. The incidence of and risk factors for complications when removing a single uterine fibroid during cesarean section: a retrospective study with use of two comparison groups. *J Matern Fetal Neonatal Med*. 2019:1–8.

67. Zaami S, Montanari Vergallo G, Malvasi A, Marinelli E. Uterine rupture during induced labor after myomectomy and risk of lawsuits. *Eur Rev Med Pharmacol Sci*. 2019;23(4):1379–1381.

68. Andonovová V, Hruban L, Gerychivá R, Janku P, Ventruba P. Uterine rupture during pregnancy and delivery: risk factors, symptoms and maternal and neonatal outcomes-Restrospective cohort. *Cescka Gynekol*. 2019;84(2):121–128.

69. Makino S, Takeda S, Kondoh E, Kawai K, Takeda J, Matsubara S, Itakura A, Sago H, Tanigaki S, Tanaka M, Ikeda T, Kanayama M. National survey of uterine rupture in Japan: Annual report of Perinatology Committee, Japan Society of Obstetrics and Gynecology. *J Obstet Gynaecol Res*. 2019;45(4):763–765.

70. Gimovsky AC, Frangieh M, Phillips J, Vargas MV, Quinlan S, Macri C, Ahmadzia H. Perinatal outcomes of women undergoing cesarean delivery after prior myomectomy. *J Matern Fetal Neonatal Med*. 2018;20:1–6.

71. RCOG: birth after previous cesarean birth. Green-top Guideline No. 45, October 2015.

72. Wachira L, De Silva L, Orangun I, Shehzad S, Kulkarni A, Yoong W. Spontaneous preterm recurrent fundal uterine rupture at 26 weeks following laparoscopic myomectomy. *J Obstet Gynaecol*. 2019;39(5):731–732.

73. Tanos V, Toney ZA. Uterine scar rupture - Prediction, prevention, diagnosis, and management. *Best Pract Res Clin Obstet Gynaecol*. 2019:115–131.

74. Tomczyk KM, Wilczak M, Rzymski P. Uterine rupture at 28 weeks of gestation after laparoscopic myomectomy – a case report. *Prz Menopauzalny*. 2018;17(2): 101–104.

75. Chao AS, Chang YL, Yang LY, Chao A, Chang WY, Su SY, Wang CJ. Laparoscopic uterine surgery as a risk factor for uterine rupture during pregnancy. *PLoS One*. 2018;13(5):e0197307.

76. Milazzo GN, Catalano A, Badia V, Mallozzi M, Caserta D. Myoma and myomectomy: Poor evidence concern in pregnancy. *J Obstet Gynaecol Res.* 2017;43(12):1789–1804.

77. Mahajan N, Moretti ML, Lakhi NA. Spontaneous early first and second trimester uterine rupture following robotic-assisted myomectomy. *J Obstet Gynaecol.* 2019;39(2):278–280.

78. Cho H. Rupture of a myomectomy site in the third trimester of pregnancy after myomectomy, septoplasty and cesarean section: A case report. *Case Rep Womens Health.* 2018;19:e00066.

79. Al-Zirqi, I, Daltveit AK, Vangen S. Infant outcome after complete uterine rupture. *Am J Obstet Gynecol.* 2018;219(1): 109.e1–109.e8.

80. Pop L, Suciu ID, Oprescu D, Micu R, Stoicescu S, Foroughi E, Sipos P. Patency of uterine wall in pregnancies following assisted and spontaneous conception with antecedent laparoscopic and abdominal myomectomies – a difficult case and systematic review. *J Matern Fetal Neonatal Med.* 2018:1–8.

81. Wu X, Jiang W, Xu H, Ye X, Xu C. Characteristics of uterine rupture after laparoscopic surgery of the uterus: clinical analysis of 10 cases and literature review. *J Int Med Res.* 2018;46(9):3630–3639.

82. Abbas A M, Michael A, Ali SS, Makhlouf AA, Ali MN, Khalifa MA. 2018. Spontaneous prelabour recurrent uterine rupture after laparoscopic myomectomy. *J Obstet Gynaecol.*, 1–2.

83. De Silva S. Perioperative care of pregnant women with previous uterine surgery. *J Perioperat Pract.* 2018;28(3):59–61.

84. Zeteroğlu S, Aslan M, Akar B, Bender RA, Başburğ A, Çalişkan E. Uterine rupture in pregnancy subsequent to hysteroscopic surgery: A case series. *Turk J Obstet Gynecol.* 2017;14(4):252–255.

85. Vimercati A, Del Vecchio V, Chincoli A, Malvasi A, Cicinelli E. Uterine rupture after laparoscopic myomectomy in two cases: Real complication or malpractice? *Case Rep Obstet Gynecol.* 2017;2017:1–5.

86. Yazawa H, Takiguchi K, Ito F, Fujimori K. Uterine rupture at 33rd week of gestation after laparoscopic myomectomy with signs of fetal distress. A case report and review of literature. *Taiwan J Obstet Gynecol.* 2018;57(2):304–310.

87. ACOG Committee on Practice Bulletins -- Obstetrics. ACOG Practice Bulletin No. 107: Induction of labor. *Obstet Gynecol.* 2009;114 (2 Pt 1):386–397.

88. Ben-Rafael Z, Perri T, Krissi H, Dicker D, Dekel A. Myomectomy during cesarean section-time to reconsider. In: Ben-Rafael Z, Diedrich K, Dudenhausen J-W et al. *Controversies in Obstetrics Gynecology and Infertility.* Israel, Oren Publisher Ltd, International Proceedings Division, 2003, 352–356.

89. Danilov A, Yurova A, Stark M Mynbaev OA, Vassilievsky Y. Towards a unified evidence-based cesarean section in the african continent-Introduction of the all-african surgical database. *Clin Obstet Gynecol Reprod Med* 2017;3: doi: 10.15761/COGRM.1000181.

90. Holmgren G, Sjöholm L, Stark M. The Misgav Ladach method for cesarean section: method description. *Acta Obstet Gynecol Scand.* 1999;78(7):615–621.

91. Cobellis L, Pecori E, Cobellis G. Hemostatic technique for myomectomy during cesarean section. *Int J Gynaecol Obstet.* 2002;79:261–262.

92. Lee JH, Cho DH. Myomectomy using purse-string suture during cesarean section. *Arch Gynecol Obstet.* 2011;283:S35–S37.

93. Younis JS, Okon E, Anteby SO. Uterine leiomyosarcoma in pregnancy. *Arch Gynecol Obstet.* 1990;247(3):155–160.

94. Hatırnaz Ş, Güler O, Başaranoğlu S, Tokgöz C, Kılıç GS. Endometrial myomectomy: A novel surgical method during cesarean section. *J Matern Fetal Neonatal Med.* 2018;31(4):433–438.

95. Tinelli A, Malvasi A, Favilli A, Gerli S, Stark M. What are the real advantages of trans endometrial myomectomy during cesarean delivery? *J Matern Fetal Neonatal Med.* 2019;32(18):3133–3134.

96. Sparić R, Kadija S, Stefanović A, Spremović Radjenović S, Likić Ladjević I, Popović J, Tinelli A. Cesarean myomectomy in modern obstetrics: More light and fewer shadows. *J Obstet Gynaecol Res.* May 2017;43(5):798–804. doi: 10.1111/jog.13294.

97. Huang SY, Shaw SW, Su SY, Li WF, Peng HH, Cheng PJ. The impact of a novel transendometrial approach for caesarean myomectomy on obstetric outcomes of subsequent pregnancy: a longitudinal panel study. *BJOG.* 2018;125(4):495–500.

98. Pandey S. Re: The impact of a novel transendometrial approach for caesarean myomectomy on obstetric outcomes of subsequent pregnancy: a longitudinal panel study: Novel transendometrial regimen for caesarean myomectomy on obstetric outcomes of subsequent pregnancy. *BJOG.* 2018;125(4):504–505.

99. Cheng PJ, Huang SY. Authors' reply re: The impact of a novel transendometrial approach for caesarean myomectomy on obstetric outcomes of subsequent pregnancy: a longitudinal panel study. *BJOG.* 2018;125(4):505-506.

100. Kongnyuy EJ, Wiysonge CS. Interventions to reduce haemorrage during myomectomy

for fibroids. *Cochrane Database Syst Rev.* 2007;1:CD005355.

101. Fletcher H, Frederick J, Hardie M Simenon D. A randomized comparison of vasopressin and tourniquet as hemostatic agents during myomectomy. *Obstet Gynecol.* 1996;87(6):1014–1018.

102. Protopapas A, Giannoulis G, Chatzipapas I, Athanasiou S, Grigoriadis T, Kathopoulis N, Vlachos DE, Zaharakis D, Loutradis D. Vasopressin during laparoscopic myomectomy: Does it really extend its limits? *J Minim Invasive Gynecol.* 2019;26(3):441–449.

103. Subedi S, Chhetry M, Lamichhane S. Myomectomy revisited: Experiences in a teaching hospital. *JNMA J Nepal Med Assoc.* Apr–June 2016;54(202):79–81.

104. Kathpalia SK, Arora D, Vasudeva S, Singh S. Myomectomy at cesarean section: A safe option. *Med J Armed Forces India.* 2016;72(Suppl 1):S161–S163.

105. Donat LC, Menderes G, Tower AM, Azodi M. A technique for vascular control during robotic-assisted laparoscopic myomectomy. *J Minim Invasive Gynecol.* 2015;22(4):543.

106. Fanny M, Fomba M, Aka E, Adjoussou S, Olou L, Koffi A, Konan P, Koné M. Prevention of bleeding during laparotomic myomectomy in Sub-Saharan Africa: Contribution to the tourniquet on the uterine isthmus. *Gynecol Obstet Fertil Senol.* 2008;46(10–11):681–685.

107. Al RA, Yapca OE, Gumusburun N. A randomized trial comparing triple versus single uterine tourniquet in open myomectomy. *Gynecol Obstet Invest.* 2017;82(6):547–552.

108. Sapmaz E, Calik H, Altungül A. Bilateral ascending uterine artery ligation vs. tourniquet use for hemostasis in cesarean myomectomy. A comparison. *J Rreprod Med.* 2003;48(12):950–954.

109. Incebiyik A, Hilali NG, Camuzcuoglu A, Vural M, Camuzcuoglu H. Myomectomy during caesarean: a retrospective evaluation of 16 cases. *Arch Gynecol Obstet.* 2014;289:569–573.

110. Kwawukume EY. Caesarean myomectomy. *Afr J Reprod Health.* 2002;6:38–43.

111. Lin JY, Lee WL, Wang PH, Lai MJ, Chang WH, Liu WM. Uterine artery occlusion and myomectomy for treatment of pregnant women with uterine leiomyomas who are undergoing cesarean section. *J Obstet Gynaecol Res.* 2010. 36:284–290.

112. Desai BR, Patted SS, Pujar YV, Sherigar BY, Das SR, Ruge JC. A novel technique of selective uterine devascularization before myomectomy at the time of cesarean section: A pilot study. *Fertil Steril.* 2010;94(1):362–364.

113. Akkurt MO, Yavuz A, Eris Yalcin S, Akkurt T, Turan OT, Yalcin Y, Seik M. Can we consider cesarean myomectomy as a safe procedure without long-term outcome? *J Matern Fetal Neonatal Med.* 2017;30(15):1855-1860.

114. Spariç R. Intraoperative hemorrhage as a complication of cesarean myomectomy: analysis of risk factors. *Vojnosanit Pregl.* May 2016;73(5):415–421.

115. Roman AS, Tabsh KM. Myomectomy at time of cesarean delivery: A retrospective cohort study. *BMC Pregnancy Childbirth.* 2004;4:14–17.

116. Levast F, Legendre G, Bouet PE, Sentilhes L. Management of uterine myomas during pregnancy. *Gynecol Obstet Fertil.* 2016. Jun;44(6):350–354.

117. Palmer SK, Zamudio S, Coffin C Parker S, Stamm E, Moore LG. Quantitative estimation of human uterine artery blood flow and pelvic blood flow redistribution in pregnancy. *Obstet Gynecol.* 1992;80(6):1000–1006.

118. Rorie DK, Newton M. Histologic and chemical studies of the smooth muscle in the human cervix and uterus. *Am J Obstet Gynecol.* 1967;99:466–469.

119. Burton GJ, Woods AW, Jauniaux E Kingdom JCP. Rheological and physiological consequences of Cconversion of the maternal spiral arteries for uteroplacental blood flow during human pregnancy *Placenta.* 2009;30(6): 473–482.

120. Hudić I, Fatušić Z, Kamerić L, Misić M, Serak I, Latifagić A. Vaginal delivery after Misgav-Ladach cesarean section--is the risk of uterine rupture acceptable? *J Matern Fetal Neonatal Med.* 2010;23(10):1156–1159.

121. Adesiyun AG, Ojabo A, Durosinlorun-Mohammed A. Fertility and obstetric outcome after caesarean myomectomy. *J Obstet Gynecol.* 2008;28: 710–712.

122. Akkurt MO, Yavuz A, Eris Yalcin S, Akkurt I, Turan OT, Yalcin Y, Sezik M. Can we consider cesarean myomectomy as a safe procedure without long-term outcome? *J Matern Fetal Neonatal Med.* 2016;9:1–6.

123. Malvasi A, Cavallotti C, Morroni M, Lorenzi T, Dell'Edera D, Nicolardi G Tinelli A. Uterine fibroid pseudocapsule studied by transmission electron microscopy. *Eur J Obstet Gynecol Reprod Biol.* 2012;162:187–191.

124. Tinelli A, Hurst BS, Hudelist G, Tsin DA, Stark M, Mettler L, Guido M, Malvasi A. Laparoscopic myomectomy focusing on the myoma pseudocapsule: Technical and outcome reports. *Hum Reprod.* 2012;27:427–435.

125. Tinelli A, Spariç R, Kadija S, Babovic I, Tinelli R, Mynabaev OA, Malvasi A. Myomas: Anatomy and related issues. *Minerva Ginecol.* 2016;68(3):261–273.

126. Tinelli A, Malvasi A, Hudelist G, Cavallotti C, Tsin DA, Schollmeyer T, Bojahr B, Mettler L. Laparoscopic intracapsular myomectomy: comparison of single versus multiple fibroids removal. An institutional experience. *J Laparoendosc Adv Sur Tech A.* 2010;20(8):705–711.

127. Spariç R, Malvasi A, Kadija S, Babović I, Nejković L, Tinelli A. Cesarean myomectomy trends and controversies: an appraisal. *J Matern Fetal Neonatal Med.* May 2017;30(9):1114–1123.

128. Tinelli A, Malvasi A, Mynbaev OA, Barbera A, Perrone E, Guido M, Kosmas I, Stark M. The surgical outcome of intracapsular cesarean myomectomy. A match control study. *J Matern Fetal Neonatal Med.* 2014;27(1):66–71.

129. Milazzo GN, Catalano A, Badia V, Mallozzi M, Caserta D. Myoma and myomectomy: Poor evidence concern in pregnancy. *J Obstet Gynecol Res.* 2017;43(12):1789–1804.

18 Adenomyomectomy

Anshumala Shukla Kulkarni and Fouzia Hayat

CONTENTS

Adenomyosis, characterized by the invasion of endometrial glands and stroma in the uterine myometrium, is a common benign gynecologic disease. Adenomyosis can be either diffuse or focal, and the etiology and pathogenic mechanism of adenomyosis are poorly understood.

The main symptoms of adenomyosis are menorrhagia, dysmenorrhea, and subfertility. Moreover, adenomyosis may be associated with recurrent abortion, premature delivery, and complications of late pregnancy, such as placenta previa.

Conservative surgical management in the form of adenomyomectomy remains the recommended treatment for those who have not completed their childbearing. The evolution of adenomyomectomy as a surgery has largely been "unexciting," and there is a general paucity of data [1]. Hyama introduced the first reported case of open adenomyomectomy in 1952 [1].

INDICATIONS

Adenomyomectomy is now at a stage where new surgical methods are being tried, but the indications for surgery differ depending on the surgeon. The indications include dysmenorrhea and hypermenorrhea that are difficult to control with medication, infertility and recurrent miscarriages, and a desire to preserve fertility or the uterus. Focal adenomyosis resection is similar to the myomectomy procedure and is very well managed with laparoscopy; however, when diffuse adenomyosis is present, one may need laparotomy. Any surgery for adenomyosis entails a risk of leaving some unexcised lesions.

Success of surgery depends on excision and ability to repair the uterine wall by suturing in layers (Figure 18.1).

INVESTIGATIONS

Two-Dimensional Ultrasonography

Two-dimensional (2D) transabdominal ultrasonography (USG) may reveal uterine enlargement or asymmetric thickening of the anterior and posterior myometrial walls [2]. USG features of adenomyosis are heterogeneity, increased echogenicity, decreased echogenicity, and anechoic lacunae or myometrial cysts [3]. In contrast to uterine fibroids, adenomyoma has a more elliptical shaped lesion with poorly defined borders and no calcifications or edge shadowing. In doubtful cases, Doppler sonography may be helpful. In the case of adenomyoma, blood vessels usually follow their normal vertical course

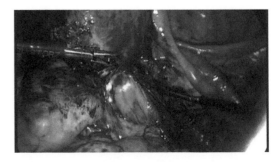

Figure 18.1 Adenomyoma with obliteration of the pouch of Douglas (POD) and adhesions. Normalizing anatomy and giving mobility is first step before adenomyomectomy.

in the myometrial areas, whereas in the case of uterine fibroid, blood vessels are usually located in the periphery [4, 5]. Three-dimensional (3D) USG improves diagnostic accuracy of adenomyosis as it allows better imaging of the junctional zone (JZ). The JZ is often visible as a hypoechogenic subendometrial halo which is composed of longitudinal and circular closely packed smooth muscle fibers.

Magnetic Resonance Imaging

Magnetic resonance imaging (MRI) is the gold-standard imaging modality for assessing the JZ in the evaluation of adenomyosis. The use of preoperative MRI is helps in mapping of the adenomyoma as well as differentiation between fibroid and focal adenomyoma.

SURGICAL TREATMENT FOR ADENOMYOSIS

The conservative surgical treatment for adenomyosis in young women was first reported in 1952. Subsequently, the partial excision of an adenomyosis, as a cytoreductive surgery, became common after the introduction of wedge resections, in which the uterine wall is excised in a V shape (Figure 18.2).

Partial Reduction Surgeries
Wedge Resection of the Uterine Wall

In this classic technique, parts of the serosa and uterine adenomyoma are removed via wedge resection. The seromuscular layer where the adenomyoma is located is incised and then an attempt is made to excise the adenomyoma. However, a part of the adenomyoma tissue may remain on one or both sides of the incision. The uterine wall defect created by the adenomyoma resection is sutured together with the remaining muscular layer and serosa. The postoperative clinical benefit on dysmenorrhea and menorrhagia is small, and recurrence occurs because of the presence of remaining adenomyomatous tissue. Reconstruction of the uterine wall

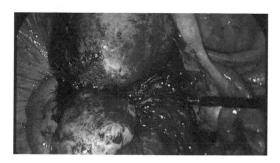

Figure 18.2 Focal adenomyoma.

involves suturing using the continuous horizontal mattress technique. The external serous layer is sutured such that the cut edges are inverted to reduce adhesion of the omentum, intestines, and peritoneum to the raw suture line. This suturing technique involves the "baseball" or continuous Lembert stitch method. In a study among 103 patients, 70 attempted to conceive during the study period. Out of 70 patients, 21 (30%) achieved clinical pregnancies and 16 (22.8%) achieved live births [6] (Figure 18.4).

Transverse H-Incision of the Uterine Wall

A report describing a modification technique on laparotomy compared five women treated with the classic method with six women undergoing modified reduction surgeries involving the transverse H-incision technique [7]. The transverse incision was made on the uterine fundus, using an electrosurgical scalpel, separating the uterine serosa from the uterine myometrium. After a wide opening of the uterine serosa on either side of the incision, the adenomyoma tissue was removed using an electrosurgical scalpel or scissors. A tension-less suturing technique was used to bring the myometrial edges together and close the wound in one or two layers. The first layer of sutures was applied to close the defect in the uterine wall and establish hemostasis. The bilateral serosal flaps resulting from the vertical incision, and the upper and lower flaps resulting from the transverse incision, were closed with a subserosal interrupted suture. In a later study by the same author, based on data collected up to 2010, out of the 41 patients who underwent the H-incision technique, 31 attempted to conceive and 12 (38.7%) achieved clinical pregnancy, 5 (16.1%) miscarried, and 7 (22.5%) reported live births [8]. Another study reported 14 women who underwent the technique mentioned above [9]. All of them wished to conceive, and 3 (21.4%) achieved pregnancy and all had healthy babies.

Complete Adenomyosis Excision
Triple-Flap Method

This adenomyomectomy technique is based on a completely new idea that differs from conventional surgical methods. The method involves reconstructing the uterine wall defect using normal uterine muscle. The technique is effective not only for diffuse uterine adenomyosis but also for nodular adenomyosis and has the potential to prevent uterine ruptures during postoperative pregnancies. The technique consists of the following three steps:

1. Complete extraction of the uterine adenomyosis by performing adenomyomectomy. Only cold-knife excision is used to perform adenomyomectomy in order to prevent thermal damage and which is considered to cause impaired healing. The incision extends from the uterine cavity to the serosa, and the adenomyoma is excised by palpation.

2. Preparation of uterine muscle flap after dissection of the adenomyoma. This uses the serosal side muscle to intervene and fill the gap.

3. Wound closure is carried out with sutures in three layers to reconstruct the uterus.

A study that examined 113 women who underwent this method demonstrated that the blood flow in the operated area had returned to normal in almost all cases (92/113, 81.4%) within 6 months [10]. Of 62 women who wished to conceive, 46 conceived and 32 delivered a healthy baby by elective cesarean section. There was no case of uterine rupture. During the 27 years of the study period, only 4 cases (3.5%) relapsed and required surgical treatment. In cases where a uterine adenomyosis resection is performed without opening the uterine cavity and the uterine wall is formed by superimposing a uterine muscle flap from the serosal side, the procedure is referred to as the double-flap method. As the excision of the adenomyoma should be carried out under palpation and delicate suturing by hand is required, the laparoscopic approach may be difficult and hence open surgery is preferable. However, following the steps of open surgery, some authors have described the same surgery as laparoscopically assisted adenomyomectomy [6, 11].

Asymmetric Dissection Method

This procedure involves asymmetric dissection of the uterus longitudinally, using a round-type loop electrode and a high-frequency cutter, followed by retracting the uterine fundus upward using a silk suture and then cutting the uterine adenomyoma into slices. From the incision, the myometrium is dissected diagonally as if hollowing out the uterine cavity. It is followed by a transverse incision to open the uterine cavity. As the index finger is inserted into the uterine cavity, the adenomyosis lesion is excised to more than 5 mm of the inner myometrium. The lesion is then excised to more than 5 mm of the serosal myometrium on the left uterine side. Afterward, the uterine cavity is sutured and closed, followed by uterine reconstruction, and

the left side covers the right side. The serosa is continuously sutured using the same suture to rejoin the uterus. To date, 1349 patients have undergone this technique. Postoperative spontaneous uterine rupture was seen in five cases in this series [12].

Laparoscopic Approach to Adenomyosis

Although the laparoscopic approach gives minimal access advantage to the patients, the limitations of movements of the instruments and reduced haptics are disadvantages to the surgeon performing adenomyomectomy surgery. Focal adenomyoma owing to a nodular appearance allows laparoscopic surgery similar to that used for uterine fibroids. Diffuse-type lesions require extensive resection and complicated suturing, necessitating difficult operations involving advanced suturing techniques.

The laparoscopic method involves a longitudinal or transverse incision along the adenomyoma, followed by dissection using a monopolar needle or cold knife. The defect is sutured in two or three layers. The suture of choice would be a delayed absorbable suture with interrupted U-shaped sutures. This reduces tension on the tissue and allows good approximation. The serosal layers can be closed using a barbed suture with baseball suture techniques that buries the stitch line [13]. Finally, removal of the adenomyotic mass may be accomplished using a morcellator but only in a contained bag system to prevent dispersal throughout the abdomen [14].

Some reports suggest that ultrasonic guidance is useful when the intraoperative recognition of the adenomatous lesion is difficult. Morita et al. reported a series of three women with focal adenomyosis who underwent excisions of adenomyoma with a surgical technique similar to those used for laparoscopic myomectomies [15]. There were no complications, and the average length of hospital stay was 3 days. In the report, the authors concluded that accurate diagnoses and preoperative MRI evaluations of the adenomyosis were the most important indicators of successful surgery [15].

POSTOPERATIVE PREGNANCY OUTCOMES

Post-adenomyomectomy improvements in dysmenorrhea and hypermenorrhea vary but are recognized. The postoperative pregnancy rate also varies between 17.5% and 72.7%. However, artificial reproductive technology largely contributes to the relatively high pregnancy rate. In total, 2365 uterine adenomyomectomies have been reported from 18 facilities worldwide. Of these, 2123 procedures have been performed at 13 facilities in Japan, constituting 89.8% of the global total. Among these, 449 pregnancies have been confirmed and 363 (80.8%) resulted in deliveries, including 2 cases of stillbirths. There were 13 (3.6%) cases of uterine ruptures. An additional 11 cases of uterine rupture have been reported.

UTERINE RUPTURE RISK

The frequency of uterine rupture in non-scarred uteri is 0.005% but increases to 0.04–0.02% in women with scarred uteri, and vaginal births after cesarean sections further increase the risk to 0.27–0.7% [6]. The risk of uterine rupture due to pregnancy, after removal of a uterine adenomyosis, is more than 1.0% [16] compared with 0.26% in pregnancies following myomectomy [10].

FACTORS CAUSING UTERINE RUPTURES

The factors that can potentially cause uterine ruptures in a subsequent pregnancies include the method of adenomyosis removal (e.g., cold knife, powered instruments), degree of extirpation of the adenomyosis (adenomyosis remnants in the tissue), extent and size of the uterine muscle defect, method of reconstructing the uterine cavity and the uterine wall, postoperative wound infection and postoperative hematoma formation, the period of contraception prior to postoperative pregnancy, and the skill of the surgeon.

CONTRACEPTION PERIOD BEFORE PLANNING PREGNANCY AFTER ADENOMYOMECTOMY

Counseling regarding time period to start planning conception after adenomyomectomy varies by surgeon preference. Some recommend conception within 3 months after surgery, but most recommended contraception for 6–12 months and then plan pregnancy. Vascularity of the operated area has been used as a criterion by some authors. They used color Doppler or MRI contrast to confirm resumption of blood flow. In this group, blood flow resumed in 92 cases (81.4%) within 6 months. However, when the uterine wall was largely resected, the resumption of blood flow could be delayed as much as 2 years [6].

LAPAROTOMY VERSUS LAPAROSCOPIC SURGERY

No study has shown a statistically significant difference in outcomes of adenomyomectomy carried out via laparotomy or laparoscopy or robot-assisted surgery. Nezhat et al. [17] found laparoscopic myomectomy and adenomyomectomy to be a safe alternative to open surgery. In another report, Nezhat et al. [18] found that a large percentage of patients with symptomatic adenomas and adenomyosis had concurrent endometriosis.

CHALLENGES FACED WITH ADENOMYOMECTOMY AND MODIFICATIONS

Diagnosis

Often, focal adenomyoma is misdiagnosed as fibroid and detected intraoperatively. When a patient presents with dysmenorrhea not correlating with fibroids, an MRI should be advised to determine the presence of adenomyoma. This influences the way in which patients are counseled preoperatively and affects patients' outcomes achieved through surgery.

Extent of Removal

Uncertainty in defining the site and extent owing to a lack of surgical plane makes it difficult to determine the extent of complete excision. One constantly needs to balance between inadequate removal of the adenomyoma versus excessive healthy myometrial excision that is detrimental to wound integrity.

Technical Difficulties

The excision of ill-defined tough adenomyotic tissue via laparoscopy is often difficult owing to a lack of tactile feedback. Robust suturing is also needed to close the defect while preventing the tearing of tissues. Techniques that have been recommended to enhance the strength of the sutures include the use of monofilament sutures, taking deep bites of the myometrium to prevent dead space formation and using interrupted sutures to reduce tension on the wound.

Associated Complications

Potential complications of adenomyomectomy include intraoperative hemorrhage, postoperative formation of intra-abdominal adhesions that may cause pain or contribute to infertility, uterine rupture in future pregnancies, and recurrence of the pathology.

Preoperative Gonadotropin-Releasing Hormone Agonists

Preoperative gonadotropin-releasing hormone agonists have been used for the treatment of adenomyoma-related diseases, resulting in a reduction in uterine size and symptomatic improvement. This is primarily used preoperatively to decrease the size of the lesion, facilitate resection, and reduce intraoperative bleeding. Morita et al. [15] had documented an average of 53.3 mL of blood loss when GnRH agonist was used prior to resecting the adenomyomas.

Vasopressin

Vasopressin acts by constricting the smooth muscle in the walls of capillaries, small arterioles, and venules. The role of vasopressin has been well established in myomectomies. Injecting vasopressin diluted in normal saline prior to making the incision on adenomyoma helps to decrease bleeding from the incision for about 20 min. However, it has been mentioned in the literature that possible drawbacks of the use of vasopressin in laparoscopic myomectomy include bleeding from the needle puncture sites, which often persists throughout the procedure, requiring later electrosurgical coagulation, and delayed bleeding in the myometrium. One needs to maintain vigilance in achieving hemostasis even when using vasopressin because of the risk of delayed bleeding, thereby rendering a false sense of security (Figure 18.3).

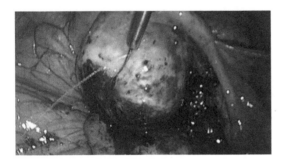

Figure 18.3 Vasopressin infitration to reduce bleeding.

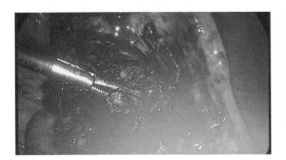

Figure 18.4 Wedge resection using monopolar.

Defect Closure

Meticulous and quick suturing for closure by experienced surgeons is the most definitive way to lessen intraoperative blood loss after adenomyomectomy. The key idea is to close up all the dead spaces so that hematoma formation does not occur. A useful trick is to approximate the edges with U-shaped sutures. This approximation serves to reduce tearing of the tissue and reduce tension prior to definitive closure. The simple explanation could be that the central stitch helped reduce the blood loss through a tamponade effect almost immediately (Figures 18.5–18.8).

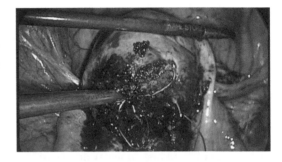

Figure 18.5 Multiple layer closure with interrupted sutures.

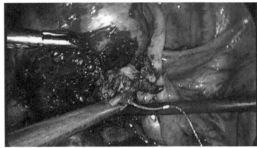

Figure 18.6 Serosal flap with myometrium created during dissection to close the gap.

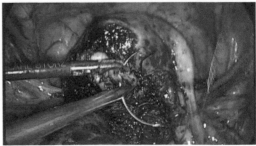

Figure 18.7 Serosal flap with myometrium created during dissection to close the gap.

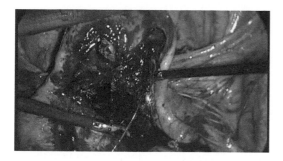

Figure 18.8 Dead space obliterated.

Laparoscopic Uterine Artery Occlusion or Ligation

Uterine artery ligation prior to myomectomy is well established. The similar analogy can be applied to adenomyomectomy as well. The uterine arteries can be ligated by an anterior approach or posterior approach. In the anterior approach, the uterovesical fold of the peritoneum is first opened and the bladder is pushed down, moving the ureters laterally to prevent them from being included in the sutures. The uterine vessels are identified on either side and ligated. In the posterior approach, the uterine artery can be ligated at its origin from the anterior division of the internal iliac after opening the triangle enclosed by the round ligament, external iliac artery, and infundibulopelvic ligament. A retrospective cohort study published by Kang et al. [8] looked at the role of uterine artery occlusion in laparoscopic adenomyomectomy. Thirty-seven patients were treated with uterine artery occlusion via the posterior approach, combined with partial resection of adenomyosis via laparoscopy. No severe complications were noted during the surgical procedure or follow-up. The mean blood loss was 90.0 ± 35.2 mL (range of 50–150 mL). At 6 months after surgery, the volume of the uterus shrank 24.7% compared with preoperative volume, and the shrinkage rate was 59.2% at 12 months after surgery. Studies on uterine artery embolization have stated the possibility of ovarian failure following the procedure. Other studies suggest that, unlike uterine artery embolization, uterine artery occlusion is a selective procedure and does not cause decreased ovarian reserve. However, in cases of fertility preservation, uterine artery occlusion is best avoided to maintain good blood flow to the ovaries and endometrium.

Timing of Surgery

Currently, no studies are looking at the relationship between timing of adenomyomectomy with regard to the menstrual cycle and intraoperative blood loss. However, surgery in the follicular phase can reduce blood loss and prevent surgery in an undiagnosed luteal pregnancy. One postulation is that vaginal and pelvic microvessels exhibit increased vascular reactivity during the follicular phase, which allows for better contraction of these microvessels and better hemostasis.

ADHESIONS

There are no data to validate use of adhesion barriers to prevent postoperative adhesions. In our practice, anti-adhesion agents such as Interceed and Seprafilm are still widely used in various types of gynecological surgeries.

Combined Surgical Medical Treatment

Adenomyomectomy should not be the be-all and end-all in managing adenomyomas. Prior to making a decision to undertake operative adenomyomectomy, one should consider whether conservative medical treatment may alleviate the patient's symptoms without subjecting her to the risks of surgery. In cases where adenomyomectomy has been deemed to be the best management option, consideration should be given to the use of adjuvant medical therapy postoperatively to improve patient outcomes. A variation of adenomyoma can be seen as multiple cystic adenomas. This is a rare form of adenomyoma. It presents as multiple cystic spaces in myometrium usually subserosal and contains endometrial tissue. These cystic spaces are actually cavitated lesions usually more than a cm and contain chocolate fluid. (Figures 18.9–18.12).

Robotic Adenomyomectomy

Following the first case report, robotic adenomyomectomy widens the options available for excision of localized adenomyosis. At present, robot technology helps in bridging the learning-curve gap between the open and laparoscopic approach. However, aside from

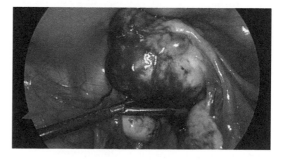

Figure 18.9 Multiple adenomyomas.

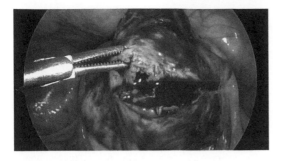

Figure 18.10   Multiple adenomyomas.

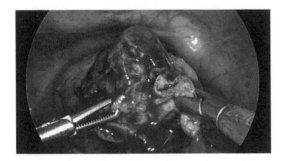

Figure 18.11   Multiple adenomyomas.

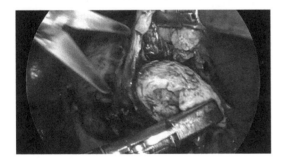

Figure 18.12   Multiple adenomyomas.

the additional drawback of increased operative costs, the challenges inherent in laparoscopy as highlighted earlier are still not fully addressed in robotic surgeries [19].

FOLLOW-UP

Surgical efficacy is evaluated by rating the levels of serum CA125, the size of the uterus, and the severity of dysmenorrhea and hypermenorrhea before and after surgery as well as the presence of pregnancy after surgery [20].

CONCLUSION

Traditionally, laparoscopic adenomyomectomy is performed via wedge resection where the part of the seromuscular layer where the

adenomyoma is located is removed. In this procedure, some of the adenomyotic tissue may remain on either side of the incision. Part of the muscle layer is then sutured, the tumor cavity is closed with absorbable sutures, and the residual seromuscular layer is sutured. Surgical modifications to the traditional wedge resection have been developed to decrease complications and intraoperative blood loss, and the surgical techniques involved in laparoscopic modified adenomyomectomy are some of these modifications.

REFERENCES

1. Hyama LL. Adenomyosis: Its conservative surgical treatment (hysteroplasty) in young women. *N Y J Med.* 1952;52:2778–2783.

2. Reinhold C, Atri M, Mehio A, Zakarian R, Aldis AE, Bret PM. Diffuse uterine adenomyosis: Morphologic criteria and diagnostic accuracy of endovaginal sonography. *Radiology.* 1995;197(3):609–614.

3. Dueholm M, Lundorf E. Trans vaginal ultrasound or MRI for diagnosis of adenomyosis. *Curr Opin Obstet Gynecol.* 2007;19(6):505–512.

4. Chiang CH, Chang MY, Hsu JJ, Chiu T-H, Lee K-F, Hsieh T-T, et al. Tumor vascular pattern and blood flow impedance in the differential diagnosis of leiomyoma and adenomyosis by color Doppler sonography. *J Assisted Reproduct Genet.* 1999;16(5):268–275.

5. Van den Bosch T, Dueholm M, Leone FP, Valentin L, Rasmussen CK, Votino A, et al. Terms, definitions and measurements to describe sonographic features of myometrium and uterine masses: A consensus opinion from the Morphological Uterus Sonographic Assessment (MUSA) group. *Ultrasound Obstetet Gynecol.* 2015;46(3):284–298.

6. Saremi AT, Bahrami H, Salehian P, Hakak N, Poolad A. Treatment of adenomyomectomy in women with severe uterine adenomyosis using a novel technique. *Reprod Biomed Online* 2014;28:753–760.

7. Fujishita A, Masuzaki H, Khan KN, Kitajima M, Ishimaru T. Modified reduction surgery for adenomyosis. A preliminary report of the transverse H incision technique. *Gynecol Obstet Invest.* 2004;57:132–138.

8. Kang L, Gong J, Cheng Z, Dai H, Hu L. Clinical application and midterm results of laparoscopic partial resection of symptomatic adenomyosis combined with uterine artery occlusion. *J Minim Invasive Gynecol.* 2009;16:169e173

9. Nishimoto M, Nabeshima H. Shikyusenkinkakushutsujutu. [Adenomyomectomy.]. *J Obstet Gynecol Pract (Tokyo).* 2011;60:1001–1007.

10. Sizzi O, Rossetti A, Malzoni M, Minelli L, Grotta FL, Soranna L, et al. Italian multi-center study on complications of laparoscopic myomectomy. *J Minim Invasive Gynecol.* 2007;14:453–462.

11. Kim JK, Shin CS, Ko YB, Nam SY, Yim HS, Lee KH. Laparoscopic assisted adenomyomectomy using double flap method. *Obstet Gynecol Sci.* 2014;57:128–135.

12. Nishida M, Otsubo Y, Ichikawa R, Arai Y, Sakanaka S. Shikyusenkinshokakushutsujutsu-go ninshin-ji no shikyuharetsu-yobo ni tsuite (Prevention of uterine rupture during pregnancy after adenomyomectomy). *Obstet Gynecol Surg, Medical View, Tokyo.* 2016;27:69–76.

13. Kitade M, Kumakiri K, Kuroda J, Jinushi M, Ujihira Y, Ikuma K, et al. Shikyusenkinsho gappei-funin ni taishite fukukukyoka-shikyu-onzon-ryoho wa yukoka? jutsugo-ninshinritsu to senko-shujutsu no umu ni yoru shusanki-yogo no kento [Is laparoscopic uterine preservation surgery effective against infertility associated with uterine adenomyosis? A study of perinatal prognosis by postoperative pregnancy rate and the presence of prior surgery]. *J Jpn Soc Endometriosis.* 2017;38:70.

14. Nabeshima H, Murakami T, Terada Y, Noda T, Yaegash N, Okamura K. Total laparoscopic surgery of cystic adenomyoma under hydroultrasonographic monitoring. *J Am Assoc Gynecol Laparosc.* 2003;10:195–199.

15. Morita M, Asakawa Y, Nakakuma M, Kubo H. Laparoscopic excision of myometrial adenomyomas in patients with adenomyosis uteri and main symptoms of severe dysmenorrhea and hypermenorrhea. *J Am Assoc Gynecol Laparosc.* 2004; *11*:86–89; Ofir K, Sheiner E, Levy A, Katz M, Mazor M. Uterine rupture: differences between a scarred and an unscarred uterus. *Am J Obstet Gynecol.* 2004;191:425–429.

16. Dubuisson JB, Fauconnier A, Deffarges JV, Norgaard C, Kreiker G, Chapron C. Pregnancy outcome and deliveries following laparoscopic myomectomy. *Hum Reprod.* 2000;15:869–873.

17. Nezhat C, Nezhat F, Bess O, Nezhat CH, Mashiach R. Laparoscopically assisted myomectomy: a report of a new technique in 57 cases. *Int J Fertil Menopausal Stud.* 1994;39:39–44.

18. Nezhat C, Li A, Abed S, Balassiano E, Soliemannjad R, Nezhat A. Strong association between endometriosis and symptomatic leiomyomas. *JSLS.* 2016;20:e2016.00053.

19. Shim JI, Jo EH, Kim M, Kim MK, Kim ML, Yun BS, et al. A comparison of surgical outcomes between robot and laparoscopy-assisted adenomyomectomy. *Medicine (Baltimore).* 2019 May;98(18):e15466.

20. Saremi AT, Bahrami H, Salehian P, Hakak N, Poolad A. Treatment of adenomyomectomy in women with severe uterine adenomyosis using a novel technique. *Reprod Biomed Online.* 2014;28:753–760.

19 Morcellation Techniques for Fibroid Uterus

Prakash Trivedi, Soumil Trivedi, Anjali Sonawane, and Aditi Parikh

CONTENTS

INTRODUCTION

With the advancement of laparoscopic surgery, the removal of large fibroids or multiple fibroids-uterus was always an issue. In parous women, colpotomy, which has the disadvantage of loss of pneumoperitoneum, limitation in size of fibroid, and occasionally dyspareunia, was used by few. The other option of widening the port size is nearly a minilaparotomy. These methods did not give all the benefits of laparoscopic minimal access surgery.

ERA OF MORCELLATORS

In 1993, Steiner et al. [1] introduced the first handheld power device with a grasper within two cylindrical tubes. The inner tube was sharp and rotates on a foot-switch control. This converts fibroids into long strips of 1–1.5 cm. The only drawback is that tissues spill around and they are to be picked up.

After Steiner's, Power morcellator, Sawalhe's I–II, Gyrus bipolar morcellator, Rotocut, Versator (Figure 19.1) came as a reusable or disposable morcellator. From 1994, when the morcellator was approved by the US Food and Drug Administration (FDA) [2], hundreds of thousands of removals of fibroid took place. The types of morcellator, size, torque, power of extracting a good volume of tissue with a blunt trocar for insertion, and a bevel or hood at the tip to protect the cutting blade are important.

The best port for entry of morcellator was widening the left lower port to 12–15 mm since it allows the morcellation tip to be continuously under vision for safety. Pneumoperitoneum pressure could be increased during insertion of the morcellator and can be maintained in contained bag morcellation.

VARIATIONS AND AREAS OF CONCERN IN MORCELLATION OF FIBROIDS

Fibroids varied in size from 3 to 20 cm and more, were 1–18 or more in number, and had anterior, posterior, lateral, broad ligament, isthmic, and cervical locations. Furthermore, fibroids can be degenerated, firm, angioleiomyoma, leiolipoma, and stony hard. All of these have to be tackled by proper dissection. Finally, to park and then accommodate for morcellation without missing any and reducing spillage of tissues. With conventional uncontained morcellation, scattering of tissues was always an issue [3].

Unfortunately, spillage of tissues led to leiomyomatosis, occasional spread of leiomyosarcoma [3], and port-site fibroid [4]. In April 2014, a serious concern was raised by the FDA on restricting use of morcellation because of the risk of spreading tumor or sarcoma [5]. A black-box warning was necessary for morcellation, stating that uterine tissue or myoma may contain unsuspected cancer. Insurance claims for morcellations were cancelled. Litigations grew up from patients to companies, consultants, and hospitals.

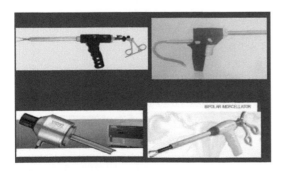

Figure 19.1 Different morcellators.

THE PHASE BEYOND THE MORCELLATION CONTROVERSY

The contained bag systems are of different varieties and have unique ways of adjusting morcellation. Multiple punctures on the bag or widening the port to accommodate optics, morcellator, and insufflation is cumbersome. Cold-knife blind morcellation in a bag had high bag puncture rates and tissue spread. The Ecosac, anchor retrieval system, Endocatch, Morsafe, Isolation bag, and many more are in clinical use today. (Figure 19.2). The hand-assisted system is essentially a laparotomy with increased risk of hernia.

TOTAL HEALTH-CARE TECHNIQUE OF CONTAINED VISUAL IN-BAG MORCELLATION OF FIBROIDS - UTERUS

After laparoscopic morcellation for fibroid and large uterus was accepted [2], a controversy erupted with one case of leiomyosarcoma in a patient with laparoscopic hysterectomy after morcellation leading to spread of sarcoma with significant morbidity [2]. This immediately led to a halt to laparoscopic morcellation. Due to black box warning issued by FDA in 2014, today it is acceptable to use in bag electro mechanical morcellation after infroming the risks and taking patient's consent. [2].

Although the risk of myomectomy or removal of large uterus involves many steps before morcellation, which are the same with open or laparoscopic surgery, morcellation is blamed for the spread of cells.

In view of the FDA caution with the main objective of acceptance and safety, a comparative study was done at the Total Health Care Centre (Mumbai, India) to evaluate the role of laparoscopic contained bag morcellation of myomas and uterus with myoma. The study period of in bag morcellation was from

May 2015 to August 2019 and included 426 cases. This was then compared with 430 cases of uncontained morcellation over a four year period from May 2011 to April 2015 (control group).

The steps of laparoscopic myomectomy–hysterectomy were the same; except for multiple large fibroids of more than 12 cm, an additional port on right side may be added for manipulation.

After separation of fibroids - uterus, contained bag morcellation was carried out as follows.

SURGICAL STEPS OF CONTAINED BAG MORCELLATION

The polyurethane stomach-shaped specially designed bag (Figure 19.3) is used. It is available in three sizes, namely small, medium and large, which have mouth openings of 13, 15, and 17 cm and volumes of 1.6, 2.1, and 2.6 L, respectively. Undiluted 0.5% sensorcaine is injected around the left lower port, which is widened to 1.5 cm, and then the blunt trocar of a 15-mm morcellator was passed to widen this port in its entirety. A plastic open trocar comes with the sterile bag for morcellation. The mouth of the bag is held to fit in the open plastic trocar, inserted from the left lower port. An assistant holds the edge of the bag's mouth (Figure 19.4), and the surgeon removes the plastic open trocar. In a series of horizontal pulls on the bag by the surgeon and assistant, the whole bag is now in the abdomen. At this moment, the left lower port is replaced by a 10-mm cannula with reducer; if gas leaks, a towel clip is applied on the skin. The mouth of the bag is opened slides into the pelvis. The assistant stabilizes a 12 o'clock position of the dual-colored bag, and the surgeon stabilizes a 6 o'clock position to keep the mouth open facing toward the camera. At this moment, the Trendelenburg position is

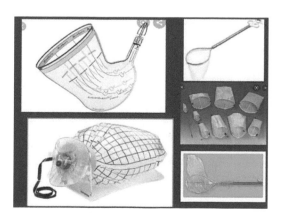

Figure 19.2 Different tissue retrieval bags.

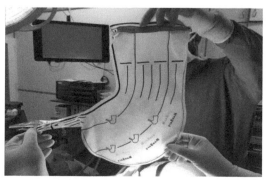

Figure 19.3 MorSafe: Stomach shaped bag with earlike tail.

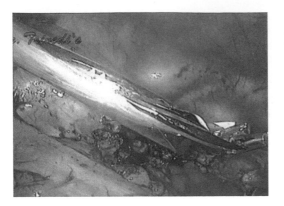

Figure 19.4 Bag edge introduced with sheath through left lower port held.

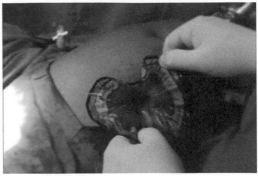

Figure 19.6 Flower-like mouth of bag retrieved through left lower port.

removed and the surgeon holds the fibroid or uterus with a single-toothed tenaculum and puts the specimen inside the bag. With this same tenaculum, another fibroid is put into the bag. In this fashion, multiple fibroids can be put into the bag (Figure 19.5). However, if the fibroid is large (more than 15 cm) or the uterus is too big, then with tenaculum the pressure is maintained on the specimen toward the pelvis and the margins of the mouth opening of the bag are elevated circumferentially. Once all the fibroids or uterus and tubes are in, the edges of the mouth of the bag are held closed from the assistant's to surgeon's side. Last, the lateral edge of the mouth close to the morcellation port is held and brought out, pulling a part of the bag outside. The mouth of the bag is pulled out of the abdomen (Figure 19.6). Next, the duodenum-shaped tail is inserted in a railroad fashion into the umbilical or primary cannula (Figure 19.7). Thus, the mouth is out of the left lower port and the tail end is out of the umbilicus or primary port. This tail has an opening and a 10-mm cannula is inserted through it (Figure 19.8) once the

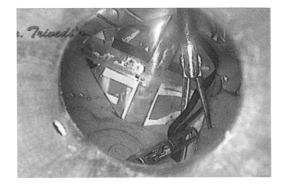

Figure 19.7 Ear shaped tail rail-roaded into umbilical cannula.

pneumoperitonium is created, and the carbon dioxide (CO_2) through the primary cannula distends the bag. Optics is passed and shows the specimen in the bag. The entire peritoneal cavity and abdominal structures are outside the bag. A 15-mm morcellator with a blunt trocar is introduced through the left lower port, the trocar is removed, and the grasper is introduced.

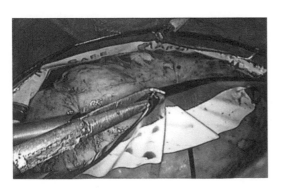

Figure 19.5 Specimen placed into bag and bag edges drawn over the specimen.

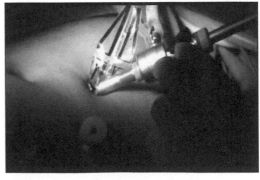

Figure 19.8 Cannula re-introduced into opening in the tail and insufflation started.

The entire specimen can be morcellated now (Figures 19.9 and 19.10).

With contained bag morcellation in 426 cases, up to 2100 g uterus (Figure 19.11), 17 fibroids, and a fibroid of 20 cm were removed.

The morcellator is removed and the primary cannula is withdrawn. A knot is tied at the tail end of the bag below the opening through which the optics passed (Figure 19.12). Pneumoperitoneum is removed, and by pulling the mouth of the bag from the left lower port, the entire bag is removed (Figure 19.13). There is no peritoneal spillage after morcellation as it is contained. In all 365 cases, bag integrity has been checked with 1.5 L of diluted methylene blue instilled in the bag (Figure 19.14).

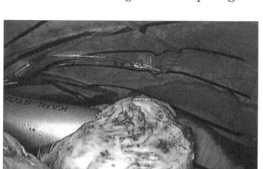

Figure 19.9 Morcellation of myoma or uterus done within bag which replaces peritoneal cavity (Storz Rotocut Morcellator).

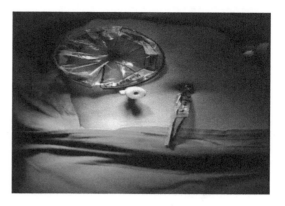

Figure 19.12 Opening in tail secured with knot below and bag can be withdrawn.

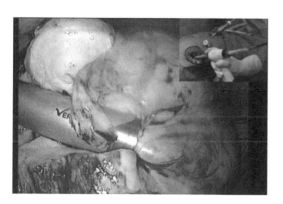

Figure 19.10 Morcellation of multiple myoma in bag (Versator Morcellator).

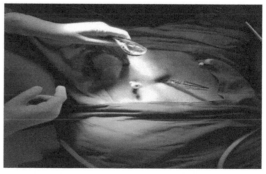

Figure 19.13 Bag being pulled from left lower port with tail receding into the umbilicus.

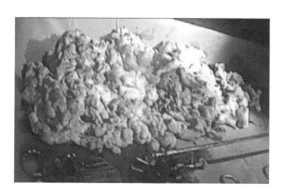

Figure 19.11 Large specimen of 1.83 kg post morcellation in bag.

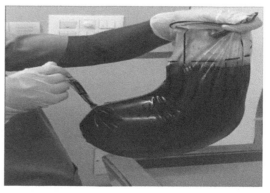

Figure 19.14 Bag filled with methylene blue to test for spillage and integrity check.

Next, hemostasis is checked and the morcellation port is closed with a port closure needle with two stitches. All patients were discharged in 48 h and follow-up was carried out clinically, and sonography and magnetic resonance imaging were carried out after 6 months and 1 year in 85% of cases.

RESULTS

In the study and control groups, parameters like duration of surgery, blood loss, and complications were comparable, and contained bag morcellation added the safety of avoiding spillage of tissues and improved patient parameters during morcellation as CO_2 goes in the bag and not in the circulation. No case of leiomyosarcoma or leiomyomatosis or port-site fibroid was reported in either group.

DISCUSSION

The prevalence of fibroids is high in many subgroups, and the need of myomectomy or hysterectomy for large fibroids (39%) with morcellation is an essential part of laparoscopic surgery.

Although the initial steps of myomectomy or hysterectomy are the same by open or laparoscopic route. Morcellation became controversial when there was spread in a case of leiomyosarcoma followed by restriction on the use of electromechanical morcellator by FDA.

The prevalence of leiomyosarcoma was 0.02% out of 10,731 uteri morcellated [6]. The Agency of Human Research and Quality - ACOG (American College of Obstetricians and Gynecologists) 1, 36, 195 cases with 160 meta-analysis reveals very low risk of leiomyosarcoma (from 0.02 to 0.08%) [7].

A key question that remains unanswered is the clear evidence of leiomyoma progressing to leiomyosarcoma.

A study of their cases over 24 years from Vienna Oncology hospitals revealed that, out of 71 cases of leiomyosarcoma back-traced, none started as a fibroid [8].

It is understood that leiomyosarcoma is due to selective genes suppression and fibroids develop due to gene expression. Hence, it is unlikely for a fibroid to become a leiomyosarcoma [9].

A study by Pados et al. found that, out of 2582 unsuspicious laparoscopic myomectomy, there was no case of leiomyosarcoma, but 6 cases of atypical myomas were found in 1216 subjects who underwent morcellation (ages of 18–45 years) [10]. The prevalence of leiomyosarcoma was 0% and atypical myoma 0.6%, and six atypical bizarre and one mitotically active leiomyoma were reported [10].

In bag morcellation also addresses to a major concern of leiomyomatosis which is huge liability after uncontained laparoscopic morcellation of fibroids, far more than rare leiomyosarcoma.

CONCLUSION

Laparoscopic morcellation of fibroid was thought to be a great breakthrough in 1994 and then it brought one of the biggest controversy in 2014. However, the whole understanding is based on connection or no connection of fibroids with leiomyosarcoma.

The fundamental steps of myomectomy or hysterectomy open or laparoscopic are the same and can lead to the spread of disease, but as morcellation was made out to be the culprit, our study on contained visual in-bag morcellation suggests the following:

1. Pre operative Diagnosis of leiomyosarcoma is not possible with certainty. The unexpected incidence of leiomyosarcoma is exceedingly low.

2. Further if one operates on an unexpected leiomyosarcoma, it will spread by any approach and could already have pre-existing intravascular spread.

3. The Vienna Oncology group's 24-year study on leiomyosarcoma suggests that none actually started from a fibroid.

4. Genetic evidence suggests that leiomyosarcoma is due to selective gene suppression and fibroids are the expression. Therefore, leiomyosarcoma progressing from a leiomyoma is an unlikely event.

5. Finally, contained visual bag morcellation should be the norm not only to address the concern of leiomyosarcoma, but also to prevent iatrogenic parasitic fibroids.

Research, controversy, and advances will continue.

REFERENCES

1. Steiner RA, Wight E, Tadir Y, Haller U. Electrical cutting device for laparoscopic removal of tissue from the abdominal cavity. *Obstet Gynecol*. 1993;81(3):471-474.

2. The Morcellation Controversy: A Timeline – Medscape, Apr 24, 2014.

3. *Journal of Minimally Invasive Gynecology* May/June 2018;25(4):544.

4. Oindi FM, Mutiso SK, Obura T. Port site parasitic leiomyoma after laparoscopic myomectomy: A case report and review of the literature. *J Med Case Rep*. 2018;12:339.

5. Oindi et al. *J Med Case Rep*. 2018;12:339; *Food Drug Adm*. 2014;17:4. FDA discourages use of Laparoscopic power morcellation for removal of uterus or uterine fibroids. (US FDA, http://www.fda.cov/medical devices/safety/alerts and notices/393576.htm, 2014).

6. Bojahr B, De Wilde RL, Tchartchian G. Malignancy rate of 10,731 uteri morcellated during laparoscopic supracervical hysterectomy (LASH). *Arch Gynecol Obstet*. 2015;292:665–672.

7. ACOG Committee Opinion No. 770. Uterine morcellation for presumed leiomyomas. *Am Col Obstet Gynecol Obstet Gynecol*. 2019;133:e238–e248.

8. Mayerhofer K, Obermair A, Windbichler G, et al. Leiomyosarcoma of the uterus: a clinicopathologic multicenter study of 71 cases. *Gynecol Oncol*. 1999;74(2):196–201.

9. Quade BJ, Wang TY, Sornberger K, et al. Molecular pathogenesis of uterine smooth muscle tumors from transcriptional profiling. *Genes Chromosomes Cancer*. 2004;40:97–108.

10. Pados G, Tsolakidis D, Theodoulidis V, Makedos A, Zaramboukas T, Tarlatzis B. Prevalence of occult leiomyosarcomas and atypical leiomyomas after laparoscopic morcellation of leiomyomas in reproductive-age women. *Hum Reproduct*. 2017;32(10):2036–2041.

20 Parasitic Fibroids

Rooma Sinha and Bana Rupa

CONTENTS

INTRODUCTION

Fibroids that derive nourishment from an extra-uterine source are known as parasitic fibroids. Uterine fibroids are common uterine tumors, but parasitic fibroids are rare tumors of uncertain etiology. Parasitic fibroids can develop *de novo* when they develop after morcellation of specimen-containing fibroids during myomectomy or hysterectomy. Then they are termed iatrogenic parasitic myomas [1]. As the popularity of minimal access surgery increased, there became an increasing need to morcellate tissues at the end of the surgery. The act of morcellation then began to create an iatrogenic situation requiring further surgical interventions. Parasitic fibroids present without a history of morcellation can develop because of hormonal or genetic factors [2].

In their paper, Nezhat and Kho classified parasitic fibroids into three broad categories [1]. One category of parasitic fibroids develops spontaneously from pedunculated fibroids that simply detach from the uterus and start growing by deriving blood from neighboring organs. The second category of parasitic fibroids develops because of restriction of blood supply to the uterus, and the third category develops following uterine surgery, especially if morcellation was carried out [1].

There is also a report of 41-year-old woman who underwent magnetic resonance imaging (MRI)-guided focused ultrasound for treatment of fibroids. Eleven months later, when she underwent surgery, she had 1.2-cm parasitic fibroids on the posterior wall of the vagina [1]. Sometimes, parasitic fibroids can also develop because of peritoneal metaplasia that are sensitive to hormonal influence and can be seen in various parts of the abdomen. Leiomyomatosis peritonealis disseminata (LPD) is the presence of multiple nodules on peritoneal surfaces and was first described in 1952 by Willson and Peale [3]. It is primarily a benign condition, where nodules are seen studded not only on surfaces of peritoneum but also on the uterus, intestines, and abdominal walls [4,5].

PATHOGENESIS

Kelley and Cullen, in their publication in 1910, described a series of 37 parasitic fibroids [6]. In their article, the authors mention that the development of parasitic fibroids was "inherent in the myomata and not in the surrounding organs." They theorized that the uterus contracts and tries to expel intramural fibroids. As it continues to contract, these intramural fibroids become pedunculated, lose their uterine blood supply, and the pedicle separates. At this point, the omentum, adjoining bowel, or even bladder provides a blood supply to these detached fibroids for its sustenance [6].

The pathogenesis described by Kho and Nezhat is the displacement of myoma from the original site of attachment [7]. This can be seen in cases that receive gonadotropin-releasing hormone, which restricts the blood supply to the fibroids. A pedunculated fibroids restricts the blood supply, detaches, and parasitizes to an adjacent organ [7].

Another popular theory for the development of parasitic fibroids is unconfined morcellation during gynecological surgeries and can be seen in about 1% of cases [8]. The first case of a parasitic fibroids after use of the laparoscopic morcellation was reported in 1997 by Ostrzenski [9]. In fact, the prevalence of uterine sarcoma and morcellation has been the focus of most discussions in recent times. However, benign sequelae are much more common than the presence of sarcoma in the morcellated tissues. The US Food and Drug Administration quoted the presence of sarcoma in fibroids that are surgically removed to be 1 in 350 cases in 2014 [10]. However, a meta-analysis by Pritts et al. [11] reported a much lower incidence (1 in 2000). Though not as sinister as sarcoma, benign sequelae are more common and may need another surgical intervention following the initial surgery where morcellation was used. These are seen more with unconfined morcellation with electromechanical device, which was the norm until recent times. A systematic review by Van der Meulen (2016) included 44 studies and reported that the incidence of iatrogenic parasitic fibroids was 0.12–0.94% [12]. The total number of patients included was 69, and the time of presentation from the primary surgery was an average of 4 years. The mean number of parasitic fibroids was 2.9 (range of 1–16), most frequently seen after myomectomy; 21.7% of patients were asymptomatic in this review. Most patients with parasitic fibroids present with abdominal discomfort, fatigue, backache, dyspareunia, and urinary/bowel complaints [12].

The pathogenesis of iatrogenic parasitic fibroids is still not clearly understood. It is seen that fibroids greater than 6.5 cm have a higher incidence of abnormal karyotypes (75% vs. 34%) than fibroids less than 6.5 cm [13]. Thus, if morcellation is carried out for fibroids greater than 6.5 cm, it has a higher tendency to implant in peritoneal cavity and grow over time. In a review by Darii et al., 29% of cases with parasitic fibroids underwent laparoscopic myomectomies for fibroids greater than 6 cm, and only in two cases was the fibroid size less than 6 cm [14]. Fibroids located in the posterior wall of the uterus are difficult to reach and operate during surgery, and small fragments may be left behind. It is possible that this is a contributing factor in the development of parasitic fibroids.

Electromechanical morcellator has a coring knife inside a rapidly circulating cylinder. An electromechanical device rotates this cylinder as it cuts the tissue in long strips and then is removed from the abdominal cavity through the cannula. This mechanism creates different sizes of tissue both macroscopic and microscopic that can spread into the peritoneal cavity. The extremely small fragments can go unnoticed by the surgeon. These tissue fragments of various sizes remain in the abdominal cavity and sometimes at the trocar sites. They then get a blood supply from neighboring structures and start to grow as iatrogenic parasitic fibroids.

Though not common with open abdominal surgery, morcellation through the vagina can also be associated with parasitic fibroids. Large masses are removed via small vaginal openings. Vaginal morcellation in a bag, though feasible, can be cumbersome and challenging. A 140-g parasitic myoma at the vault was reported 3 months after vaginal hysterectomy and vaginal morcellation [15].

Figure 20.1a,b show MRI of a previously unreported case from our institution that presented with a fibroid of approximately 5 cm at the vaginal vault a year after surgery. This 43-year-old patient had undergone total laparoscopic hysterectomy for multiple fibroids with vaginal morcellation.

In their review, Van der Meulen described the duration of steroid exposure as a risk factor for development of parasitic fibroids. [12]. Morcellation in premenopausal patients has a higher likelihood to develop parasitic fibroids as compared with women in the postmenopausal age group [12]. That the histology of the parasitic fibroids is usually consistent with the original fibroids in these patients suggests a biologically plausible relationship [16]. The molecular genetic analysis further confirms the relationship between parasitic fibroids and LPD nodules within the original fibroids in the patient [17]. Fibroids in locations other than the uterus could also originate from the remains of the Müllerian or Wolffian ducts [18].

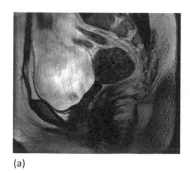
(a)

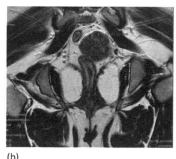
(b)

Figure 20.1 (a and b) Parasitic fibroid at the vault after vaginal morcellation.

LOCATION

The most common locations of parasitic fibroids are in the pelvis. The location and number of parasitic fibroids can depend on the type of morcellation. If mechanical morcellation is used, the number of parasitic fibroids is usually single and they are confined to the pelvis. If electromechanical morcellator is used, the resultant parasitic fibroids are multiple and the location can be anywhere in the peritoneal cavity. This could be explained by the fact that larger fragments during mechanical morcellation can be picked up easily but the electromechanical morcellation creates very small fragments that get dispersed into the peritoneal cavity. The size of the parasitic fibroids is reported to be from 3 mm to 30 cm. During surgery, bits of morcellated tissues can be deposited in the rectus muscle and subcutaneous tissue, where they grow with the adjacent blood supply. Minimal access surgery can cause trocar site deposits and the development of iatrogenic parasitic fibroids. Small fragments of fibroids can stick on the cannula sleeve, and when the sleeve is pulled, these fragments are trapped in the port sites as the cannulas are being withdrawn. These then grow into large fibroids with the effect of circulating estrogen and blood supply.

We describe a case of a 38-year-old woman who underwent laparoscopic myomectomy 6 years ago. Her previous surgical notes confirmed the use of unconfined electromorcellation. She then presented with recurrent uterine fibroids along with large abdominal masses. The parasitic fibroids were found in the abdominal wall, intraperineally in both the paracolic gutters, some attached to the omentum. She underwent laparotomy with excision of all the parasitic fibroids and total hysterectomy (Figure 20.2a–c).

Parasitic fibroids have been reported in almost every part of the abdominal cavity, like the omentum, intestinal serosa, appendix, paravesical space, and pararectal or paracolic fossa. Sinha et al. reported the presence of parasitic fibroids under the diaphragm [19]. We describe a patient who while undergoing a robotic-assisted multiple myomectomy was found to have a parasitic fibroid from the lateral pelvic wall at our unit at Apollo Hospitals. Figure 20.3 from this patient shows a parasitic myoma arising from the right pelvic wall close to the external iliac vessels (Figure 20.3a,b). Another case at our center that was planned for total laparoscopic hysterectomy revealed a fibroid arising from the rectum (Figure 20.4). This patient did not have any history of pelvic surgery.

A 50-year-old patient at our center was advised to have a total laparoscopic hysterectomy for urinary symptom and pelvic pain. Both clinical examination and transvaginal ultrasonography confirmed enlarged uterus with anterior wall fibroid. On laparoscopy, the uterus was of normal size and separate from a large fibroid seen anterior to uterus arising from the space of Retzius (Figure 20.5a,b). There are similar reports of fibroids seen in the space of Retzius in the literature [20].

Primary ovarian fibroids are a rare solid tumor of the ovary. Only 0.5–1% of benign ovarian neoplasms are ovarian fibromas [21]. About 75 cases have been reported in the literature. They are usually unilateral and often present along with uterine fibroids. We present a case of a 28-year-old patient presenting with secondary infertility. Her ultrasound imaging showed multiple fibroids. During robotic-assisted myomectomy, one of the fibroids was seen arising primarily from the left ovary (Figure 20.6). The pathogenesis of these ovarian fibroids is from the smooth muscle cells in hilar

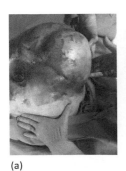
(a)

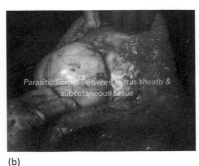
(b)

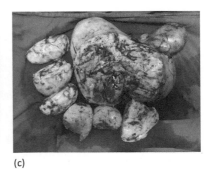
(c)

Figure 20.2 (a) External picture showing large multiple parasitic fibroids of the abdominal wall. (b) Parasitic fibroid seen between the rectus sheathe and subcutaneous tissue in the abdominal wall. (c) Multiple fibroids removed by laparotomy in the same patient.

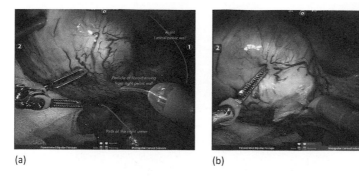

(a)   (b)

Figure 20.3   (a) Parasitic fibroid from the right lateral wall. (b) Robot-assisted excision of the parasitic fibroid from the lateral wall of the pelvis.

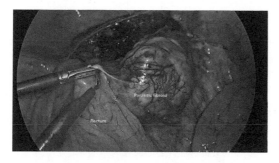

Figure 20.4   Fibroid arising from rectum without any previous history of surgery.

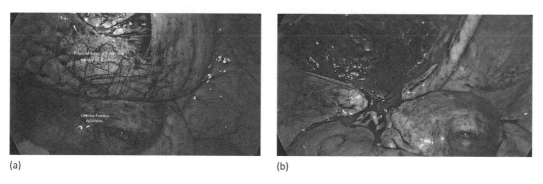

(a)   (b)

Figure 20.5   (a) Fibroid arising from the space of Retzius, a separate and normal size uterus can be seen below the fibroid. (b) large peritoneal dissection seen in the space of Retzius after the fibroid was removed. A normal size uterus can be seen.

blood vessels or they develop from the metaplasia of smooth muscles of ovarian stroma or ovarian ligaments [22].

The presence of fibroids in the urinary bladder is another unusual presentation of parasitic fibroids. About 250 cases of bladder fibroids have been reported to date and they constitute less than 0.5% of all bladder tumors [23]. It can present as intravesical, intramural, or extravesical. These are typically benign, and small ones can be removed with transurethral resection. Large ones need surgical removal along with partial cystectomy. We describe a case of a 36-year-old woman with dysuria and frequency presenting with a large intravesical fibroid. Open surgical excision of fibroid was carried out with partial cystectomy (Figure 20.7a–c).

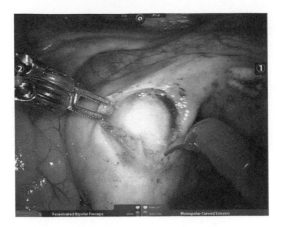

Figure 20.6 Primary parasitic ovarian fibroid from the left ovary.

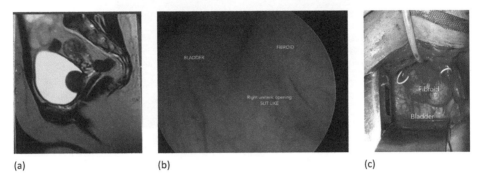

(a)　　　　　　　　　　(b)　　　　　　　　　　(c)

Figure 20.7 (a) Magnetic resonance imaging (MRI) showing intravesical myoma. (b) Cystoscopy of the same patient shows presence of fibroid from the posterior wall of the bladder. The right ureteric orifice opening can be seen like a slit on the fibroid. (c). Laparotomy view of the open bladder with the fibroid. Ureteric catheters in both ureteric orifices.

TREATMENT

The challenge in managing cases of parasitic fibroids is to make a precise preoperative diagnosis. Identifying the location before surgery is important to plan the approach of surgical excision. Differentiation of parasitic fibroids from malignant tumors like leiomyosarcoma can pose a difficulty during the workup. MRI or 3D ultrasound is the most useful technique for preoperative evaluation. Histopathology gives the final diagnosis, and additional immunohistochemical tests can be carried out in case of doubtful masses. Management offered can be both medical and surgical. Medical castration of smaller parasitic fibroids can be tried with or without resection. The clinical course is usually benign. However, the risk of malignant transformation is higher than regular uterine fibroids (2–5%). Owing to this fact, close surveillance is mandatory or surgical removal should be carried out if parasitic fibroid is detected [24]. Surgical excision of the parasitic fibroids is carried out with or without hysterectomy. Laparotomy is commonly used, but laparoscopic management of parasitic fibroids is safe and feasible. More than half the cases in the literature and most of our cases discussed here were diagnosed and managed laparoscopically.

CONCLUSION

Parasitic fibroids, though rare, need surgical management most of the time. The pathogenesis of their development in the absence of a history of surgery is still not clear. Fragments that are left during mechanical or electromechanical morcellation deposit in the peritoneal cavity, survive, and grow as iatrogenic parasitic fibroids. In-bag contained morcellation might decrease their incidence. Meticulous morcellation technique and a systematic survey of the entire peritoneal cavity at the end of the procedure are recommended. Efforts must be made to meticulously remove all fragments to reduce this iatrogenic problem.

REFERENCES

1. Nezhat C, Kho K. Iatrogenic myomas: New class of myomas? *J Minim Invasive Gynecol.* 2010;17(5):544–550.

2. Al-Talib A, Tulandi T. Pathophysiology and possible iatrogenic cause of leiomyomatosis peritonealis disseminata. *Gynecol Obstet Invest.* 2010;69(4):239–244.

3. Willson JR, Peale AR. Multiple peritoneal leiomyomas associated with a granulosa-cell tumor of the ovary. *Am J Obstet Gynecol.* 1952;64(1):204–208.

4. Sharma P, Chaturvedi KU, Gupta R, Nigam S. Leiomyomatosis peritonealis disseminata with malignant change in a post-menopausal woman. *Gynecol Oncol.* 2004;95(3):742–745.

5. Thian YL, Tan KH, Kwek JW, Wang J, Chern B, Yam KL. Leiomyomatosis peritonealis disseminata and subcutaneous myoma-a rare complication of laparoscopic myomectomy. *Abdom Imaging.* 2009;34(2):235–238.

6. Kelley-Cullen. Myomata of the uterus. *South Med J.* 1910;3(3):213.

7. Kho K, Nezhat C. Parasitic myomas: Report of the largest case series. *J Minim Invasive Gynecol.* 2009;16(6):S48–S49.

8. Tulandi T, Leung A, Jan N. Nonmalignant sequelae of unconfined morcellation at laparoscopic hysterectomy or myomectomy. *J Minim Invasiv Gynecol.* 2016;23:331–337.

9. Ostrzenski A. Uterine leiomyoma particle growing in an abdominal-wall incision after laparoscopic retrieval. *Obstet Gynecol.* 1997;89(5 II suppl):853–854.

10. US Food and Drug Administration. Laparoscopic uterine power morcellation in hysterectomy and myomectomy: FDA safety communication. http://www.fda.gov/MedicalDevices/Safety. 2014.

11. Pritts EA, Vanness DJ, Berek JS, Parker W, Feinberg R, Feinberg J, et al. The prevalence of occult leiomyosarcoma at surgery for presumed uterine fibroids: a meta-analysis. *Gynecol Surg.* 2015;12:165–177.

12. Van Der Meulen JF, Pijnenborg JMA, Boomsma CM, Verberg MFG, Geomini PMAJ, Bongers MY. Parasitic myoma after laparoscopic morcellation: A systematic review of the literature. *BJOG: An Int J Obstet Gynaecol.* 2016;123:69–75.

13. Rein MS, Powell WL, Walters FC, Weremowicz S, Cantor RM, Barbieri RL, et al. Cytogenetic abnormalities in uterine myomas are associated with myoma size. *Mol Hum Reprod.* 1998;4(1):83–86.

14. Darii N, Anton E, Doroftei B, Ciobica A, Maftei R, Anton SC, et al. Iatrogenic parasitic myoma and iatrogenic adenomyoma after laparoscopic morcellation: A mini-review. *J Adv Res.* 2019;20:1–8.

15. Agostini A, Vejux N, Capelle M, Ronda I, Blanc B. Laparoscopic removal of a remaining myoma after vaginal hysterectomy: A case report. *J Minim Invasive Gynecol.* 2005;12(4):372–373.

16. Takeda A, Mori M, Sakai K, Mitsui T, Nakamura H. Parasitic peritoneal leiomyomatosis diagnosed 6 years after laparoscopic myomectomy with electric tissue morcellation: Report of a case and review of the literature. *J Minim Invasive Gynecol.* 2007;14(6):770–775.

17. Carter J, McCarus S. Time savings using the Steiner morcellator in laparoscopic myomectomy. *J Am Assoc Gynecol Laparosc.* 1996; 3(4):S6.

18. Fasih N, Shanbhogue AKP, Macdonald DB, Fraser-Hill MA, Papadatos D, Kielar AZ, et al. Leiomyomas beyond the uterus: Unusual locations, rare manifestations. *Radiographics.* 2008;28(7):1931–1948.

19. Sinha R, Sundaram M, Lakhotia S, Kadam P, Rao G, Mahajan C. Parasitic myoma after morcellation. *J Gynecol Endosc Surg.* 2009;1(2):113–115.

20. Niwa N, Yanaihara H, Horinaga M, Asakura H. Leiomyoma in Retzius' space: An unusual location. *Can Urol Assoc J.* 2013;7(9–10):E612–E613.

21. Van Winter JT, Stanhope CR. Giant ovarian leiomyoma associated with ascites and polymyositis. *Obstet Gynecol.* 1992;80(3):560–563.

22. Fallahzadeh H, Dockerty MB, Lee RA. Leiomyoma of the ovary: Report of five cases and review of the literature. *Am J Obstet Gynecol.* 1972;113:394–398.

23. Mendes JE, Ferreira AV, Coelho S, Gil C. Bladder leiomyoma. *Urol Ann.* 2017;9(3):275–277.

24. Halama N, Grauling-Halama SA, Daboul I. Familial clustering of Leiomyomatosis peritonealis disseminata: An unknown genetic syndrome? *BMC Gastroenterol.* 2005;5:33. Published 2005 Oct 13. doi:10.1186/1471-230X-5-33.

21 Laparoscopic Hysterectomy in the Setting of Large Fibroids

Alphy S. Puthiyidom

CONTENTS

When it comes to large and multiple fibroids, especially in perimenopausal women, the most commonly opted surgical treatment is hysterectomy. A large uterine size has traditionally been considered a contraindication to laparoscopic and vaginal hysterectomy procedures. With the passage of time, surgical techniques have been refined and laparoscopic instruments have improved, making laparoscopic hysterectomy a safe and effective procedure for large uteri.

Although the numbers of laparoscopic hysterectomies have been increasing, this surgical procedure is still under-used when it comes to the large uterus.

Total laparoscopic hysterectomy in a uterus enlarged with multiple fibroids can pose several challenges that can result in increased operating time, increased blood loss, and a risk of injury to surrounding structures. These obstacles include limited visualization, less freedom to manipulate a larger uterus, distortion of normal anatomy, and greater vascularity. The challenges of laparoscopic hysterectomy warrant a modified approach tailored to addressing the distinctive pathology.

In this chapter, we will discuss the following:

1. Prerequisites

2. Surgical technique
   - Port placement
   - Methods to reduce intraoperative blood loss
   - Uterine manipulation
   - Specimen retrieval

PREREQUISITES FOR A SMOOTH SURGERY

Along with routine laparoscopic instruments, proper uterine manipulators and electrosurgery equipment are key items for any difficult surgeries. In hysterectomy for large fibroid uterus, proper use of the manipulator and a 30° angle scope allow proper visualization of the uterine isthmus and the lateral and posterior fornices. These eliminate the visual impairment caused by the large fibroid uterus and create a familiar operative field that is very similar to that seen in a normal-sized uterus, thus inspiring confidence and safety. The availability of vessel sealing and ultrasonic devices plays a key role in tackling the varicosities and adhesions. Equipment used should be functional and there must be a backup plan in place to cover any unanticipated malfunction.

Patient Position

These procedures are performed under general anesthesia with endotracheal intubation. The legs are placed in a low lithotomy position with the hips extended to around 140° to 150°. Allen stirrups or knee braces that are adjustable to each patient are recommended. The arms are tucked at the sides to allow free movements for the surgeons and to avoid brachial plexus injury (Figures 21.1 and 21.2).

Once the primary trocar is in place and the pneumoperitoneum is created, the patient is placed in a steep Trendelenburg position. A tilt of 30° or more can provide a better view into the deep pelvis, which is very important while ligating lower pedicles and opening the vaginal vault. A shoulder support can help prevent the patient from sliding on a tilted operating table and avoid injuries.

PORT PLACEMENT

Trocar positioning is the first and most important step for laparoscopic surgery. Correct

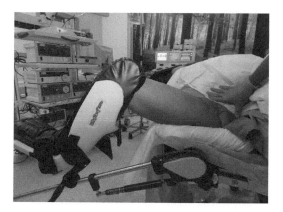

Figure 21.1 Low lithotomy position with hips extended.

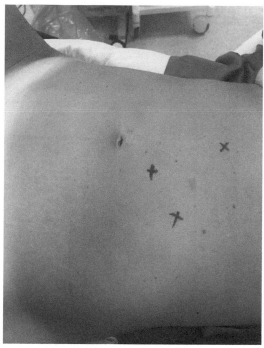

Figure 21.3 Suggested sites for primary port placement.

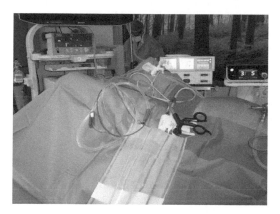

Figure 21.2 Optimum patient low lithotomy position for laparoscopic hysterectomy.

trocar positioning provides a sufficient view of the operation field and adequate range of motion for instruments, facilitating the surgery. Generally, the higher the primary trocar is, the better the visualisation of the operative field. The distance between the primary trocar and the uterine fundus should be at least 5 to 8 cm to allow an adequate view and space for operation during uterine manipulation, without interference by masses. Thus, the primary trocar should be placed at least at the midpoint between the umbilicus and the xiphoid process (Lee–Huang point) [1], Palmer's point, or a point above the umbilicus (in the) midline or in the left upper quadrant, depending on the size of the uterus. As for ancillary trocars, the numbers and positions vary, depending on the uterine size, location of fibroids, and complexity of the surgery.

Generally, three accessory ports of 5 mm are sufficient. They should be placed at the level of the umbilicus or above the level of cornual structures to easily approach the opposite side of the utero-ovarian ligament and the broad ligament without obstruction by the fundus during uterine manipulation.

Routine use of nasogastric tube decreases small bowel distension and diminishes the chance of trocar injury to the stomach. This is particularly important as the primary trocar placement will be at a higher level than usual (Figures 21.3 and 21.4).

METHODS TO REDUCE INTRAOPERATIVE BLOOD LOSS

Increased intraoperative blood loss is the major concern in laparoscopic hysterectomies for large uteri and also the main reason that many surgeons hesitate to perform this surgery. Therefore, reducing intraoperative blood loss, decreasing the need for blood transfusion, and the related morbidities are important issues.

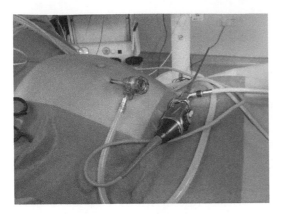

Figure 21.4 Primary port in a 16-week size uterus.

Preoperative Methods

Administration of gonadotropin-releasing hormone (GnRH) analogues prior to the operation can significantly decrease both the myoma size and uterine volume. Lethaby et al. [2] reviewed the role of pretreatment with GnRH analogues for women with uterine fibroid and found both uterine and fibroid volume reduced after GnRH analogue therapy. Hysterectomies appeared to be easier with shortening of operation time and decreasing the blood loss. Duration of hospital stay was also decreased. The authors concluded that the use of GnRH analogues for 3 to 4 months prior to surgery had benefits in reducing surgery-related morbidities.

Perioperative Methods

Misoprostol has been shown to reduce blood loss and the post operative drop in hemoglobin in a large number of well-designed but small randomized controlled trials [3–5].

Intravenous infusion of oxytocin during surgery causes uterine contractions and decreased uterine perfusion, resulting in less blood loss intraoperatively. Oxytocin 20 U was added to 1000 mL of saline solution running at the rate of 40 mU/min during the course of surgery [6].

The beneficial effects of oxytocin remain suspicious given the lack of significant oxytocin receptor expression in human myometrium outside of late gestation [7] and comparable messenger RNA expression between a leiomyoma and a normal myometrium in multiple studies [8, 9]. However, beneficial effects remain plausible in light of immunohistochemistry results showing wide oxytocin receptor expression in human leiomyoma cells but not the myometrium [10].

Vasopressin injection into the lower uterine segment helps in decreasing blood loss without increasing morbidity [11]. Injection of vasopressin 10 units diluted in 100 mL normal saline helps to reduce bleeding especially while using a myoma screw to manipulate the uterus.

Intraoperative

Devascularization of the uterus by clipping or coagulating the uterine artery can decrease the uterine perfusion; hence, a reduction in intraoperative blood loss can be achieved. Uterine vessels may be ligated at their origin, at the site where they cross the ureter, or where they enter the uterus. Blocking uterine arteries requires the opening of the pararectal space, tracing the lateral umbilical ligaments till their connection with the internal iliac arteries [12], and identification of the ureters [13] to enable safe coagulation or clipping of uterine arteries. The method of clipping the uterine artery with identification of the ureter in addition to reducing the intraoperative bleeding helps to prevent ureteric injury in cervical and broad ligament fibroid. Selective ligation of the uterine artery without adjacent vein gives the uterus a chance to return its blood supply to the general circulation. It also results in a less voluminous uterus for morcellation. Complete devascularization includes coagulation of uterine arteries, utero-ovarian ligaments if adnexa are preserved, or infundibulo-pelvic ligaments if adnexectomies are performed.

UTERINE MANIPULATION

Adequate uterine manipulation and good visualization are important factors for a successful laparoscopic hysterectomy in large uteri. The uterine manipulator is used to get a good retraction of the uterus, surgical exposure, tissue tension, and identification of essential anatomy. Lateralization of the ureter by manipulating the uterus also minimizes the risk of injury to vital structures and promotes case efficiency. Uterine manipulation can be achieved by using a vaginal uterine manipulator or a myoma screw or both. These two instruments each have their benefits and disadvantages.

Vaginal Uterine Manipulator

A variety of vaginal manipulators are available on the market, and the surgeon should choose the one that gives good uterine manipulation for his or her dexterity and comfort. Each manipulator should come with its attached colpotomizer cup and vaginal occluding sleeve.

A vaginal manipulator is beneficial:

- To clearly identify and distend the vaginal fornices to enable a circular incision on the vaginal fornices,

- To elevate and define the cervicovaginal junction to enable a safer dissection of the vesico-uterine fold and fascia, and

- To maintain a regular pneumoperitoneum after opening of the vaginal vault (Figures 21.5 and 21.6).

Myoma Screw as Manipulator

A 5-mm myoma screw can be used as an excellent uterine manipulator, especially in the very large uterus that is irregularly enlarged with multiple fibroids and impacted in the pelvis. It can be used through the right port so that the other two accessory ports are available for insertion of the energy source and other instruments. With a vaginal manipulator, it may not be possible to lift a very large uterus adequately to reveal the posterior fornix. In these cases, the myoma screw helps to dislodge and lift up the uterus from the pelvis and gives adequate traction and makes it easier to access the pelvic spaces around the uterovaginal junction.

For the larger uterus, the position of the myoma screw on the uterus often needs to be changed midway through the procedure to a more suitable site to get adequate traction. While the position of the myoma screw is being changed, there can be bleeding from the initial site and this can make the surgery field bloody. A good way to avoid excessive bleeding here is to inject diluted vasopressin to the fundus and the anterior wall of the uterus.

Also, while pushing the uterus with a myoma screw to get traction, one should be careful not to perforate through the uterus and hit on bowel or major vessels, which can happen very rarely, especially while taking the right-side pedicles.

In certain cases, we can consider using both a myoma screw and a vaginal manipulator, depending on the surgeon's experience and comfort (Figure 21.7).

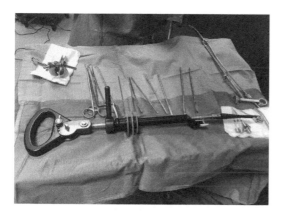

Figure 21.5 Clermondt-Ferrand Uterine Manipulator.

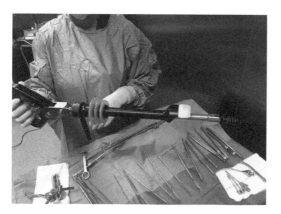

Figure 21.6 Clermont-Ferrand Uterine Manipulator.

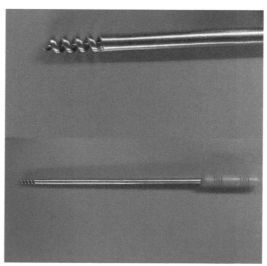

Figure 21.7 Myoma screw.

DIVISION OF CERVICOVAGINAL ATTACHMENTS AND CULDOTOMY

In the large uterus, it is often difficult to open the vagina from above as the cervix may be elongated and deep. Usage of a vaginal colpotomizer allows the vaginal fornices to be pushed up so that a distinct endpoint for dissection is created. Use of a 30° scope is essential for proper visualization, especially in the uterus with fibroids in the lower segment. After the uterine vessels and cardinal ligaments are secured on either side, the vaginal vault can be opened anteriorly or posteriorly near the cervicovaginal junction, over the colpotomizer cup with a monopolar hook or other energy source. Circumferential culdotomy is carried out with the delineator as a back stop. Excessive coagulation of the vaginal vault should be avoided as it can cause poor healing and increases the risk of vault dehiscence.

When the myoma screw is used as a manipulator, the vaginal vault can be opened in any of the following ways:

1. To open the vault, the uterosacral ligament should be incised exactly at the point of insertion at the cervicovaginal junction and the vault is opened laterally. One should be careful not to cut into the cervix.

2. Sometimes, with the above method, we may find it difficult to open the vault. In that case, it is useful to place a sponge on a holder in the vagina and push the lateral vaginal fornix. Incising laparoscopically from inside the abdomen over the resulting bulge helps to easily open the vaginal vault.

3. The third option is to place a reusable vaginal delineator tube, which helps to outline the cervicovaginal junction circumferentially. These types of vaginal tube prevent the loss of pneumoperitoneum.

Unlike the cuffed uterine manipulators that prevent the loss of gas from the abdomen when the vagina is incised, using the myoma screw as the manipulator has the drawback of not maintaining the pneumoperitoneum once the vagina has been opened, and allowing a route for the gas to escape. To overcome this difficulty, a wet pack or a pack inside a surgical glove can be placed in the vagina. Alternatively, the assistant standing in between the legs of the patient to hold the myoma screw can close the vagina with the other gloved hand.

SPECIMEN RETRIEVAL

After all the vessels and the ligaments of a uterus are cut, the method of removal of the large specimen determines the rest of the operation time. The specimen can be removed more efficiently by many techniques for volume reduction, including transvaginal volume reduction, laparoscopic morcellation, a combination of vaginal and laparoscopic procedures, and minilaparotomy [14].

Vaginal Morcellation

Generally, the transvaginal technique is preferred, except in women with morbid obesity, narrow vaginal cavity, or round and firm uteri prohibiting downward extraction. During the transvaginal procedure, bisection, morcellation, myometrial coring, vaginal myomectomy, and wedge resection are used to facilitate the process of removing the specimen.

A curved clockwise or counterclockwise incision with a #10 blade on a long knife handle under direct vision can be made along the deepest uterine wall simultaneously with rotation and traction of the uterus. The myometrium is incised circumferentially parallel to the axis of the uterine cavity with the scalpel tip always inside the myomatous tissue and pointed centrally, away from the surrounding vagina. If the remaining specimen was stuck in the pelvis because of the large mass or irregular configuration of the uterus, the uterus should be pushed inward a little followed by traction again to keep the largest portion presenting in the vagina. The incision procedure should be repeated until the whole uterus is extracted completely. Under the protection of the vaginal wall, with the bladder and bowels held back by two retractors, two tenaculum forceps may be used for downward traction of the cervix (Figures 21.8 and 21.9).

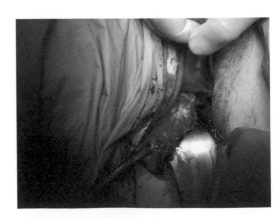

Figure 21.8 Vaginal morcellation.

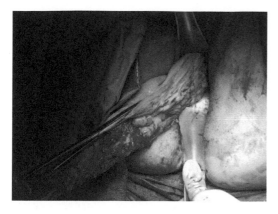

Figure 21.9 Vaginal morcellation.

Bisection

Bisection can be carried out in a uterus that is not very big. The cervix is grasped with two tenaculum forceps on both sides and a scalpel is used to make successive cuts on the uterus in an anterior–posterior direction. After each cut on the uterus, the tenaculum forceps are repositioned closer to the upper part of the incision and, with the rotation of the proximal part toward the pubic arch, help the incision to progress to eventually reach the fundus. When the fundus has been reached or when posterior bisection is difficult, the uterus is repositioned in the correct orientation and bivalving continues anteriorly in a similar way. After bisection, one half of uterus is delivered through the vagina, followed by the other half.

Myomectomy

Vaginal myomectomy is usually combined with the other techniques. Once the capsule is opened, the smaller myomas can be easily removed. Larger myomas are removed in smaller pieces. To avoid a sudden re-ascending of the uterus, a tenaculum should always be holding the residual uterine bulk. Otherwise, with re-ascending, there is the risk that the surgeon may to blindly grasp the uterus inside the abdomen and this can be dangerous for other abdominal structures.

Laparoscopic Morcellation

Morcellation with electromechanical power morcellation increases the risk of tissue dissemination during morcellation. In benign diseases, it can cause iatrogenic parasitic leiomyomas, inoculated endometriomas, upstaging, and metastasis in possible unknown malignancy.

In-bag morcellation should be attempted in all possible cases planned for laparoscopic power morcellation. Different types of morcellation bags are available in different sizes varying from 1500 to 5000 mL, which can accommodate a uterine size up to 15 cm. In case in-bag morcellation or vaginal morcellation is not possible, the option is to perform a minilaparotomy to remove the specimen [15].

Minilaparotomy

A minilaparotomy can be performed by enlarging one of the existing abdominal ports or creating a new incision, typically at either the umbilical or the suprapubic location. Depending on the size of the specimen to be extracted, this incision may be 1.5 to 4 cm; larger incisions allow easier extraction. A self-retaining circular retractor is inserted in the minilaparotomy. Manual morcellation of the uterine specimen can be carried out if needed, preferably in a bag. The specimen is grasped, pulled upward, and morcellated by hand with a scalpel in smaller pieces or strips. The blade can be maneuvered in a curvilinear manner or with a paper roll technique to create long strips of tissue, coring, or wedging of the uterine specimen (Figure 21.10).

POINTS TO REMEMBER

- Appropriate port placement is based on the size of the uterus.

- Adequate uterine manipulation with good tissue stretch makes the procedure simpler.

- Upper pedicles should be coagulated and cut 1 to 1.5 cm from the uterine body to prevent retrograde bleeding.

- The uterine artery should be coagulated and cut only after opening the uterovesical fold of the peritoneum and pushing the bladder down.

- The pedicles from the uterine artery and below should be taken very close to the uterus. This helps to prevent thermal injury to the ureter and gives a safe margin for

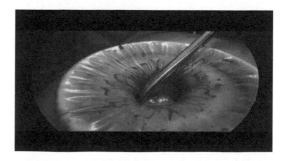

Figure 21.10 Minilaparotomy morcellation.

coagulation in case of bleeding from the pedicles.

- In case of cervical and broad ligament fibroids, opening the pelvic side wall to identify the ureter and clipping the uterine artery at the origin make the procedure safer by helping to avoid injury to the ureter.

- Care should be taken not to use excessive thermal energy on the vaginal vault. When the vault is being sutured, it is preferred to take thick bites to prevent vault dehiscence and secondary vault bleeding. Including uterosacral ligaments and pubocervical facia in the suture bites helps to prevent vault prolapse to some extent.

- While the specimen is being removed, contained in-bag morcellation should be considered wherever feasible, whether the morcellation be abdominal or vaginal.

Below are the steps of total laparoscopic hysterectomy using myoma screw as manipulator in a uterus with 12-cm posterior wall fibroid

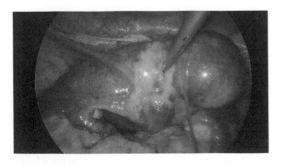

Figure 21.11 Patient positioning and placement of primary trocar.

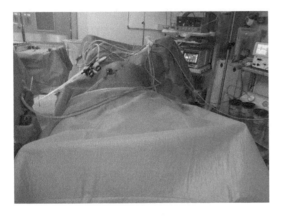

Figure 21.12 Diluted vasopressin injected to reduce bleeding.

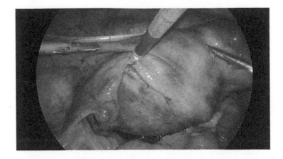

Figure 21.13 Myoma screw placement.

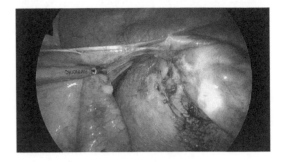

Figure 21.14 Adequate tissue stretch obtained on left side with manipulation of myoma screw.

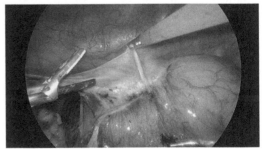

Figure 21.15 Dissecting bladder down, in case of previous lower segment caesarean section.

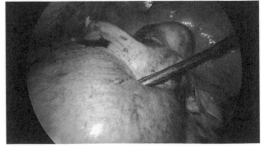

Figure 21.16 Myoma screw placed on the posterior fibroid, dislodged, and pulled up from pelvis which allows a proper visualization of left uterine artery.

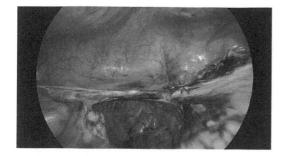

Figure 21.17 Left uterine artery and parametrium clearly seen with adequate stretch.

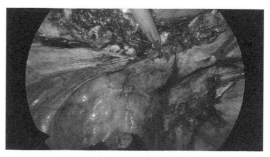

Figure 21.21 Dissection of uterosacral ligament at level of attachment to the cervix.

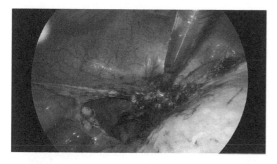

Figure 21.18 Left uterine artery is desiccated and divided.

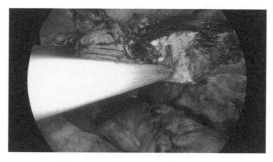

Figure 21.22 Colpotomy of the left lateral vaginal fornix.

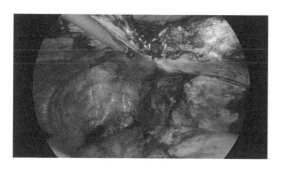

Figure 21.19 Clear visualization of parametrium and pouch of Douglas is facilitated by the use of a 30° scope.

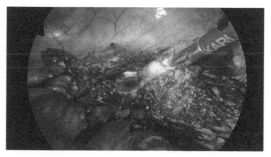

Figure 21.23 Colpotomy incision extended to the opposite side.

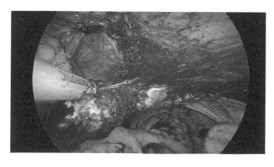

Figure 21.20 Dissection of the left Mackenrodts and uterosacral ligaments.

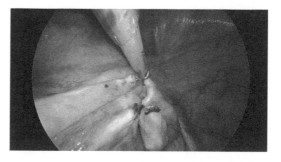

Figure 21.24 Myoma screw removed and reinserted in the uterine fundus toward the right. Pushing the myoma screw to left gives an adequate stretch to visualize the right pedicles.

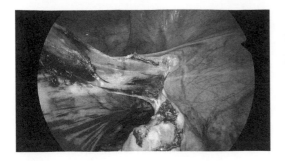

Figure 21.25 Posterior peritoneum should be incised to the direction of right uterosacral ligament.

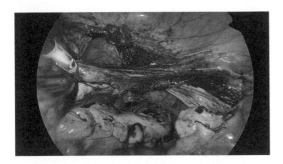

Figure 21.26 Right uterine artery is coagulated and cut followed by cutting the cardinal ligament to complete the hysterectomy.

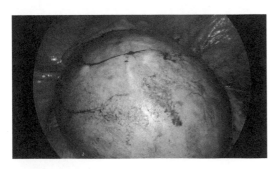

Figure 21.27 View after completion of hysterectomy before specimen removal.

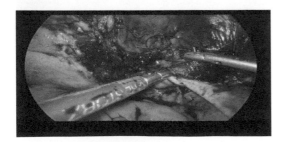

Figure 21.28 Vaginal vault closure using 2-0 V-Loc including the uterosacral ligament.

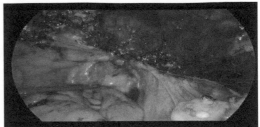

Figure 21.29 Final view of vault after suturing.

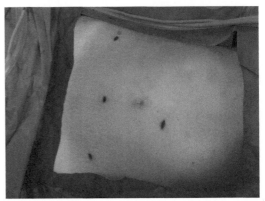

Figure 21.30 View of the port site after removal of trocars.

REFERENCES

1. Lee CL, Huang KG, Jain S, Wang CJ, Yen CF, Soong YK. A new portal for gynecologic laparoscopy. *J Am Assoc Gynecol Laparosc.* 2001;8:147–150.

2. Lethaby A, Vollenhoven B, Sowter M. Efficacy of pre-operative gonadotrophin hormone releasing analogues for women with uterine fibroids undergoing hysterectomy or myomectomy: A systematic review. *BJOG.* 2002;109:1097–1108.

3. Makled AK, Alsaied A, Ismail O, Farhan S. Effect of sublingual miso- prostol on intraoperative blood loss during abdominal hysterectomy: Randomized controlled trial. *Egypt J Hosp Med.* 2017;69:1692–1697.

4. Nankali A, Fakheri T, Hematti M, Noori T. Pre-operative sublingual misoprostol and intra-operative blood loss during total abdominal hys- terectomy: A randomized single-blinded controlled clinical trial. *World Fam Med.* 2017;15:35–39.

5. Tabatabai A, Karimi-Zarchi M, Meibodi B, Vaghefi M, Yazdian P, Zeidabadi M, et al. Effects of a single rectal dose of misoprostol prior to abdominal hysterectomy in women with symptomatic leiomyoma: A randomized double-blind clinical trial. *Electron Physician.* 2015;7:1372–1375.

6. Wang CJ, Yuen LT, Yen CF, Lee CL, Soong YK. A simplified method to decrease operative blood loss in laparoscopic-assisted vaginal hysterectomy for the large uterus. *J Am Assoc Gynecol Laparosc* 2004;11:370–373.

7. Wing DA, Goharkhay N, Felix JC, Rostamkhani M, Naidu YM, Kovacs BW. Expression of the oxytocin and V1a vasopressin receptors in human myometrium in differing physiologic states and following misoprostol administration. *Gynecol Obstet Invest.* 2006;62:181–185.

8. Arslan AA, Gold LI, Mittal K, et al. Gene expression studies provide clues to the pathogenesis of uterine leiomyoma: New evidence and a systematic review. *Hum Reprod.* 2005;20:852–863.

9. Busnelli M, Rimoldi V, Vigano P, Persani L, Di Blasio AM, Chini B. Oxytocin-induced cell growth proliferation in human myometrial cells and leiomyomas. *Fertil Steril.* 2010;94:1869–1874.

10. Sendemir A, Sendemir E, Kosmehl H, Jirikowski GF. Expression of sex hormone-binding globulin, oxytocin receptor, caveolin-1 and p21 in leiomyoma. *Gynecol Endocrinol.* 2008;24:105–112.

11. Okin CR, Guido RS, Meyn LA, Ramanathan S. Vasopressin during abdominal hysterectomy: A randomized controlled trial. *Obstet Gynecol.* 2001;97:867-872.

12. Chang WC, Torng PL, Huang SC, Sheu BC, Hsu WC, Chen RJ, et al. Laparoscopic-assisted vaginal hysterectomy with uterine artery ligation through retrograde umbilical ligament tracking. *J Minim Invasive Gynecol.* 2005;12:336-342.

13. Roman H, Zanati J, Friederich L, Resch B, Lena E, Marpeau L. Laparoscopic hysterectomy of large uteri with uterine artery coagulation at its origin. *JSLS.* 2008;12:25-29.

14. O'Shea RT, Cook JR, Seman EI. Total laparoscopic hysterectomy: A new option for removal of the large myomatous uterus. *Aust N Z J Obstet Gynaecol.* 2002;42:282-284.

15. Nisse V. Clark MD.Tissue extraction techniques during laparoscopic uterine surgery. *J Minimal Invas Gynecol.* 2018;25(2):251–256.

22 Robotic Hysterectomy in Fibroid Uterus

Anupama Bahadur

CONTENTS

Hysterectomy is one of the most commonly performed gynecological surgery. Established surgical techniques for hysterectomy include abdominal (open/minimally invasive), vaginal, for prolapse uterus and non-descent vaginal hysterectomy [1]. Selection of the route of hysterectomy for benign diseases of the uterus can be influenced by the size and shape of the uterus, accessibility, previous surgery, need for a concurrent procedure, surgeon's training and experience, existing facilities in the hospital setup, whether it is an emergency or a routine procedure, and patient's preference. Choosing a minimally invasive technique (laparoscopy/robotic approach) over laparotomy allows a reduction of trauma to the patient's body by facilitating smaller surgical incision, less blood loss, less pain, faster recovery, shorter hospital stay, and reduced patient morbidity [2].

The first total laparoscopic hysterectomy was performed in 1989 in a patient where vaginal approach was not feasible; since then, laparoscopic hysterectomy has gained popularity with patients and surgeons alike [3]. In 2005, the US Food and Drug Administration approved the da Vinci surgical system (Intuitive Surgical, Sunnyvale, CA, USA) for gynecological surgeries. Since then, minimally invasive surgery has won a great deal of enthusiasm, and greater numbers of patients prefer the robotic route and surgeons prefer to operate robotically for both complex and malignant gynecological conditions [4]. The spectrum of diseases of benign uterine conditions includes myomectomy, hysterectomy, endometriosis, cystectomy, tubal recanalization, vesico-vaginal fistulas, and sacrocolpopexy.

The da Vinci surgical system consists of three components: a surgeon's console, a patient side cart with four robotic arms manipulated by the surgeon, and a high-definition three-dimensional (3D) vision cart [5].

Articulating surgical instruments are mounted on robotic arms, which are introduced into the patient's body through specially designed cannulas with a remote center [6]. The robotic system provides a steady 3D image, and the articulating tip of robotic instruments allows 7 degree of movement, thereby surpassing mobility of the human wrist and facilitating better endo-suturing, especially in myomectomies. In addition, control at the surgical console eliminates human hand tremor, making surgical maneuvers much easier than laparoscopy, particularly in the narrow confines of the human pelvis [7]. Patients operated robotically have less blood loss and report less pain with subsequently less morbidity and lower requirement for analgesia as compared with patients operated laparoscopically. The conversion rate to open surgery is less with robotic assistance when compared with laparoscopy. Since the advent of the da Vinci surgical system in 2005, there has been mounting evidence of the safety and feasibility of robotic surgery in benign gynecology disease [4]. However, the main disadvantages of the robotic surgical system, including its high cost, special training of surgeons and staff, and lack of tactile sensation during surgery, should not be overlooked.

Fibroids or leiomyomas are monoclonal tumors originating from uterine musculature [8]. It is difficult to predict the actual incidence of leiomyoma since most women having fibroids are asymptomatic and hence only a small fraction of them present to a gynecologist. However, in premenopausal women, the incidence of fibroid has been estimated to be around 30 to 70%, which increases with age [8]. Various modalities for the treatment of fibroids have been proposed. The medical approach is usually the first line of management and consists of mainly hormonal. Non-hormonal medical treatment can give symptomatic relief [9]. The surgical approach for fibroids is recommended in patients with abnormal uterine bleeding (AUB) or with pressure symptoms or failed medical management. In subfertile women where fibroid is a contributing factor, myomectomy may improve fertility.

The definitive management for fibroids in patients who do not desire future fertility is hysterectomy, which has high rates of patient satisfaction. In a prospective study by Carlson et al. which included 311 patients, it was seen that satisfaction rates were greater than 90% in patients undergoing hysterectomy for fibroid uterus with significant improvements in urinary symptoms, pelvic pain, and sexual dysfunction [10]. Studies comparing morbidity between myomectomy and hysterectomy demonstrated similar perioperative risks for both laparoscopic and abdominal approaches [11, 12]. It is interesting to note that the risk of recurrence of fibroid 5 years postoperatively after myomectomy ranges between 20% and 40% [13]. A large number of fibroids, increase in size, large uterine size, and increased age are certain risk factors for recurrence [14]. The surgical approach is chosen carefully depending upon individual patient factors, like uterine size, body habitus, and fibroid number, type, and size. The benefits of a minimally invasive approach should be balanced with the potential morbidity associated with increased intraoperative time.

INDICATIONS FOR SURGICAL THERAPY OF UTERINE FIBROIDS

- AUB disorders
- Failed medical management for AUB-L
- Pressure symptoms
- Primary or secondary infertility and recurrent pregnancy loss

TREATMENT OF FIBROID IN WOMEN CONTEMPLATING PREGNANCY [15]

- Single intramural/subserosal fibroid: If the patient is asymptomatic, no intervention is required unless there is growth/desire for fertility.
- Intramural distorting cavity/submucosal fibroid: Women who presented with complaints of infertility or recurrent pregnancy loss or AUB-L and were keen on conception were offered myomectomy.
- Multiple myomas (more than 3) or myoma of size greater than 5 cm and uterus less than 18 weeks, or number of myomas less than 3,

size less than 5 cm: If there are complaints of infertility with or without AUB, then myomectomy (open/minimally invasive approach) is considered.

SURGICAL PROCEDURE
ROBOTIC HYSTERECTOMY

- A detailed preoperative assessment, including history and physical examination, is to be carried out. All preoperative investigations are done. Feasibility of robotic approach is assessed based on the patient's body mass index, associated comorbidities, pulmonary and cardiac functions, which may impact the ability to tolerate steep Trendelenburg positioning and ventilation.

- After induction of general anesthesia, the patient is positioned in low lithotomy with a maximum Trendelenburg position. Padding is applied in popliteal fossa to prevent common peroneal nerve injury. Shoulder pads are applied to prevent nerve compression injuries. After cleaning and draping, bladder catheterization is done and finally uterine manipulator is inserted.

- A Veress needle is used to create pneumoperitoneum and then the camera port is created about 15 to 20 cm above the symphysis pubis. Operating and assistant ports are created under visualization 8 cm lateral to each other. The Da Vinci Xi system is docked after that.

- Uterus with bilateral fallopian tubes and ovaries are visualized. Round ligaments are coagulated and divided (Figure 22.1).

- Utero-vesical fold opened and dissected and bladder pushed down (Figure 22.2).

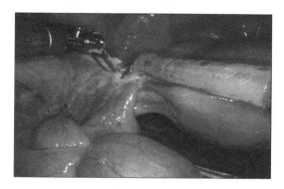

Figure 22.1 Round ligament being coagulated and divided.

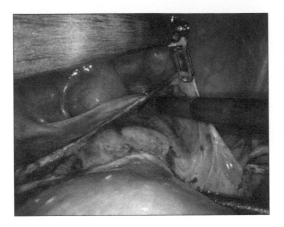

Figure 22.2 Utero-vesicle fold dissected and bladder pushed down.

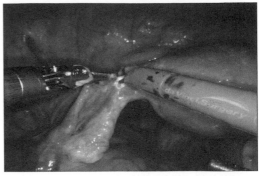

Figure 22.3 Tubo-ovarian ligament being coagulated and divided.

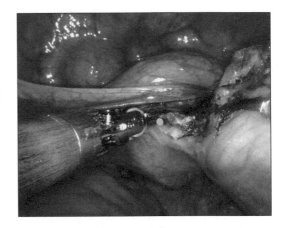

Figure 22.4 Uterine artery skeletonized, coagulated, and divided.

- The ureter should be identified and kept in view throughout critical portions of the hysterectomy procedure. It may be possible to identify the ureter transperitoneally along the lateral pelvic sidewall. If this cannot be seen, then a retroperitoneal dissection to identify the ureter is performed by incising the peritoneum parallel to the infundibulo-pelvic ligament at the level of the pelvic brim. A combination of sharp and blunt dissection is performed until the ureter is in view, and the dissection may be continued inferiorly toward the ischial spine as needed.

- If salpingo-oophorectomy is planned, ovarian vasculature is coagulated and cut. If adnexae are to be preserved, utero-ovarian ligaments are coagulated and divided.

Traditionally, the teaching was to remove ovaries in women undergoing hysterectomy in post-reproductive years. However, in contemporary practice, concerns have been raised about adverse health outcomes of premenopausal women undergoing oophorectomy. There is increasing interest in the role of salpingectomy for risk reduction of ovarian cancer. Data suggest that the fallopian tube may be a primary site for cancers that present with an ovarian mass [16] (Figure 22.3).

- Uterine artery is coagulated and divided after skeletonization. Uterine vessels are coagulated at the level of the colpotomy ring of the uterine manipulator (Figure 22.4).

- Circumferential colpotomy done and uterus with cervix is delivered through the colpotomy vaginally and morcellated if the specimen is large. (Figure 22.5).

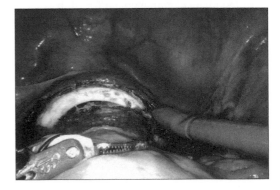

Figure 22.5 Colpotomy done over manipulator cuff.

- Vaginal angles are secured and the cuff is closed by running or interrupted absorbable sutures, placed 1 cm back from the edge of the vagina to minimize cuff dehiscence (Figure 22.6).

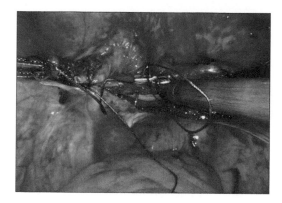

Figure 22.6 Vault closure by single-layer continuous absorbable suture.

- The surgical field is inspected for hemostasis. Observation under low intraperitoneal pressure is done to confirm hemostasis at the vault.

- Abdominal wall fascial defects over 10 mm are sutured to avoid port-site herniation [17]. The skin incisions are closed.

- After desufflation of the abdomen, it is useful to have the anesthesiologist administer five forced respirations to encourage carbon dioxide expulsion as residual carbon dioxide in the peritoneal cavity can lead to irritation and referred pain in the shoulder (shoulder tip pain) [18].

As uterine size increases, the ability to perform a hysterectomy by the vaginal route and also minimally invasive route decreases. Traditionally, a uterus size greater than 12 weeks has been considered an indication for laparotomy over laparoscopy [19]. Other studies have set an upper limit for large uterine size as being more than 16 weeks' period of gestation size or weight of more than 500 g [19]. However, surgeon expertise comes into play when dealing with bigger uteri. Difficulties with enlarged uteri are limited access to uterine vascular pedicles depending on the size and location of myomas and thus a high risk of intraoperative hemorrhage. There may also be distortion of normal anatomy with a large uterus and multiple fibroids, especially ureters and uterine vessels. As large uterus results in a significantly distorted anatomy along with poor exposure there is an increase in the risk of bladder, ureteric, and bowel injury. The difficulty in extracting the uterus vaginally by morcellation, increases the duration of the procedure [19]. Therefore, it has often been suggested that grossly enlarged

uteri are a relative contraindication for minimally invasive routes.

COMPLICATIONS

The common complications encountered during robotic hysterectomy, especially in uteri with large or multiple fibroids:

- Conversion to laparotomy
- Hemorrhage requiring blood transfusion
- Bowel injury
- Urinary tract injury (bladder and ureter)
- Vaginal cuff dehiscence

COMPLICATION RATES IN ROBOTIC VERSUS LAPAROSCOPIC APPROACH [20]

- *Ureteric injury*: 0.08% (robotic), 0.10% (laparoscopic)
- *Bladder injury*: 0.11% (robotic), 0.08% (laparoscopic)
- *Bowel injury*: 0.03% (robotic), 0.03% (laparoscopic)
- *Conversion to open*: 2.67% (robotic), 2.66% (laparoscopic)

ROBOTIC VERSUS LAPAROSCOPIC APPROACH

Liu et al., in a 2014 Cochrane review that included six randomized controlled trials, compared robotic and laparoscopic hysterectomy for benign conditions [21]. The authors reported a longer operative time, which was not statistically significant, and the mean difference was 16.33 min [21]. A trend toward lower rates of intraoperative and postoperative complications was also observed. Also, no statistical differences were found between complications and readmission rates. When it comes to cost-analysis, robotic-assisted hysterectomy is more costly despite stratifying analyses by length of hospital stay, age, and conversion to laparotomy. Numerous factors contribute to this increased cost. First, robotic instruments have a limited number of uses. Expense of instrument replacement is higher compared with laparoscopy since the latter has largely reusable consumables [22]. Furthermore, along with its expensive acquisition fee, the sum of its maintenance and repair costs represents 10% of the capital acquisition cost.

In another Cochrane review (2015), Aarts et al. compared different modalities of hysterectomy [23]. It was reported by patients that average days for return to normal activities was observed to be much shorter in vaginal and laparoscopic hysterectomy than in abdominal hysterectomy. However, there was no statistically significant difference between the mean days to return to normal activities between the two modalities. Urinary complications like injury to urinary tract, involving ureters and bladder, were found to be more in the laparoscopic than in the abdominal approach and the difference was statistically significant. There were no statistically significant differences on comparing laparoscopic with vaginal or vaginal with abdominal approach. On comparing laparoscopic with abdominal and vaginal hysterectomy, risk of bowel injury, vascular injury, and bleeding was not found to be statistically significant. No difference was noted in intraoperative vascular and visceral injuries, postoperative infection rates, need for transfusion, and return to normal activities between robotic versus laparoscopic hysterectomy. This was assessed by comparing two small randomized controlled trials in this study; however, the operative time was significantly greater in robotic hysterectomy by 32 min [23].

CONCLUSION

Both laparoscopic and robotic-assisted hysterectomies for fibroid uterus are safe surgical modalities with negligible complication rates. Robotic hysterectomy is associated with a lower blood loss and postoperative requirement of analgesia. Hysterectomy for Large uterus with multiple fibroids is surgically challenging due to compromised vision, difficulty in reaching pedicles, controlling hemorrhage and increased risk of adjacent organ damage. The approach to vaginal vault opening and subsequent removal of a large uterus needs surgical expertise. However, with use of robotic assistance and improved surgical skill the above factors can be handled more easily thus increasing the chance of completion of hysterectomy for large uterus safely by minimal access surgery. This ultimately reduces need for open surgery for large fibroid uterus giving the advantage of early recovery to patients.

REFERENCES

1. Raju KS, Papadopoulos AJ, Khan MS, Dasgupta P. A pilot study to assess the feasibility, safety and cost of robotic assisted total hysterectomy and bilateral salpingo-oophorectomy. *J Robotic Surg*. 2010;4(1):41–44.

2. Raju KS, Auld BJ. A randomised prospective study of laparoscopic vaginal hysterectomy versus abdominal hysterectomy each with bilateral salpingoooophorectomy. *Br J Obstet Gynaecol*. 1994;101(12):1068–1071

3. Orady M, Hrynewych A, Nawfal AK, Wegienka G. Comparison of robotic-assisted hysterectomy to other minimally invasive approaches. *JSLS: J Soc Laparoendosc Surg*. 2012;16(4):542–548.

4. Sinha R, Sanjay M, Rupa B, Kumari S. Robotic surgery in Journal of gynecology. *Minim Access Surg*. 2015;11(1):50–59.

5. Silasi DA, Gallo T, Silasi M, Menderes G, Azodi M. Robotic versus abdominal hysterectomy for very large uteri. *J Soc Laparoendosc Surg*. 2013;17(3):400–406.

6. Macciò A, Chiappe G, Kotsonis P, Nieddu R, Lavrva F, Serra M, et al. Surgical outcome and complications of total laparoscopic hysterectomy for very large myomatous uteri in relation to uterine weight: a prospective study in a continuous series of 461 procedures. *Arch Gynecol Obstet*. 2016;294:525.

7. Wattiez A, Soriano D, Fiaccavento A, Canis M, Botchorishvili R, Pouly J, et al. Total laparoscopic hysterectomy for very enlarged uteri. *J Am Assoc Gynecol Laparosc*. 2002;9:125–130. [PubMed].

8. Okolo S. Incidence aetiology and epidemiology of uterine fibroids. *Best Pract Res Clin Obstet Gynaecol*. 2008;22(4):571–88.

9. Billow MR, El-Nashar SA. Management of abnormal uterine bleeding with emphasis on alternatives to hysterectomy. *Obstet Gynecol Clin North Am*. 2016;43(3):415–30.

10. Carlson KJ, Miller BA, Fowler Jr FJ. The Maine women's health study: II. Outcomes of nonsurgical management of leiomyomas, abnormal bleeding, and chronic pelvic pain. *Obstet Gynecol*. 1994;83(4):566–72.

11. Lemyre M, Bujold E, Lathi R, Bhagan L, Huang JQ, Nezhat C, et al. Comparison of morbidity associated with laparoscopic myomectomy and hysterectomy for the treatment of uterine leiomyomas. *J Obstet Gynaecol Can*. 2012;34(1):57–62.

12. Odejinmi F, Maclaran K, Agarwal N. Laparoscopic treatment of uterine fibroids: A comparison of peri-operative outcome in laparoscopic hysterectomy and myomectomy. *Arc Gynecol Obstet*. 2015;291(3):579–84.

13. Radosa MP, Owsianowski Z, Mothes A, Weisheit A, Vorwergk J, Asskaryar FA, et al. Long-term risk of fibroid recurrence after laparoscopic myomectomy. *Eur J Obstet Gynecol Reprod Biol*. 2014;180:35–9.

14. Buckley VA, Nesbitt-Hawes EM, Atkinson P, Won HR, Deans R, Burton A, et al. Laparoscopic myomectomy: Clinical outcomes and comparative evidence. *J Minim Invasive Gynecol*. 2015;22(1):11–25.

15. Alkatout I, Mettler L, Günther V, Maass N, Eckmann-Scholz C, Elessawy M, et al. Safety and economical innovations regarding surgical treatment of fibroids, *Minim Invasiv Ther Allied Technol*. 2016; 25(6):301–313. doi: 10.1080/13645706.2016.1190380.

16. Przybycin CG, Kurman RJ, Ronnett BM, Shih I-M, Vang R. Are all pelvic (nonuterine) serous carcinomas of tubal origin? *Am J Surg Pathol*. 2010;34:1407.

17. Chiong E, Hegarty PK, Davis JW, Kamat AM, Pisters LL, Matin SF, et al. Port-site hernias occurring after the use of bladeless radially expanding trocars. *Urology*. 2010;75:574.

18. Phelps P, Cakmakkaya OS, Apfel CC, Radke OC. A simple clinical maneuver to reduce laparoscopy-induced shoulder pain: A randomized controlled trial. *Obstet Gynecol*. 2008;111:1155.

19. Borahay MA, Tapısız ÖL, Alanbay İ, Kılıç GS. Outcomes of robotic, laparoscopic, and open hysterectomy for benign conditions in obese patients. *J Turkish German Gynecol Assoc*. 2018;19(2):72–77. doi:10.4274/jtgga.2018.0018.

20. Tina Ngan TY, Zakhari A, Czuzoj-Shulman N, Tulandi T, Abenhaim HA. Laparoscopic and robotic-assisted hysterectomy for uterine leiomyomas: A comparison of complications and costs. *J Obstet Gynaecol Can*. 2018;40(4):432–439. https://doi.org/10.1016/j.jogc.2017.08.005.

21. Lawrie TA, Liu H, Lu DH, Dowswell T, Song H, Wang L, et al. Robot-assisted surgery in gynaecology. *Cochrane Database Syst Rev*. 2014;12:CD011422.

22. Korsholm M, Sorensen J, Mogensen O, Wu C, Karlsen K, Jensen PT. A systematic review about costing methodology in robotic surgery: Evidence for low quality in most of the studies. *Health Econ Rev*. 2018;8(1):21. https://doi.org/10.1186/s/13561-018-0207-5.

23. Nieboer TE, Johnson N, Lethaby A, Tavender E, Curr E, Garry R, et al. Surgical approach to hysterectomy for benign gynaecological disease. *Cochrane Database Syst Rev*. 2015;8:CD003677.

Index

Page numbers in *italics* refer to content in *figures*; page numbers in **bold** refer to content in **tables**.